T0122464

Studies in Big Data

Volume 86

Series Editor

Janusz Kacprzyk, Polish Academy of Sciences, Warsaw, Poland

The series "Studies in Big Data" (SBD) publishes new developments and advances in the various areas of Big Data- quickly and with a high quality. The intent is to cover the theory, research, development, and applications of Big Data, as embedded in the fields of engineering, computer science, physics, economics and life sciences. The books of the series refer to the analysis and understanding of large, complex, and/or distributed data sets generated from recent digital sources coming from sensors or other physical instruments as well as simulations, crowd sourcing, social networks or other internet transactions, such as emails or video click streams and other. The series contains monographs, lecture notes and edited volumes in Big Data spanning the areas of computational intelligence including neural networks, evolutionary computation, soft computing, fuzzy systems, as well as artificial intelligence, data mining, modern statistics and Operations research, as well as self-organizing systems. Of particular value to both the contributors and the readership are the short publication timeframe and the world-wide distribution, which enable both wide and rapid dissemination of research output.

The books of this series are reviewed in a single blind peer review process.

Indexed by zbMATH.

All books published in the series are submitted for consideration in Web of Science.

More information about this series at http://www.springer.com/series/11970

Hasmat Malik · Nuzhat Fatema · Jafar A. Alzubi
Editors

AI and Machine Learning Paradigms for Health Monitoring System

Intelligent Data Analytics

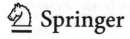 Springer

Editors
Hasmat Malik 🄳
National University of Singapore (NUS)
BEARS
Singapore, Singapore

Nuzhat Fatema
Universiti Sultan Zainal Abidin (UniSZA)
Kampung Gong Badak, Malaysia

Jafar A. Alzubi
Wake Forest University
Winston Salem, NC, USA

ISSN 2197-6503   ISSN 2197-6511 (electronic)
Studies in Big Data
ISBN 978-981-33-4414-3   ISBN 978-981-33-4412-9 (eBook)
https://doi.org/10.1007/978-981-33-4412-9

This Springer imprint is published by the registered company Springer Nature Singapore Pte Ltd.
The registered company address is: 152 Beach Road, #21-01/04 Gateway East, Singapore 189721,
Singapore

Preface

Data analytics helps businesses improve their performances. When it is implemented in the business model of an organization, it can reduce costs by analyzing better way of running business and storing a very large amount of data. Data analytic techniques basically enable researchers to take raw data and discover patterns to bring out valuable insights from it. Data scientists and analysts are using data analytic techniques in their research and businesses to take decisions. Data analysis is assisting organizations to better understand their customers, evaluate their ad campaigns, personalize content, create content strategies and develop products. It can be said that businesses are using data analytics to increase their business performance and improve their bottom line.

Artificial intelligence and machine learning, data management, data mining and predictive analytics are some of the technologies that make today's data analytics the most powerful strategy.

Machine learning and artificial intelligence (AI) is the field of developing and utilizing computer systems which can simulate human intelligence to perform different tasks. Precisely, machine learning (ML) is a subset of AI that is significant for data analytics and involves algorithms that can learn on its own. ML enables applications to utilize data and analyze it to predict outcomes without knowing system parameters to harness the useful information. Machine learning algorithm is being trained on a small sample of data, and the system will continue to learn by its own as it accumulates more data, turning into more accurate as time passes.

Big data analytics describes the large volume of data, maybe structured or unstructured data, which deals a business. It is essential to recognize how this data is being utilized by different organization. Big data is being analyzed for insights that lead to better decisions and strategic business improvements. Big data is creating new growth opportunities and entirely new categories of companies that can combine and analyze industry data. These organizations have plenty of information about the various products and services, all buyers and suppliers, and consumer choices that can be analyzed. Every organization uses data in its own way; the more efficiently an organization uses its data, the more it grows by cost saving, time reductions by taking fast decisions, by understanding the market scenarios early and correctly, by controlling reputation by receiving continuous feedback, by observing customer behavior and loyalty and by solving advertisers' problem and making to offer marketing insights. Moreover, big data analytics is a major driver of innovations and product development. Big data analytics is implemented in both public and private sectors, such as advertising, education, health care, insurance, manufacturing or banking. Big data is serving to deliver benefits in many surprising areas.

This book is comprised of 34 different chapters divided into three main parts covering almost the entire domain of AI and machine learning paradigms for health monitoring system, which covers intelligent data analytics.

- *Brief Introduction of AI and Machine Learning (AIML) and Its Applications*
- *AIML Applications for Monitoring System in Health and Management*
- *AIML Applications for Monitoring System in Engineering and Automation*

The first part reviews the brief introduction of AI and ML and its applications. This part represents the optimization solution for demand-side management (DSM), insight tools and softwares used, security enhancement and monitoring of data-sensing network, cuckoo search algorithm, routing protocols and particle-swarm-optimization-based applications.

The second part presents the applications of AIML for monitoring system in health and management. This part represents the studies related to knee injuries, COVID-19 and its past and future preventions, loyalty management of the customers, EEG signal monitoring and traffic noise prediction.

The third part shows the applications of AIML for monitoring system in engineering and automation. This section includes 22 studies, such as price forecasting, economic load dispatch monitoring, EV charging planning, LPG leakage detection, load monitoring, grid converter, energy storage, transformer FDD, PV monitoring and control, MPPT, load frequency control, and design and monitoring of permanent magnet BLDC motor.

Chapter "Optimization Solutions for Demand Side Management and Monitoring" provides the optimization solutions for demand-side management (DSM) and monitoring, which includes reviews and discusses the framework of DSM on the basis of modes and programs. Several residential DSM systems have been discussed with categorization of loads and constraints.

Chapter "An Insight into Tool and Software Used in AI, Machine Learning and Data Analytics" represents the insight information regarding tool and software used in the areas of AI, ML and intelligent data analytics. This chapter shows the need for and importance of the open access software. Authors survey the various kinds of open-source tools available on the Internet to take up projects in this field. Besides elucidating the application domains in which these analytics tools can be used, author also validates the results using a case study performed to detect fraudulent transactions. Moreover, authors review data analytics tools, libraries and software, what they are typically used for, what points of interest and inconveniences they offer to choose from them based on his convenience.

Chapter "Security Enhancement and Monitoring for Data Sensing Networks Using a Novel Asymmetric Mirror-Key Data Encryption Method" presents security enhancement and monitoring for data-sensing networks using a novel asymmetric mirror-key data encryption method. This chapter proposes a semi-asymmetric mirror-dual encryption approach. Here, the encrypted key is appended along with the data, but even the intruder collects the data or the key; then, they cannot hack the key or the data because of the mirroring cryptographic technique. This method is safer because it does not transfer the actual data, nor the actual key for encryption. This technique is secure than other symmetric key encryption because it is neither transmitting the actual data nor the encryption actual key as in conventional methods.

Chapter "Introduction to Cuckoo Search and Its Paradigms: A Bibliographic Survey and Recommendations" shows the introduction to cuckoo search and its paradigms. This chapter includes a bibliographic survey and recommendations of metaheuristic algorithms and its application for monitoring and control along with its latest developments as well as recommendation for the applications in various disciplines. The presented survey analyzes the algorithm search insight, its Lévy flight strategy and search mechanism efficiency. Despite being capable of solving various complex and multi-modal problems, the researcher further improves cuckoo search algorithm performance due to its immature convergence.

Chapter "Routing Protocols for Internet of Vehicles: A Review" represents an introduction of routing protocols for internet of vehicles for better insight information about the modern vehicles that they should be able to commutate a tremendous amount of data and information within their neighbourhood.

Chapter "Introduction to Particle Swarm Optimization and Its Paradigms: A Bibliographic Survey" shows the introduction to particle swarm optimization (PSO) and its paradigms. However, swarm stagnation and dynamic environments are still identified as significant challenges for future development. With more than 10,000 contributions in the IEEE database alone, PSO seems to show no sign of slowing down even after 25 years of the first appearance. This chapter enlists and discusses in brief the major developments in PSO along with the area of successful application in a concise form.

Chapter "Classification and Monitoring of Injuries Around Knee Using Radiographs Based Deep Learning Algorithm" represents classification and monitoring of injuries around knee using radiograph-based deep learning algorithm, which diagnoses the various types of fractures around the knee. Bone, tibial plateau, tibial shaft, fibula head, fibula shaft, patellae and femur distal end have been fed. Before feeding these images to the deep learning algorithm, all the images were reoriented, rotated and resized to a size of 600×300 pixels. These images are then populated to create a dataset for each type of fracture. This chapter is novel in approach, and all types of fractures around the knee are identified with the highest accuracy using the proposed deep learning algorithm.

Chapters "Artificial Intelligence: It's Role in Diagnosis and Monitoring Against COVID-19" and "Predicting Future, Past and Misinterpreted COVID-19 Cases Using Bidirectional LSTM Model for Proper Health Monitoring: Advances in Data Analytics" present the application of AI in the current pandemic situation diagnosis. This chapter shows the role of AI in diagnosis and monitoring against COVID-19. In the chapter "Artificial Intelligence: It's Role in Diagnosis and Monitoring Against COVID-19", authors aim to review the recent successes. Lastly, after introducing different applications, author underlines the common problems and limitations of the AI systems in COVID-19. In this short communication, authors discussed the presence of AI to combat against the novel COVID-19 and its limitations. In the chapter "Predicting Future, Past and Misinterpreted COVID-19 Cases Using Bidirectional LSTM Model for Proper Health Monitoring: Advances in Data Analytics", predicting future, past and misinterpreted COVID-19 cases using bidirectional LSTM model for proper health monitoring has been presented for the point of advances in data analytics.

Chapter "Data Driven Analysis to Identify the Role of Relational Benefit in Developing Customer Loyalty and Management: A Case Study" represents the data-driven analysis to identify the role of relational benefit in developing customer loyalty and management. This is a case study from the industry. The purpose of this study was to examine the relationship in between the relationship benefit and confidence-benefit in developing customer loyalty.

Chapter "Interpretation of EEG Signals During Wrist Movement Using Multi--depth Wavelet Features for BCI Application" represents the interpretation of EEG signals during wrist movement using multi-depth wavelet features for BCI application. The proposed signal-processing approach investigates the effectiveness of wavelet transforms in classifying different motion attributes using non-invasive MEG recording for brain–computer interface applications.

Chapter "Validation of Road Traffic Noise Prediction Model CoRTN for Indian Road and Traffic Conditions" shows the validation of road traffic noise prediction model, CoRTN, for Indian road and traffic conditions. The standard deviation between monitored and predicted level of noise before and after applying correction factor has been found to be in the range from 0.62 to 4.99 and 0.06 to 3.47, respectively, which shows the high acceptability rate.

Chapter "Deep Learning and Statistical Based Daily Stock Price Forecasting and Monitoring" represents the deep learning and statistical-based daily stock price forecasting and monitoring. Generally, financial time series data is highly dynamic in nature and makes it difficult to analyze through statistical methods. Recurrent neural network (RNN)-based long short-term memory (LSTM) networks were able to capture the patterns of the sequence data; meanwhile, statistical methods tried to generalize by memorizing data instead of recognizing patterns. The experimental results of this study show that LSTM networks outperformed traditional statistical methods like ARIMA, MA and AR models.

Chapter "Intelligent Modelling of Renewable Energy Resources based Hybrid Energy System for Sustainable Power Generation and Monitoring" represents the intelligent modeling of renewable energy resource-based hybrid energy system for sustainable power generation and monitoring. The present research focuses on the optimal design and sizing of hybrid energy system based on renewable energy resources, including solar photovoltaic (SPV), wind energy system, biomass and biogas with battery to electrify the rural areas of India's Haryana state. Different models of hybrid energy systems have been chosen and optimized using different intelligent approaches.

Chapter "Economic Load Dispatch Monitoring and Optimization for Emission Control Using Flower Pollination Algorithm: A Case Study" proposes an economic load dispatch monitoring and optimization for emission control using flower pollination algorithm. The electrical energy market has historically not been that complex, and focus was put solely on optimizing the energy dispatch costs. Since last few years, environmental pollution is the eye-catching issue, and government is making tough regulations to control it. Reducing the toxic pollution generated by the operations of thermal-based power generation plants becomes equally important. To overcome these two main problems, author presented a study which comprises in a form of a case study.

Chapter "Planning and Monitoring of EV Fast Charging Stations Including DG in Distribution System Using Particle Swarm Optimization" presents the planning and monitoring of EV fast-charging stations including DG in distribution system using particle swarm optimization. This work presents an innovative method for the optimal planning of charging stations with distributed generations (DGs) to establish an efficient charging infrastructure by considering the novel parameters, such as power losses, voltage, reliability and economic parameters in the proposed modified radial distribution network of the study area. Moreover, proposed multi-objective function is utilized for the optimal planning of DGs and the electric vehicle charging stations considering the network performance parameters as objectives variables. In this chapter, the case study for Durgapur, WB, India, is presented for a particular network section in city center area with modified IEEE-33 bus radial distribution system.

Chapter "IOT Based LPG Leakage Detection System with Prevention Compensation" shows the IoT-based LPG leakage detection system with prevention compensation. This chapter provides the strategy for security to all the people around the world from LP gas leakage by equipping them with an economical and effective alarming system which not only can detect this menace threat but also can automatically control it by its safety line of action.

Chapter "Short-Term Scheduling of Hydrothermal Based on Teaching Learning Optimization" presents short-term scheduling of hydrothermal based on teaching learning optimization. This chapter proposes an optimization technique based on teaching-learning (TLBO) for short-period scheduling of thermal and hydropower generation systems known as short-term hydrothermal scheduling (STHTS).

Chapter "Simulation and Analysis of Rectifier Based Four Level Grid-Connected Inverter Using Genetic Algorithm" presents a simulation and analysis of rectifier-based four-level grid-connected inverter using genetic algorithm. In the present work, four-level single-phase grid-connected converter is proposed and mathematically analyzed. Grid power, power factor and line current THD are controlled by controlling the firing angle of switches. The GA is used to optimize the line current THD in terms of switching angles.

Chapter "Vector Control of Dual 3-φ Induction Machine Based Flywheel Energy Storage System Using Fuzzy Logic Controllers" presents the vector control of dual 3-φ induction-machine-based flywheel energy storage system using fuzzy logic controllers. This chapter proposes the exploitation of multi-phase machines' reliability features in FESS applications. The FLC ensures fast and smart vector control that suits the nature of critical applications.

Chapter "Hotspot Detection in Distribution Transformers Using Thermal Imaging and MATLAB" shows the condition monitoring of the power transformer. This chapter includes the hotspot detection in distribution transformers using thermal imaging and MATLAB.

Chapter "An Innovative Fuzzy Modeling Technique for Photovoltaic Power Generation Farm's Failure Modes and Effects Analysis" presents an innovative fuzzy modeling technique for photovoltaic power generation farm's failure modes and effects analysis using FMEA model. The fuzzy-based FMEA approach improves the reliability and performance of the system and overcomes the drawback of conventional FMEA method.

Chapter "Analysis and Application of Nine Level Boost Inverter for Distributed Solar PV System" describes the analysis and application of nine-level boost inverter for distributed solar PV system. A nine-level multi-level topology based on the switched-capacitor technique which is capable of boosting the output voltage to twice the input voltage is presented for distributed solar PV system without using an external balancing circuit as the topology.

Chapter "Performance Evaluation of a 500 kWp RoofTop Grid Interactive SPV System at Integral University, Lucknow: A Feasible Study Under Adverse Weather Condition" presents the performance evaluation of a 500 kwp rooftop grid-interactive SPV system at Integral University Lucknow. This study has been performed under adverse weather condition in every month of January for the last 3 years, because maximum variation of temperature and insolation takes place.

Chapter "Fuzzy Logic Based Cycloconverter for Cement Mill Drives" shows the fuzzy-logic-based cycloconverter for cement mill drives that has been developed. The fuzzy logic controller is used to control the output of the converter. This chapter shows how to get variable voltage and frequency to control the cement mill drives with the help of a fuzzy-based controller.

Chapter "Comparative Control Study of CSTR Using Different Methodologies: MRAC, IMC-PID, PSO-PID and Hybrid BBO-FF-PID" shows the comparative control study of CSTR using different methodologies: MRAC, IMC-PID, PSO-PID and hybrid BBO-FF-PID. This paper presents different control methodologies for CSTR, i.e., continuously stirred tank reactor. More broadly, two control methodologies, i.e., model-based controllers and optimization-based controllers, are used.

Chapter "Performance Analysis of Nine Level Packed E Cell Inverter for Different Carrier Wave PWM Techniques" represents the performance analysis of nine-level Packed E-Cell Inverter for different carrier-wave PWM techniques. Multi-level inverter topology has been investigated.

Chapter "PSO Based Selective Harmonics Elimination Method for Improving THD in Three-Phase Multi-level Inverter" investigates PSO-based selective harmonic elimination method for improving THD in three-phase multi-level inverter. A three-phase five-level MLI is proposed which involves a lesser number of switches as compared with other topologies present in the literature. The proposed MLI involves a single DC source and two capacitors along with ten switches.

Chapter "Optimized Controller Design for Fast Steering Mirror Based Laser Beam Steering Applications" shows the optimized controller design for fast-steering-mirror-based laser beam steering applications that has been developed. This chapter presents the dynamic modeling and control configuration design of FSM in azimuth direction. The ultimate objective of control configuration design is to obtain the faster input command response and isolate the line-of-sight movement from any kind of internal or external disturbances.

Chapter "Comparison of Metaheuristic and Conventional Algorithms for Maximum Power Point Tracking of Solar PV Array" presents the comparison of metaheuristic and conventional algorithms for maximum power point tracking of solar PV array. In this chapter, the metaheuristic algorithms have been used in order to track the maximum power among various available peaks. Also, the comparison between different metaheuristic algorithms is done to show the best algorithm for maximum power point tracking (MPPT) applications.

Similar to the above discussed chapter, the chapter "Artificial Neural Network Based Maximum Power Point Tracking Method with the Improved Effectiveness of Standalone Photovoltaic System" represents the artificial-neural-network-based maximum power point tracking method with the improved effectiveness of standalone photovoltaic system.

Chapter "Analysis on Various Optimization Technique Used for Load Frequency Control" shows the analysis on various optimization techniques used for load frequency control that has been developed. This chapter provides an overview of the different LFC technique which is based on different controller.

Chapter "Optimal Design of Permanent Magnet Brushless DC (PMBLDC) Motor Using PSO Algorithm" presents optimal design of permanent magnet brushless DC (PMBLDC) motor using PSO algorithm. The motor characteristic has been expressed as its geometrical functions. The optimal function is combination of its cost, losses and volume. In this optimization procedure mainly four design variables (i.e., l_{sr}: axial length of stator/rotor, r_{ro}: radius of rotor, l_{mag}: thickness of magnet, and l_{wd}: thickness of winding) are being utilized.

Chapter "A Novel Lossless Image Cryptosystem for Binary Images Using Feed–Forward Back-Propagation Neural Networks" represents the application of AIML for lossless image cryptosystem for binary images for communication system monitoring using feed-forward back-propagation neural networks. The proposed methodology works by encrypting individual sets of binary values for enhanced security with no loss in image quality. The presented approach yields more security than the existing methods, which simply generate the cipher using neural networks by performing mix operations on the plaintext.

Due to the simplicity of the intelligent data analytics methods and flexibility, readers from any field of study can employ them for any type of problems. The book shall serve as a viable source on how to design, adapt and evaluate the algorithms, which would be beneficial for the readers interested in learning and developing AI/ML algorithms for intelligent data analytics. The book will find adaptability among researchers and practicing engineers alike. This single volume encompasses a wide range of subject area with fundamental to advanced level information.

We thank all the contributors of this book for their valuable effort in producing high-class literature for research community. We are sincerely thankful to the Intelligent Prognostic Private Limited India (iPrognostic.com) to provide the all type of technical and non-technical facilities, cooperation and support in each stage to make this book in reality.

We wish to thank our colleagues and friends for their insight and helpful discussion during the production of this edited book. We would like to highlight the contribution of Prof. Atif Iqbal, Qatar University at Doha; Prof. Sukumar Mishra, IIT Delhi at India; Prof. Imtiaz Ashraf, Aligarh Muslim University, India; Prof. M. S. Jamil Asghar, Aligarh Muslim University, India; Prof. Salman Hameed, Aligarh Muslim University, India; Prof. A. H. Bhat, NIT Srinagar, India; Prof. Kouzou Abdellah, Djelfa University, Algeria; Prof. Jaroslaw Guzinski, Gdansk University of Technology; Prof. Akhtar Kalam, Victoria University of Technology, Australia; Prof. Mairaj Ud Din Mufti, NIT Srinagar, India; Prof. Y. R. Sood, NIT Hamirpur (HP), India; Prof. A. P. Mittal, NSUT Delhi, India; Prof R. K. Jarial, NIT Hamirpur (HP), India; Prof. Rajesh Kumar, GGSIPU, India; Prof. Anand Parey, IIT Indore, India; and Prof Yogesh Pandya, PIEMR, Indore, India.

We would like to express our gratitude to our love and affection to our family members for their intense feeling of deep affection.

Woodlands, Singapore/New Delhi, India   Dr. Hasmat Malik
Woodlands, Singapore/UniSZA, Malaysia   Dr. Nuzhat Fatema
Winston Salem, NC, USA   Dr. Jafar A. Alzubi

Contents

Editors and Contributors

About the Editors

Dr. Hasmat Malik (M'16) received Diploma in Electrical Engineering from Aryabhatt Govt. Polytechnic Delhi, B.Tech. degree in electrical & electronics engineering from the GGSIP University, Delhi, M.Tech degree in electrical engineering from National Institute of Technology (NIT) Hamirpur, Himachal Pradesh, and Ph.D in power system from Electrical Engineering Department, Indian Institute of Technology (IIT) Delhi, India. He is currently a Postdoctoral Scholar at BEARS, University Town, NUS Campus, Singapore. He is a chartered Engineer [IEI]. He is a Life Member of Institute of Engineers (India) (IEI), Indian Society for Technical Education (ISTE), Institution of Electronics and Telecommunication Engineering (IETE), International Association of Engineers (IAENG), Hong Kong, International Society for Research and Development, London (ISRD) and Member of the Institute of Electrical and Electronics Engineers (IEEE), USA and Mir Labs, Asia. He has published more than 100 research articles, including papers in international journals, conferences and book chapters. He is a Guest Editor of Special Issue of Journal of Intelligent & Fuzzy Systems, 2018, 2020 (SCI, Impact Factor 2020:1.851), (IOS Press). He received the POSOCO Power System Award (PPSA-2017) for his Ph.D work for research and innovation in the area of power system. He has received best research papers awards at IEEE INDICON-2015, and full registration fee award at IEEE SSD-2012 (Germany). He has supervised 23 PG students. He is involved in several large R&D projects. His principal area of research interests is artificial intelligence, machine learning and big-data analytics for renewable energy, smart building & automation, condition monitoring and online fault detection & diagnosis (FDD).

Dr. Nuzhat Fatema has 10 years of experience in intelligent data analytics using AI & Machine learning for hospital and health care management. Dr. Fatema is the Co-founder of the Intelligent Prognostic Private Limited. Dr Fatema speaks nationally and internationally about the importance and power of data in hospital and healthcare systems.

Dr. Fatema a BAMS graduated from Maharashtra University of Health Sciences, India. She has cured many patients with her skills of medicinal knowledge. Later to go beyond the clinical skills, she has achieved post-graduation in hospital management from International Institute of Health Management Research (IIHMR), Delhi. This was the platform where she has utilized her clinical skills with her managerial skills using artificial intelligence (AI), Machine Learning (ML) and Data Analytics. She has worked as a research associate at National Board of Examinations (NBE) India and dealt with the accreditation process for post graduate courses in different multi-specialty hospitals in the country. She has authored one book describing a trouble free tool prepared by using different standardized manuals of medicines in different countries for usage of the most complicated drug like Warfarin. She has published several research papers in renowned international journals and conferences. Presently she is associated with UniSZA, Malaysia.

Her area of interest is AI, ML and intelligent data analytics application in healthcare, monitoring, prediction, forecasting, detection & diagnosis where she believes that it's a data driven world with stockpile of database in the industry which is to be used to extract value to make better informed, more accurate decisions in diagnosis, management and better outcomes in industry care. Simply throwing the numbers by analyzing any data has zero value; therefore she has produced narratives using data for decision making. She has been doing research study by spotting patterns in data and setting up infrastructure in the real-time industrial monitoring domain.

Jafar A. Alzubi is Associate Professor at Al-Balqa Applied University, School of Engineering, Jordan. He received Ph.D. degree in Advanced Telecommunications from Swansea University, Swansea, UK (2012), Master of Science degree (Hons.) in Electrical and Computer Engineering from New York Institute of Technology, New York, USA (2005), And Bachelor of Science degree (Hons.) in Electrical Engineering, majoring in Electronics and Communications, from the University of Engineering and Technology, Lahore, Pakistan (2001). Jafar works and researches in multi- and interdisciplinary environment involving machine learning, classifications and detection of Web scams, the Internet of things, wireless sensor networks, cryptography and using Algebraic–Geometric theory in channel coding for wireless networks. As part of his research, he designed the first regular and first irregular block turbo codes using Algebraic–Geometry codes and investigated their performance across various computer and wireless networks. He managed and directed few projects funded by the European Union. He has a cumulative research experience for over ten years, resulted in publishing more than forty papers in highly impacted journals.

Currently, he is serving as Editor for IEEE Access Journal and wireless sensor networks area Editor for Turkish Journal of Electrical Engineering and Computer Sciences. In addition, he is Editorial Board Member and Reviewer in many other prestigious journals in computer engineering and science field. He also managed several special issues in high impacted journals.

Contributors

Ehtesham Abbasi Green Economics Institute, Reading, UK; Sustainable Urban Development, Kellogg College University of Oxford, Oxford, UK

S. S. Afsar Department of Civil Engineering, Jamia Millia Islamia, New Delhi, India

Gulfam Ahamad Department of Computer Sciences, Baba Ghulam Shah Badshah University, Rajouri, Jammu & Kashmir, India

Anzar Ahmad Department of Electrical Engineering, AMU, Aligarh, UP, India

Kafeel Ahmad Department of Civil Engineering, Jamia Millia Islamia, New Delhi, India

Umme Aiman Electrical Engineering Department, Aligarh Muslim University, Aligarh, India

Farhana Ajaz Department of Computer Sciences, Baba Ghulam Shah Badshah University, Rajouri, Jammu & Kashmir, India

Iram Akhtar Department of Electrical Engineering, Faculty of Engineering & Technology, New Delhi, India

Nasim Akhtar CSIR, CRRI, New Delhi, India

Md Shahbaz Alam Electrical Engineering Department, Aligarh Muslim University, Aligarh, India

Pervez Alam Department of Civil Engineering, Jamia Millia Islamia, New Delhi, India

Rashid Alammari Electrical Engineering Department, College of Engineering, Qatar University, Doha, Qatar

Mohammad Ali Department of Electrical Engineering, Z.H.C.E.T, Aligarh Muslim University, Aligarh, India

Wahid Ali Department of Chemical Engineering Technology, College of Applied Industrial Technology (CAIT), Jazan University, Jazan, Kingdom of Saudi Arabia

Priyanka Anand Department of Electronics and Communication Engineering, B.P.S. Mahila Vishwavidyalaya, Sonipat, Haryana, India

Mu Anas Department of Electrical Engineering, AMU, Aligarh, UP, India

Khursheed B. Ansari Department of Chemical Engineering, Zakir Husain College of Engineering and Technology, Aligarh Muslim University, Aligarh, India

Md Nishat Anwar Department of Electrical Engineering, National Institute of Technology Patna, Patna, India

Shefali Arora Department of Computer Science, NSUT, Delhi, India

Mohammed Asim Department of Electrical Engineering, Integral University, Lucknow, India

Sarabjeet Kaur Bath Department of Electrical Engineering, Giani Zail Singh Campus College of Engineering and Technology, Bathinda, Punjab, India

M. P. S. Bhatia Department of Computer Science, NSUT, Delhi, India

Gargi Bhattacharjee Information Technology, Veer Surendra Sai University of Technology, Burla, Odisha, India

Bharat Bhushan Delhi Technological University, New Delhi, India

Aashish Kumar Bohre Electrical Engineering Department, National Institute of Technology (NIT) Durgapur, Durgapur, WB, India

Himanshu Chaudhary Department of Electrical Engineering, Jamia Millia Islamia University, New Delhi, Delhi, India

Rajeev Kumar Chauhan Department of EN, IMS Engineering College, Ghaziabad, UP, India

Vinay Kumar Reddy Chimmula Electronics Systems Engineering, University of Regina, Regina, SK, Canada

Sherly Daniel Mar Thoma College of Science and Technology, Kollam, Kerala, India

Mohamed Daoud Department of Electrical Engineering, Qatar University, Doha, Qatar

R. Dhanasekaran ECE, Saveetha School of Engineering, SIMATS, Chennai, India

Omar Farooq Aligarh Muslim University, Aligarh, India

Shoeb Azam Farooqui Department of Electrical Engineering, Aligarh Muslim University, Aligarh, India

Mashhood Hasan Department of Electrical Power Engineering Technology, College of Applied Industrial Technology (CAIT), Jazan University, Jazan, Kingdom of Saudi Arabia

Magray Abrar Hassan Department of Electronics and Communication Engineering, BGSB University, Rajouri, J&K, India

Atif Iqbal Electrical Engineering Department, College of Engineering, Qatar University, Doha, Qatar;
Department of Electrical Engineering, Qatar University, Doha, Qatar

Marium Jalal Fatima Jinnah Women University, Rawalpindi, Pakistan;
Department of Electrical Engineering, Lahore College for Women University, Lahore, Pakistan

Rajanish Kumar Kaushal EED, Punjab Engineering College, Chandigarh, India

Mohd Rizwan Khalid Electrical Engineering Department, Aligarh Muslim University, Aligarh, India

Asim Iqbal Khan Department of Electrical Engineering, Aligarh Muslim University, Aligarh, India

Mohammad Asfar Khan Department of Electrical Engineering, ZHCET, Aligarh Muslim University, Aligarh, India

Mohammad Ehtisham Khan Department of Chemical Engineering Technology, College of Applied Industrial Technology (CAIT), Jazan University, Jazan, Kingdom of Saudi Arabia

Mohd Shariq Khan Department of Chemical Engineering, Dhofar University, Salalah, Oman

Qamar Rayees Khan Department of Computer Sciences, Baba Ghulam Shah Badshah University, Rajouri, Jammu & Kashmir, India

Rashid Ahmed Khan Department of Electrical Engineering, Aligarh Muslim University, Aligarh, India

Shahbaz Ahmad Khan Department of Electrical Engineering, Z.H.C.E.T, Aligarh Muslim University, Aligarh, India

Neha Khanduja Delhi Technological University, New Delhi, India

Shahida Khatoon Department of Electrical Engineering, Jamia Millia Islamia University, New Delhi, Delhi, India

Sheeraz Kirmani Department of Electrical Engineering, Faculty of Engineering & Technology, New Delhi, India

Sumitra Kisan Computer Science & Engineering, Veer Surendra Sai University of Technology, Burla, Odisha, India

Pragya Kuchhal Department of Information Technology, NSUT, Delhi, India

Abhinay Kumar Electronics Engineering, Sreenidhi Institute of Science & Technology—SNIST, Hyderabad, India

Raj Kumar Department of Electrical Engineering, National Institute of Technology Patna, Patna, India

Rajesh Kumar Department of Electrical Engineering, NIT Hamirpur, Hamirpur, HP, India

Amit Kumar Yadav Electrical Engineering, National Institute of Technology (NIT), Sikkim, Ravangla, India

Moonyong Lee School of Chemical Engineering, Yeungnam University, Gyeongsan, South Korea

Deepesh Mali Department of Electrical Engineering, MNIT, Jaipur, Rajasthan, India

Hasmat Malik Electrical Engineering, Indian Institute of Technology (IIT) Delhi, New Delhi, India

Mohammad Abas Malik Department of Electronics and Communication Engineering, BGSB University, Rajouri, J&K, India

Ahmad Faiz Minai Integral University, Lucknow, India

Ruchi Mittal Department of Computer Science and Engineering, Ganga Institute of Technology and Management, Jhajjar, Haryana, India

Mohd. Naseem Department of Computer Sciences, Baba Ghulam Shah Badshah University, Rajouri, Jammu & Kashmir, India

Monaem Ibn Nasir Department of Electrical Engineering, ZHCET, Aligarh Muslim University, Aligarh, India

Ashish Pandey Defence Research and Development Organization, New Delhi, Delhi, India

Atul Jaysing Patil Department of Electrical Engineering, NIT Hamirpur, Hamirpur, HP, India

Gulnar Perveen Defence Research and Development Organisation, Metcalfe House Annexe, Delhi, India

Imran Pervez Department of Electrical Engineering, ZHCET, Aligarh Muslim University, Aligarh, India

C. V. Praharsha Musculoskeletal Clinical Physiotherapist, Defence Research and Development Organization, Secunderabad, India

Mohammad Obaid Qamar Department of Civil Engineering, Yeungnam University, Gyeongsan, South Korea

Muhammad Abdul Qyyum School of Chemical Engineering, Yeungnam University, Gyeongsan, South Korea

Nidal Rafiuddin Aligarh Muslim University, Aligarh, India

Nazia Rehman Electrical Engineering Department, Aligarh Muslim University, Aligarh, India

Ahmed Riyaz Department of Electrical Engineering, BGSB University, Rajouri, India

Mohammad Rizwan Department of Electrical Engineering, College of Engineering, Qassim University, Buraydah, Qassim, Saudi Arabia;
Department of Electrical Engineering, Delhi Technological University, Delhi, India

Harsha Vardhan Sahoo Computer Science & Engineering, Veer Surendra Sai University of Technology, Burla, Odisha, India

Monika Sahu Department of Electrical Engineering, NIT Hamirpur, Hamirpur, HP, India

Asif Sanaullah Department of Business Management, UNiSZA, Kuala Terengganu, Malaysia;
Department of Business Management, Karakoram International University, Gilgit-Baltistan, Pakistan

Mohammad Sarfraz Department of Electrical Engineering, Aligarh Muslim University, Aligarh, India

Adil Sarwar Department of Electrical Engineering, AMU, Aligarh, UP, India;
Department of Electrical Engineering, Z.H.C.E.T, Aligarh Muslim University, Aligarh, India;
Electrical Engineering Department, Aligarh Muslim University, Aligarh, India

D. Saxena Department of Electrical Engineering, MNIT, Jaipur, Rajasthan, India

Adnan Shafi Department of Electronics and Communication Engineering, BGSB University, Rajouri, J&K, India

Zeeshan Ali Shah Department of Electrical Engineering, College of E&ME, National University of Sciences and Technology (NUST), Rawalpindi, Pakistan

Abdulla Shahid Mazaya Group, Dammam, Saudi Arabia

Saurabh Ranjan Sharma Department of Electrical Engineering, NIT Hamirpur, Hamirpur, HP, India

Sparsh Sharma Department of Computer Engineering, College of Engineering and Technology, Baba Ghulam Shah Badshah University, Rajouri, Jammu & Kashmir, India

Arush Singh Department of Electrical Engineering, NIT Hamirpur, Hamirpur, HP, India

Dhiraj Kumar Singh Electrical Engineering Department, National Institute of Technology (NIT) Durgapur, Durgapur, WB, India

Ravindra Singh Defence Research and Development Organization, New Delhi, Delhi, India

Yog Raj Sood Department of Electrical Engineering, NIT Hamirpur, Hamirpur, HP, India

Pullabhatla Srikanth Scientist D, DRDO, Defence Research and Development Organization, Secunderabad, India

Syed Mohd Subhan Department of Electrical Engineering, ZHCET, Aligarh Muslim University, Aligarh, India

Mohd Tariq Department of Electrical Engineering, AMU, Aligarh, UP, India; Department of Electrical Engineering, Z.H.C.E.T, Aligarh Muslim University, Aligarh, India

Tilak Thakur EED, Punjab Engineering College, Chandigarh, India

Linoy A. Tharakan Mar Thoma Institute of Information Technology, Kollam, Kerala, India

Vivek Kumar Tripathi Department of Electrical Engineering, NIT Hamirpur, Hamirpur, HP, India

Azhar Ul-Haq Department of Electrical Engineering, College of E&ME, National University of Sciences and Technology (NUST), Rawalpindi, Pakistan

Deepak Upadhyay Department of Electrical Engineering, Z.H.C.E.T, Aligarh Muslim University, Aligarh, India

T. Usmani Integral University, Lucknow, India

Yusuf Uzzaman Khan Aligarh Muslim University, Aligarh, India

Archana Verma Department of Electrical Engineering, Integral University, Lucknow, India

Mohd Wahab Arizona State University, Tempe, AZ, USA

Mohammad Zaid Department of Electrical Engineering, AMU, Aligarh, UP, India

Lei Zhang Electronics Systems Engineering, University of Regina, Regina, SK, Canada

Brief Introduction of AI and Machine Learning (AIML) and Its Applications

Optimization Solutions for Demand Side Management and Monitoring

Zeeshan Ali Shah, Azhar Ul-Haq, Rashid Alammari, Atif Iqbal, and Marium Jalal

Abstract For the last couple of decades, power consumption has been growing exponentially. The traditional power grids are experiencing various challenges such as reliability and sustainability. Due to limited energy resources and budget with increase in load demand, conventional energy management techniques are getting failed. In this case, demand side management (DSM) technique is one of the best solutions ensuring reliable and economical power flow. Demand side management consists of the activities or technologies which are used on demand side to optimize power consumption for achieving desired objectives including energy balancing and cost reduction etc. This chapter reviews and discusses the framework of demand side management on the basis of modes and programs. Demand side management techniques are differentiated on the basis of their implementation and usage, which has not been reported in the previous literature. Residential DSM system is discussed with categorization of loads and constraints. During the organization of the chapter, different optimizing models are also reviewed for the implementation of DSM programs.

Keywords Demand side management · Optimization solutions · Monitoring

Z. A. Shah · A. Ul-Haq (✉)
Department of Electrical Engineering, College of E&ME, National University of Sciences and Technology (NUST), Rawalpindi 46000, Pakistan
e-mail: azhar.ulhaq@ceme.nust.edu.pk

R. Alammari · A. Iqbal
Electrical Engineering Department, College of Engineering, Qatar University, Doha, Qatar

M. Jalal
Fatima Jinnah Women University, Rawalpindi 46000, Pakistan

Department of Electrical Engineering, Lahore College for Women University, Lahore 54000, Pakistan

Nomenclature

E_{c,T_L}	Total energy consumption in a day
ς_{R_a,T_L}	Energy consumed by regularly operated devices
ς_{S_a,T_L}	Energy consumed by shift-able operated devices
$\varsigma_{\varepsilon_a,T_L}$	Energy consumed by elastic operated devices
$\rho_{R_a}^{T_L}$	Cost per day of regularly operated devices
$\rho_{S_a}^{T_L}$	Cost per day of shift-able devices
$\rho_{\varepsilon_a}^{T_L}$	Cost per day of elastic devices
ε	Signal of electricity pricing
ζ	ON-OFF states of devices
DSM	Demand side management
SSM	Supply side management
L.F.	System's load factor
$P_{(i,j)}$	Demand of load type i at time interval number j
N	Total number of load demand types
J	Total number of time intervals
$P_{TO(j)}$	The total demand for all the loads types from $j = 1$ to $j = J$ over the time interval number j
k	The number of time interval at which the maximum demand occurs for all the load types numbers from $i = 1, N$ over all the time duration from $j = 1, J$ occurs
C	Total cost of the electrical demand and energy consumption
$ce_{(i,j)}$	Energy cost for load type i at time interval number j
$cd_{(i,j)}$	Demand cost for load type i at time interval number j
R_a	Regularly used devices
S_a	Shiftable devices
ε_a	Elastic appliances
DLC	Direct load control
DSI	Demand side integration
VSS	Variable subscription service
ADS	Active distribution systems
DR	Demand response
PV	Photovoltaic
RTO	Regional transmission organization
ISO	Independent system operator

1 Introduction

In recent times, power consumption requirements are changing constantly. A modern power system must be reliable with quality and must be environmentally friendly to meet those requirements. Traditional power plants are being upgraded and are converted into smart grids with the invention of smart devices and systems.

A simplified power supply chain is shown in Fig. 1. In first step, all power production resources are either mined as in case of coal or collected as in case of gas, oil, water. In second step, the resources collected or mined are purified or prepared for energy generation stage. At third stage, power is generated through different methods such as hydel, thermal or coal power plants. Then in next step, power is transmitted from power station to substations through overhead cables. In next step, power supply is distributed through distribution lines. Power distributed is supplied to end-users for utilization in last stage.

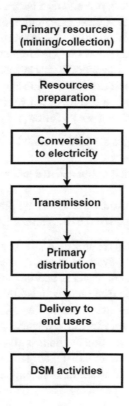

Fig. 1 Power supply chain

There are challenges in meeting electricity demands due to the increase in population which, as a result, lead to the increase in load demand. The International Energy Agency has estimated that in 2030, load demand will be higher than 50% than the load demand at present. Usually, power systems are designed in such a way that when there is surge in load demand curve, the power system is able to sustain that surge and meets the load demand. In traditional power systems, power generation is increased to cope up with the increase in load demand. But, this practice is expensive and can not be implemented due to limited or unavailability of fuel and resources. Power plants can be extended upto a certain limit until there comes a point where this practice can no longer be economical. After years of hard work, researchers and engineers have come up with a new concept called as demand side management (DSM) which improves the power system in order to meet load demands [1]. DSM is described as the actions taken to manage the usage of energy by users in such a way that the required changes in the load curve are achieved.

Many authors have explained the framework of DSM with different expressions and techniques. Most of the work presented in the past is based on a certain aspect of the DSM framework. They lack clear explanation on DSM programs and modes. Techniques cannot be distinguished from each other given in the previous literature. This chapter presents a detailed review on DSM framework covering each and every aspect. DSM is compared with conventional energy management system. Techniques are classified with respect to their implementation and usage. Residential DSM system is discussed in detail. This is a review-based work.

Key contributions of this chapter are as follows;

1. DSM programs and strategies are differentiated with respect to their implementations and usage.
2. Residential DSM framework is explained in detail with categorization of domestic loads.
3. Objective functions and constraints of DSM are presented in equation form.
4. Few efficient models are discussed to implement DSM techniques.

The overview of the chapter is given in Fig. 2. The chapter consists of the following sections; introduction to power systems is given in Sect. 1. Section 2 consists of conventional energy management systems and demand side management. Section 3 contains the work done in the past on demand side management implementation. DSM techniques and programs are given in Sect. 4. Residential DSM system is explained in Sect. 5. Architecture of the residential DSM is described in Sect. 6. Problem formulation for exact solution methods is given in Sect. 7. Section 8 consists of objective functions and constraints of DSM. Different modeling techniques are given in Sect. 9. Advantages and limitations in implementing DSM techniques are given in Sect. 10 and Sect. 11, respectively. Then, this chapter is concluded in Sect. 11.

Fig. 2 Overview of the chapter

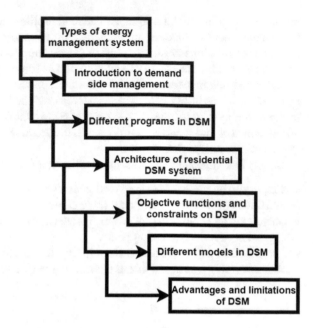

2 From Conventional Energy Management to Demand Side Management

There are two major techniques in power systems which are used to encounter predicted load demand, supply side management (SSM) and demand side management (DSM), as shown in Fig. 3 [2].

2.1 Supply Side Management SSM

SSM is defined as the measures that are taken to ensure reliable generation, transmission and distribution of power. SSM is usually associated with power generation only, but it also includes the measures that concern supply of power generation

Fig. 3 Techniques in power systems

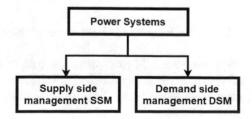

resources including coal, fossil fuels. The load profile can be improved when supply side management techniques are implemented to ensure smooth operation of generation, transmissions or distributions of power supply. In SSM, on-site generation techniques are also used to ensure smooth power supply [3].

After the implementation of SSM techniques, power systems become efficient and expenditure of the utility companies is decreased. The installed generating capacity of the power system increases as a result of SSM which in return decreases energy production cost and reduces environmental emission per unit. The reliability of the system also increases due to SSM.

Supply side management consists of following activities [3];

- Supply and utilization of energy resources: It consists of environmentally friendly substitutes of fuel and use of renewable energy.
- Generation and conversion of power: It consists of improvements in operation and upgrading of units in existing plants.
- Transmission and distribution of electricity: It consists of reduction in line losses after reforming transmission and distribution networks [3].

2.1.1 Advantages of SSM

The advantages of SSM are as following [1];

- Supply side management ensures efficient and low cost energy production, thus maximizing consumers' value.
- SSM enables the power systems to balance the supply and load demand without addition of unnecessary infrastructure.
- SSM minimizes the environmental impact by efficient operation of power system.

2.1.2 Disadvantages of Supply Side Management

However, there are some disadvantages too which greatly affect this scheme, and are listed below;

- Sometimes, load demand surpasses the power supply. Hence, power systems cannot meet the load demand.
- SSM sometimes cannot be implemented due to lack or unavailability of resources such as finance or fuel.

2.1.3 Challenges and Constraints of SSM

SSM consists of all those actions which are taken to make power system efficient and reliable by managing generation, transmission and distribution of electricity. Usually, users show interest toward demand side management rather than SSM because it is an old technique.

The are many challenges in adopting SSM. First, technical staff need comprehensive data to implement SSM for a particular situation. In many cases, it is responsibility of the customers to take such measures to ensure smooth power operation that could result positively in the favor of the customer. Sometimes, balancing customers and supplier interests are very difficult due to the capital investment. Investors sometimes need incentives to take actions which result in increase in profit, and also effect on environment is decreased.

Second is lack of capital funds to implement SSM. SSM, most of the times, produces significant effect on environment, but it requires to convince authorities on the expenditure. Sometimes short-term plan requires huge investment and that may or may not result in achieving long-term goal.

There is sometimes lack of managerial and technical skills for adopting SSM. Sometimes a country does not has such advance technology to implement SSM techniques such as clean coal technology. These lack of managerial or technical skills lead to poor energy performance. Sometimes, there is availability of enough funds but due to poor technical and managerial skills, plant does not produce desired results. Maintenance is another issue involved in SSM. Training is required for technical staff to take small but early steps to ensure smooth operation of power, resulting in increase in cost, but the desired results are achieved.

In some cases, there are enough funds to run a power plant. But to ensure smooth operation of plant, there is a requirement of collecting complete feedback data, so that in case of need, necessary actions are taken in time without disrupting power supply. In some cases, old machinery is replaced by new machines for implementing SSM. That requires good managerial and technical skill, that is another a major concern in adopting SSM.

2.2 Demand Side Management

SSM faces many challenges such as, increase in load demand, lack of resources, lack of data, lack of communication and security issues, which lead to a new technique called as demand side management. Installing new power plants is not the feasible solution to remove the gap between supply and demand. To cope with this problem, demand side management (DSM) is the viable solution. DSM urges load management on consumer side with respect to time and amount of use of electricity, so that there is an overall reduction in the system peak. Proper execution of DSM activity provides great help in balancing demand and supply.

2.2.1 Background of DSM

The term DSM was first introduced in 1973, after an energy crisis which took place in USA. It is also known as energy demand management with an aim to decrease peak demand of the power plant. DSM provides benefit for both utilities and consumers [2, 4].

DSM is described as the actions taken to manage the usage of energy by users in such a way that the required changes in the load curve are achieved. Demand side management facilitates consumers by providing them incentives. As, DSM deals with usage and managing electrical load, external factors do not affect this process [5].

2.2.2 Objectives of Demand Side Management

The objective of DSM is to minimize peak load demand and to promote efficient energy tasks.

Overconsumption in the electrical network can be achieved by

- Energy conservation
- Improving load profile

The aim of DSM programs is to maximize end use efficiency to replicate/delay the requirement of new generating capacity.

2.2.3 DSM Framework

Demand side management framework is given in Fig. 4. DSM objective function is defined first. Objective function attempts to maximize the output based on sets of constraints and relationship between decision variables. The constraints include resources, availability, capacity and limitation of the environments in which business is conducted.

Then, DSM alternatives are identified from energy efficiency, demand response and strategy load growth. In next step, a technique is selected to implement. The technique is implemented to get desired results. Power systems are constantly monitored for feedback data during whole process. On the basis of feedback, DSM objective function is refined in first step, if desired objectives are not achieved.

Fig. 4 DSM framework

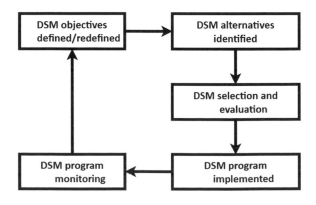

3 Literature Review

Various researchers have proposed different techniques on implementing DSM. Authors in [6] discuss different techniques to implement DSM in different environments. A wide range of techniques is presented for developing a framework for vertically integrated and restructured industry environments. A new demand side integration (DSI) technique is implemented to achieve desired load shape objectives by relating traditional form of DSM technique to the new form. A variable subscription service (VSS) method is implemented in [7] to integrate DSM into power systems. A smart grid infrastructure is discussed in reference to implementation of DSM through VSS. Authors conclude that this method proves to be a flexible tool which can balance supply and demand while providing an opportunity of decision-making between grid-purchased power and other supply alternatives. Four cases are presented in [8] to implement DSM for smart power. Three intelligent systems including storage capacity, shiftable loads and batteries are modeled. A fixed tariff, a two-tariff structure and an hourly real-time tariff structure are implemented for comparison of the performance. In [9], authors discuss the integration of network planning with DSM for planning active distribution systems (ADS). Authors in [10] discuss three key stages in development of DSM. Impact of DSM programs on power consumption and conservation influencing terminal power efficiency is discussed. With the objective of energy conservation and reduction of emission, safeguard systems and incentive mechanism of DSM are presented. Authors conclude this work by discussing polices and regulations regarding implementation of DSM in China.

Different demand response DR models under smart grid standards are given in [11]. General concept of DR is classified into two categories: wholesale and retail markets. After detailed literature review, it is concluded that DR program is dependent on prevailing electricity market conditions of a particularly region. Works presented in the literature review are academic in nature and can be extended to implement DR practically. A review is presented in [12] on issues regarding penetration of high renewables in power production. Simulations are conducted on the basis of collected field data on power consumption by refrigerators. Operation of refrigerators is scheduled with respect to the output of a small PV system. A comparison of results obtained is given in this work proving the superiority of presented work. An overview of DR on the basis of types and method from the prospective of buildings at the demand side is presented in [13].

Renewable generation resources, i.e., solar and wind power, are introduced in smart grid for smart power [14]. Forecast errors of wind speed and solar radiance are modeled in this work. A Latin hypercube sampling is implemented for plausible scenarios of renewable generators for day-ahead energy and reserve scheduling. Simulation results are obtained after implementing the suggested design in micro grid. An integrated resource planning model based on optimal DLC is presented in [15]. Aim of the presented technique is peak shaving and load shifting for cost reduction. An algorithm is presented to integrate distributed generation resources including PV, wind turbines, diesel engines, and batteries to DLC strategies. An automation generation method of optimization is discussed in [16] for orderly power utilization. A genetic algorithm is implemented to establish evaluation index system, calculation model and searching for optimization scheme. After simulations and experiments, it is concluded that the presented design can be effective in optimizing resource allocation and maximizing social benefits. A robust optimization technique is presented in [17] to derive optimal unit commitment decision for reliability unit commitment run by ISOs/TROs. The problem is formulated as a multi-stage robust mixed-integer programming problem. Results show that the suggested technique achieves the desired objective function, i.e., maximizing social benefits. A real-time pricing technique is implemented in [18] through DR management in smart grid systems. The aim of this technique is to minimize peak-to-average load ratio (PAR). The designed method solves two stage optimization problem. On one-side, each user responds to prices announced by retailer and on the other hand retailer designs real-time prices in response to forecasted user's actions. A demand response problem, whose operating conditions are modeled through mixed-integer constraints, is discussed in [19]. Operation time and energy consumption of devices are improved through demand response.

There are uncertainties in forecasting wind power, which are dealt through demand response in [20] to provide power reserve. A stochastic model consisting of generating units and responsive loads with high penetration of wind power is proposed. The designed technique is developed as two-stage stochastic programs including electricity market and actual power operation. A DR provider approach is implemented on Institute of Electrical and Electronics Engineers (IEEE) 30-bus test system over daily time horizon. The designed system reduces the operation cost and emission. A short-time hourly scheduling technique is implemented including cogeneration facility, traditional power units and heat only units in [21]. A DR program is implemented for achieving power and heat demands with cost reduction. Four cases are presented to analyze the performance of the presented program. A German balancing mechanism is analyzed in [22] to study demand response program. It is concluded that DR is undermined by three design aspects including minimum bidding volume, minimum bid duration and binding up and down bids. A home to grid DR program is presented in [23]. It uses user expected price as an indicator for differential pricing in domestic tariff. The proposed algorithm schedules the operation of electrical appliances by comparing user expected price to real-time pricing. An exponential smoothing model is used to forecast the desired amount of power, and Bayes theorem is used to determine the probability of power demand by appliances at given amount of time. A new market-based approach named contract for deferral scheme is presented in [24]. The authors present a detailed review on how need for grid capacity and defer demand-driven network investments can be reduced by integrating distributed generators, storage and demand response to network resources. A DR technique is implemented in [25] with the aim of developing framework to identify energy options for demand-supply matching and to determine which option is suitable for DR program. A DR framework is presented with combination of liquefied petroleum gas LPG-based combined heat and power CHP microgrid.

A new stochastic energy and reserve scheduling method considering different DR programs is given for microgrid [26]. Probability distribution function is used to model uncertainties caused by distribution generators. The proposed design is implemented on a microgrid consisting of different loads and generating units. In [27], DR techniques are categorized on the basis of a chosen criteria. A detailed review on DR programs is given. A hierarchical-based source-storage-load DR control system is explained in [28]. Objective of the suggested technique is to reduce the working cost. An optimal scheduling operation is introduced to optimize load curve and power output. Particle swarm optimization (PSO) method is implemented to solve the optimal problem. Simulations are performed to prove the effectiveness of the suggested model. With an aim to optimize hourly bids that microgrid aggregator submit to day-ahead market to increase its profit, a scenario-based stochastic programming framework is introduced in [29]. Due to the proposed design, DR program is integrated into microgrids through contractual agreements. The proposed design facilitates customers, microgrids operators and operation of system operator.

Different risk management strategies are discussed in [30] for retail electricity providers to deal with uncertainties in day-ahead market. It also focuses on minimizing financial losses in market. For these purposes, a two-staged stochastic programming technique. A robust DR program is proposed in [31] for commercial buildings under load prediction uncertainty. Initial control signals are obtained through conventional genetic algorithm (GA). However, optimal control signals are got through Monte Carlo method. Through dynamic pricing technique, impact of load prediction uncertainty is studied. Taking consumption shifting constraints into account, a DR program is explained in [32]. It also focuses on distributed generators DG resource management through virtual power player (VPP) aiming at minimizing operational cost.

Different modeling tools are explained in [33] for fixed and flexible loads with an aim to optimize energy dispatch. Using a case study of Corvo Island, Portugal, three different scenarios are simulated in Homer, EnergyPlan and in MATLAB. On the basis of results obtained, it is observed that modeling tools should be optimized by improving their optimization strategies to get more benefit of using DR programs. A method is proposed to balance load to determine low cost mix of DGs, DR and storage to replace conventional methods for a case study [34]. Results are obtained after implementing this technique on three different scenarios showing that by using presented technique, desirable results are achieved. A multi-timescale cost-effective power management algorithm is suggested in [35] for microgrid MG in islanded mode. The operation of MG is optimized through managing generation, storage and demand management. Batteries and electric water heaters are utilized in DR programs. First, two different ON/OFF strategies are presented for electric water heaters, and then power management algorithm is implemented to obtain optimized operation. To solve a multi-objective optimization problem for achieving optimal DR programming, artificial bee colony algorithm and quasi-static algorithm are implemented in [36]. There are some constraints regarding energy balance and operation which are taken into consideration for optimizing cost and performance of the power systems. Uncertainties are evaluated through stochastic technique to study the performance of the presented design. With the increase in use of renewable energy, there is an increase in challenge of balancing intermittent generation with demand variations. This problem is solved in [37] by introducing different demand control mechanism. A specific tariff design is proposed to get robust performances which reduces cost of energy.

A detailed review on DSM techniques, implementation and projects is given in [38]. Authors in [38] discuss the implementation of DR in China from grid, community and user prospective. Authors finally conclude this work by indicating the issues regarding implementation of DR programs in China. Three different scenarios are discussed in [39] to integrate DR programs into electricity markets. The three scenarios are optimize procurement, offer as control reserve and avoid balancing energy. The results obtained after implementing the suggested model, show that there is 3% decrease in cost. A model-based assessment energy system model is presented in [40]. In this technique, a mixed energy system model is extended by flexible load to use suggested assessment model. Results prove that DR can economically substitute upto 10GW power plant. A load scheduling algorithm is suggested after the classification of appliances into five sets with respect to their energy utilization and operational characteristics in [41]. The load scheduling algorithm adopts time-of-use pricing, controls operation time and power usage of the appliances. A generalized Benders' decomposition technique is proposed to solve mixed integer nonlinear programming. A battery-aided DR program is presented in [42] to reduce cost of energy in grid-tied systems including domestic and industrial sector. A continuous time block tariffing is suggested as pricing technique while considering nonlinear behavior of batteries. A method called as calculus of variation is also implemented to get closed form of analytical results. Results suggest that calculus of variation method gives better performance and is effective in cost reduction.

A stochastic method is proposed for scheduling industrial virtual power player (IVPP) in [43]. DR program is introduced in the power system and with the help of the proposed stochastic method, operator can choose best DR program for scheduling IVPP. In mixed-integer nonlinear programming, a suitable technique is presented to achieve desired objectives. The IEEE reliability test system is applied to the presented design to validate obtained results. The Brazilian Electrical Regulatory Agency presents a mechanism to update tariff structure of distribution companies. In [44], this mechanism and its results are analyzed in detail. DR program is introduced, and its impact on energy prices, operating prices and on end-users is studied. The presented case is based on the actual data collected from Brazilian electrical system. The authors conclude this work by giving some guidelines to improve and implement this technique. A method is proposed for demand side load shift to increase reliability and to minimize nodal price of power systems [45]. In the proposed model, conventional electricity prices are replaced by nodal prices. Demand is mutually interacted with electricity prices. Through demand-price electricity matrix, DR is modeled. Using demand- price elasticity, demand side load shifts are found. Then the load shift, which is stochastic in nature, is measured using determined load shifts under contingencies. Through optimal power flow, reliability and nodal prices are investigated. A Roy Billinton Test System (RBTS) is used for simulations to validate results. The concept of incentive payments in DR programs is explained in [46] through three different approaches considering different levels of consumer's privacy. A concept of trade-offs between consumer's privacy, resources and the reward that load aggregator get is analyzed. It is concluded that in centralized approach, resource exploitation and reward are sensitive to accuracy of load aggregator's consumer cost curves approximations.

To improve grid frequency regulation, a DLC method is presented for a dynamic model of variable speed heat pump (VSHP) [47]. To control input power of VSHP, a variable speed drive-controlled induction motor is also introduced in the system. An experimental room model is designed to analyze effect of DLC program on room temperature for two cooling systems in the room. A small signal analysis is performed on the system to study the transient behavior of VSHP and grid frequency regulation (GFR). Simulations are performed with an isolated microgrid implemented on the system designed to analyze results. In order to study grid frequency regulation, VSHP is integrated with battery energy storage systems (BEES) [48]. For this purpose, a power-hardware-in-the-loop setup is formulated in simulations to observe effect of VSHP and BEES on GFR. A new real-time GFR technique is implemented to eliminate deviations in frequency and reserve capacities of the generators. Simulation results prove that the presented VSHP and BEES can be used in effective frequency stability process. A new algorithm is presented to reduce power outages and peak average ratio [49]. To do so, forecasting of load, load shedding and DLC techniques are used. A daily schedule is formulated for intelligent electronic devices though Internet of things and stream analytics. Intelligent electronic devices are characterized on the basis of their demands, thermal comfort and load model. For implementing this algorithm, hundred different consumers are selected owning different devices. Results obtained after applying the algorithm prove the superiority of the presented design.

A quantitative technique is presented in [50] to assess the advantages of controlling load in reinforcement costs of distribution networks. The outputs obtained through initial experiments lead to development of a linear model estimating change in demand due to DLC. The impact of DLC on reinforcements cost is studied in detail. An experimental survey is conducted in [51] to investigate the willingness of consumers for participating in DLC program. A manipulative experiment is conducted by conveying two sentence message to consumers to gain their trust for participating in the program. It is concluded that their distrust in utilities leads to reduction of willingness to participate in DLC program. A robust optimization method is adopted for optimal operation of microgrid [52]. A two-stage framework is presented to reduce uncertainties in renewable resources. The two-stage framework consists of one hour ahead charging and discharging of the storage systems and quarter hour ahead working of a DLC program. For this purpose, energy storage is scheduled and a DLC program is suggested. Results obtained suggest that the designed method achieves the desired objective; maximizing profit of microgrid. Results obtained are verified through IEEE 30-bus distribution system. A dynamic agent model is presented in [53] to study its impact on profitability of generators, cost and reserve margins. This model is implemented on alternative demand curves which are suggested for Pennsylvania, New Jersey and Maryland (PJM) interconnections. It is concluded that after a sloped demand curve, the costs are low when compared to present requirements. Due to reduction of fluctuations in installed reserves, average installed capacity is less for same reliability.

In [54], authors examine the procedure and contribution of DR programs and energy efficiency EE in forward capacity markets while considering a case study in UK. It is observed that EE mechanism is heavily influenced by regulatory utilities. It is seen that target of DR and EE is end-users. While defining capacity products, needs of the system and resources potential should be kept in consideration. It is suggested that barriers should be removed in implementation of the DLC programs. A high-resolution DSM model is proposed in [55]. In this work, main module is divided into many sub-modules to ensure reliable power system while maintaining standards and needs. A multi-source DSM method is explained in [56] to reduce peak load demand. Energy cost reduction is the main objective in designing distributed DSM system using Internet of things (IoTs) presented in [57]. A review on DSM integrated with smart grid SG is given in [58]. A DSM technique is proposed in [59] which is based on PV energy resource system to deal with increase in power consumption. A new DSM method having a feature of decision making is proposed in [60] to increase power consumption. A novel DSM technique based on EV storage systems to optimize electricity cost is proposed in [61].

Table 1 shows the literature survey on techniques implemented for DSM;

4   Demand Side Management Programs and Techniques

Demand side management programs and techniques are divided into following programs; energy efficiency, demand response and strategic load growth, and are shown in Fig. 5.

4.1   Energy Efficiency (EE)

It is a long-term strategy in which energy-efficient techniques are used to reduce consumption of energy and demand of load. It includes programs like enhancement of efficiency of domestic appliances and weatherization. Weatherization is a technique in which a building is protected against external elements including wind or sunlight, etc. It also includes upgradation of building for saving energy consumption and decreasing load demand. After implementing energy efficiency programs, cost of electricity and load demand during peak hours are reduced. It also delays the plan to expand power plant capacity [1].

Table 1 Literature review with identification of features and objectives

Technique	Feature	Objectives	References
Linear programming	Scheduling of load and smart charging of the batteries	To reduce cost and peak-to-average ratio	[62]
Mixed linear and integer linear programming	Scheduling of home appliances	Optimizing peak load and cost of electricity	[63]
Multi-objective mixed integer programming	Modeling of appliances on the basis of preferences	To minimize cost of electricity while considering preferences	[64]
Double cooperative game theory	Scheduling of home appliances using electric vehicle, also scheduling appliances	Reducing cost for user and utilities	[65]
Game theoretic energy management	Scheduling of appliances through electric bicycle and energy of utilities, selling back energy to utilities	Bill reduction of users and load minimization of utilities	[66]
Quasi random process	Recursive formula for load shifting	Estimation of peak demand for residential sector	[67]
Time-of-use (TOU) based scheduling	Time and energy consumption optimization of appliances	Peak load and cost minimization	[68]
Genetic algorithm	Scheduling of electrical and thermal energy with cooperation of distribution generators	Minimizing operating cost without disturbing human comfort	[69]
Reinforcement learning	Scheduling of consumption of electricity on the basis of forecasted price and decision for domestic and commercial sector	Optimized cost and maintaining user's comfort	[70]
Greedy iterative algorithm	While considering aggregated load, scheduling of domestic appliances	Reduction of peak load, shifting of load and cost optimization	[71]
Wind-Driven optimization	Scheduling of domestic appliances while integrating renewable energy source	Reduction of cost and time	[72]

Fig. 5 DSM programs

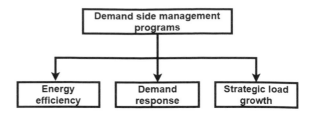

EE strategies include:

- It includes adopting energy-efficient buildings and devices.
- It includes to encourage users to adopt energy conscious behavior
- It includes improving and conducting regular maintenance of electrical equipment to reduce energy loss using modern and optimized technologies.
- It also includes improving efficiency of power transmission and distribution networks.

4.2 Demand Response (DR)

It is a manipulative short-term load program and is described as the modification in usage of electricity by end-user consumer from normal consumption in response to changes in any DR programs. As DR directly affects the load consumption, it is most used program in DSM [1, 73], which is also one of the advantages of this program. Demand response is implemented through many ways including valley filling technique in which loads are build in off-peak hours. Peak clipping is a technique in which load is reduced during peak hours. Load shifting is another technique which is the combination of both peak clipping an valley filling techniques. Peak clipping and valley filling are shown in Fig. 6.

DR program is classified into following: price-based DR, incentive/event-based DR and reduction bids. Classification of DR is shown in Fig. 7.

4.2.1 Price-Based Demand Response

In this program, customers are offered static or dynamic pricing scheme to control load profile of end-user consumers [74]. Some of the programs in price-based demand response are depicted in Fig. 8 and are given below;

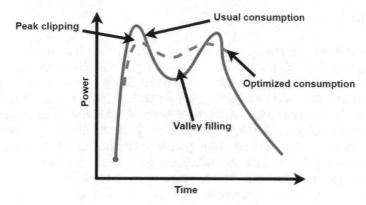

Fig. 6 DR techniques

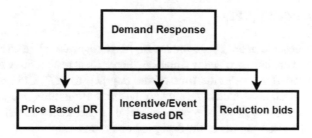

Fig. 7 DR programs

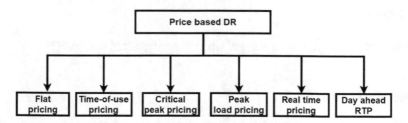

Fig. 8 Price-based DR

Flat Pricing

A technique in which unchanged prices are offered allowing consumers to consume electricity up to maximum amount, even if there is a change in load demand, is called as flat pricing. It is often termed as welfare pricing scheme. If there is change in aggregated load, users are not charged for that change. Hence, there is no financial incentive for consumers to reschedule their use of electricity. So, in case of unplanned electricity consumption, users do not have to pay high bills [74].

Time-of-Use Pricing

In traditional utility prices, price of electricity per kilowatt hour is set, which can be changed during different seasons. So, a sliding rate is introduced and is structured according to peak and off-peak time of day called as time-of-use pricing [2]. A TOU-based Monte Carlo simulation technique is implemented on smart grid pilots in China [23]. It is concluded that from the designed controller, efficient operation of smart grid is achieved. A TOU-based quadratic programming and stochastic optimization techniques are implemented in [24]. A meta-heuristic solution technique is implemented in [25] for sustainable manufacturing systems. A mixed-integer linear programming-based TOU and Gaussian mixture-model-based TOU technique are implemented in [26, 75], respectively.

Critical Peak Pricing (CPP)

When utilities observe or anticipate sudden high market prices of electricity or when power systems went into emergency situation, then critical peak pricing is introduced for critical events during specific time of the day [2]. In [27], CPP and TOU are implemented on the case study. Results show that CPP is effective than TOU in terms of cost reduction. A CPP decision model is implemented in [28]. Numerical results prove the effectiveness of the designed controller.

Peak Load Pricing

In this program, high price is charged when there is peak of the load [74].

Real-Time Pricing (RTP)

In this program, a tariffed retail is charged for delivered electrical power which vary hour to hour [2]. A RTP technique is introduced in [19] to analyze energy consumption in wind generation. A day-ahead unit commitment model is used to estimate systems operation in wind generation. A case study is presented in [76] to find the effect of RTP on the electricity supply. RTP-based DSM controllers are implemented in residential buildings [20–22].

Day-Ahead RTP

It is a type of real-time pricing in which market purchases or sells electricity at bidding ahead prices for following day [74].

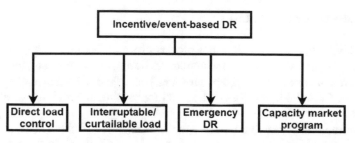

Fig. 9 Incentive/event-based DR

4.2.2 Incentive or Event-Based Demand Response

In this program, customers are offered specific DR requests and in case of acceptance of that request, customers are offered time-varying or fixed payments. Incentive-based methods are discussed in detail in [29, 30]. Incentive-based programs are implemented on load curve of peak day in Iranian power station to assess the performance of these programs [31]. Some of these programs are shown in Fig. 9 and explained below [74].

Direct Load Control

Direct load control (DLC) being a major part of DR is a technique in which operator can remotely manage the use of electricity of end-users. Thus, system operator becomes able to bring power system in normal state by applying preventive control. DLC enables utilities to remotely control the load demand by modifying appliances [1]. DLC changes the load profile by introducing a program in distribution networks or controlling user's appliances through information technology (IT). The devices that are controlled through IT include washing machine, heating ventilation and air conditioning HVAC, water heaters, etc. This program encourages customers to cooperate with utilities. DLC guarantees the reduction in load demand of utilities which as a result leads to reduction of additional production of energy. In some cases, customers face penalty for noncooperation with utilities. On the basis of time-of-use tariff, residential and small customers pay their electricity bills. From pre-specified optimization program, parameters like on-time and delay-time are obtained, which play an important role in implementing DLC.

A DLC technique based on multi-objective particle swarm optimization technique is implemented in [32]. A cooperative game DLC technique is implemented in [33]. DLC-based controlling techniques are implemented to optimize operation of air conditioning loads [34–37].

Interruptible/Curtailable Load

Interruptible program is an old relief program for utilities in which customers are provided an option to remove some appliances during emergency conditions.

However, in curtailable program, customers are asked to reduce load upon asked by utilities. Curtailable program is designed for commercial and industrial sector's customers.

In interruptible/curtailable load program, customers are offered discounts in bills in exchange for agreeing to reduce load during system contingencies. Customers can be penalized, if they do not take certain measures. Interruptible/curtailable load program is different from emergency demand response program in a way that they are proposed by electric utility and utility service has capacity to apply the program when required [1]. Interruptible programs are offered to those commercial or industrial customers who have ability to shut their appliances for small span of time or switch to other back up generators to fulfill their load demand. Customers with 1 MW load are required in this program including manufacturing plant, water treatment plant or food processing plants. The customers with backup generation capability are also included in this program, i.e., hospitals or data centers. For this effort, customers receive interruptible rates of electricity, which are lower than the normal industrial prices. Sometimes, customers receive incentives or discount for interrupted service.

Emergency Demand Response (EDR) Program

When power systems go to overload conditions, operator determines amount and time to curtail the load to bring the power system back into normal state. EDR is then implemented with certain constraints and parameters. This program will determine that which house can be added in the program so that it will not affect cost and disrupt electricity [1].

Capacity Market Program

Capacity market programs are usually considered as a form of insurance because in this program, customers are committed for providing pre-specified load curtailment when system is subjected to contingencies. A capacity market program is implemented on a case study in England [38]. A detail framework is given in for evaluation of capacity market program [39]. Capacity market program is introduced in Russia to evaluate its performance with respect to cost and quality of generation [40]. A capacity market program is implemented in China. Results show the positive impact of designed technique on power system [41].

4.2.3 Reduction Bids

Customers in reduction bids offer incentives to utility by offering reduction in load demand capacity and requested price [1]. A demand bidding program is introduced for reducing peak load. The results obtained after implementation of said program proved the effectiveness of proposed design [42]. In this program, customers are offered payments in return of reduction in load. There are two categories that are included in this program on the basis of structure of bid. Under this program, users that participate submit their bids to utility or system operator. Generally, a day-ahead bid is chosen in which a specific amount of load is shed at given time. Bids are analyzed with system forecast and supply bids by electricity market administrator. Then, the administrator determines the most economical supply and load demand options. A demand bidding program based on stochastic model is proposed in for distributed energy resources [43].

4.3 Strategic Load Growth

An increase in electrical load is called as strategic load growth. It is induced by utilities by using thermal storage and heat pumps, etc [1].

4.4 Energy Conservation (ENCON)

The aim of ENCON is to reduce the power consumption loss in power system. The methods used for end-user to improve energy consumption quality are included in ENCON. Various power-saving techniques such as use of high-efficiency motors, variable speed drivers, economizers, leak prevention and minimizing pressure drops are discussed in [10]. Multiple energy conservation techniques in cogeneration units are given in [11, 77, 78]. There is a new concept of energy recovery which is termed as energy productivity defined as for any given input of the system, the maximum output achieved is called as energy productivity. A detailed analysis of ENCON techniques with case studies is given in [12, 14]. Energy audit is an another technique in ECON, whose aim is to reduce cost of electricity and make power system environmentally friendly. Few case studies for energy audit are given in [13, 79].

5 Optimal Residential Demand Side Management Considering Renewable Energy Resources

Residential buildings have a great contribution in increasing aggregated power consumption [80]. According to statistics, buildings contribute toward 40% consumption of overall energy and also are responsible for carbon emission. Provision of reliable and uninterruptible power supply are becoming difficult challenges. To overcome these challenges, concept of smart grid (SG) emerged as a promising solution. In smart grid, DSM plays an major role in achieving required or desired results. Through DSM, the increasing load demand of consumers is managed and controlled. In DSM, consumers are encouraged to change their electricity pattern from normal pattern. Nowadays, renewable energy resources including hydroelectric, solar or wind, are being used as sources to produce energy instead of traditional power plants in which one or two generators were used to produce electricity [44]. A smart microgrid framework for residential buildings is shown in Fig. 10. A smart building system consists of generation systems, e.g., wind, PV, etc. and storage system to store electricity produced. It also consists of a grid connection which is used either in peak hours to balance load demand or it is used for selling surplus electricity.

There are many techniques offered by DSM to manage load demand such as;

1. Peak clipping
2. Valley filling
3. Load shifting

Fig. 10 Demand side management

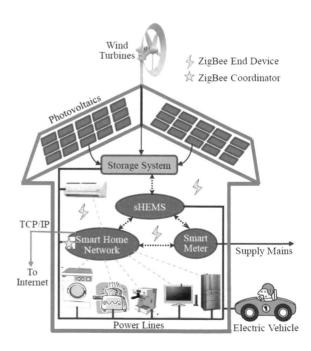

4. Strategic conservation
5. Strategic load growth.

In this architecture, there is a major component called as smart home controller (SHC) which manages devices inside the house. This device helps to obtain desired objective functions like minimizing peak load and cost based on TOU tariff, device specifications and on consumer's preferences. SHC control and manages appliances through communication networking. There are three categories of home appliances [81];

1. Time-shiftable devices: Devices whose operational hours can be shifted such as washing machine. These devices can be scheduled through SHC.
2. Power-Shiftable devices: These devices consume power in maximum and minimum range, i.e., electric vehicles. SHC decides how much energy these devices can use.
3. Non-shiftable devices: Devices which have fixed power consumption requirement, i.e., light. SHC decides their usage according to customer's preferences.

6 Architecture of Residential Demand Side Management

Architecture of residential DSM is given in Fig. 11. Basic components of DSM are given as follows [45];

1. Local generators: Local energy plants that could provide electricity and can be used either locally or injected into grid.
2. Smart devices: Electrical devices to provide data such as power consumption.
3. Sensors: Devices used to monitor data.
4. Energy storage systems: Storage devices allowing DSM to be flexible in managing electric resources.
5. Energy management unit: Manages electric resources of users based on intelligent DSM mechanisms.
6. Smart grid domains: A utility company which provides electricity to those users who pay payments. The utility company is part of market domain.

In this architecture, all components are connected through communication infrastructure. Elements within customer's domain are interconnected through home area network (HAN). Wired or wireless technologies can be used to implement HAN networks. In wired technologies, Ethernet and power line communication are used. While in wireless communication, ZigBee and low-power wireless personal area networks (LoWPAN) are brought into practice. In addition to HAN, wide area networks (WANs) is also used for connecting energy management unit to other domains of smart grid. Cellular networks are usually used as promising way of communication. Worldwide interoperability for microwave access (WiMAX) and long-term evolution (LTE) are also used for this purpose [45].

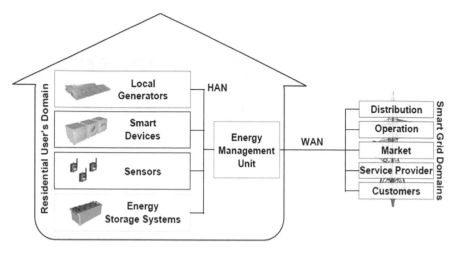

Fig. 11 Architecture of DSM

6.1 Energy Consumption Model

Suppose for energy consumption model of residential sector, a home with different appliances is shown in $A \triangleq \{a_1, a_2, a_3, \ldots\}$, while $a_1, a_2, \ldots, a_n$ represents different appliances over time $t \in T \triangleq \{1, 2, 3, \ldots, T\}$. The total energy consumption of devices is shown through Eq. 1 [5];

$$E_{C,T_L} = \sum_{t=1}^{T} \left[\sum_{j=1}^{N} E_{a_j,t} \right] \forall \, t \in T, a \in A \tag{1}$$

The energy consumed by different appliances is monitored through controller devices and the data is collected through different devices.

6.2 Categories of Load

Loads are divided into different categories according to energy consumption, user preference and their time of operating. Suppose, total load of different types of appliances can be shown through following mathematical Eq. 2 [5];

$$A_n = [R_a \cup S_a \cup \varepsilon_a] \tag{2}$$

where

R_a Regularly used devices,
S_a Shiftable devices,
ε_a Elastic appliances.

6.2.1 Regularly Operated Appliances

There are devices in daily life whose energy consumption pattern cannot be changed. Daily used appliances are denoted by R_a, aggregated energy consumed per day is represented by ς_{R_a} and power rating of R_a is denoted by $\varsigma_{R_a}^{\tau}$. The total energy consumed per day is expressed in Eq. 3 [5];

$$\varsigma_{R_a, T_L} = \sum_{t=1}^{T} \left[\sum_{R_a \in A_n} \varsigma_{R_a}^{\tau t} * \zeta(t) \right] \tag{3}$$

While the total cost is represented by Eq. 4;

$$\rho_{R_a}^{T_L} = \sum_{t=1}^{T} \left[\sum_{R_a \in A_n} \varsigma_{R_a}^{\tau t} * \varepsilon(t) * \zeta(t) \right] \tag{4}$$

where,

$\zeta(t) \in [0, 1]$ operation state of appliance
ε pricing signal.

6.2.2 Shiftable Appliances

There are some devices which can be controlled, and their time of operation can be shifted without compromising their performances called shiftable appliances denoted by S_a and their power rating is represented by v_{S_a}. The total energy is represented in Eq. 5 [5];

$$\varsigma_{S_a, T_L} = \sum_{t=1}^{T} \left[\sum_{S_a \in A_n} v_{S_a}^{t} * \zeta(t) \right] \tag{5}$$

The total cost is represented by Eq. 6,

$$\rho_{S_a}^{T_L} = \sum_{t=1}^{T} \left[\sum_{S_a \in A_n} v_{S_a}^{t} * \varepsilon(t) * \zeta(t) \right] \tag{6}$$

6.2.3 Elastic Appliances

These devices are called elastic because their time of operation and energy consumption curve can be adjusted flexibly. Elastic appliances include thermostatically controlled devices, i.e., water heater, HVAC, etc. Elastic devices are denoted as ε_a and power rating is denoted as μ_{ε_a}. The total energy is given in Eq. 7 [5],

$$\varsigma_{\varepsilon_a,T_L} = \sum_{t=1}^{T} \left[\sum_{\varepsilon_a \in A_n} \mu_{S_a}^t * \zeta(t) \right] \tag{7}$$

The total cost is given in Eq. 8,

$$\rho_{\varepsilon_a}^{T_L} = \sum_{t=1}^{T} \left[\sum_{\varepsilon_a \in A_n} \mu_{\varepsilon_a}^t * \varepsilon(t) * \zeta(t) \right] \tag{8}$$

Now, by assumption, total power consumed by all devices is given by Eq. 9,

$$\varsigma_{T_L} = \varsigma_{R_a,T_L} + \varsigma_{S_a,T_L} + \varsigma_{\varepsilon_a,T_L} \tag{9}$$

and the total cost is represented by Eq. 10 [5],

$$\rho_{T_L} = \rho_{R_a}^{T_L} + \rho_{S_a}^{T_L} + \rho_{\varsigma_a}^{T_L} \tag{10}$$

The energy consumption by appliances can be formulated through Eq. 11 [5],

$$E_c = \begin{bmatrix} \varsigma_{R_a}^{t_1} & \cdots & \varsigma_{S_a}^{t_1} & \cdots & \varsigma_{\rho_a}^{t_1} \\ \varsigma_{R_a}^{t_2} & \cdots & \varsigma_{S_a}^{t_2} & \cdots & \varsigma_{\rho_a}^{t_2} \\ \cdot & & \cdot & & \cdot \\ \cdot & & \cdot & & \cdot \\ \cdot & & \cdot & & \cdot \\ \varsigma_{R_a}^{T} & \cdots & \varsigma_{S_a}^{T} & \cdots & \varsigma_{\rho_a}^{T} \end{bmatrix} \tag{11}$$

7 Problem Formulation for the Exact Solution Methods

Problem formulation is a major step before proceeding toward solution. Problem formulation should address following concerns [45];

1. What does the model need to find?
2. What are the objectives that this model needs to be achieved?
3. What are the variables of the problem?
4. What are the constraints on the variables?

8 Objective Function and Constraints

8.1 Objective Functions

Objectives of DSM optimization model are given as follows [45];

1. Bill minimization: To decrease the cost associated with usage.
2. Minimization of discomfort: To decrease discomfort experiences by customers caused by operating devices.
3. Minimization of local generation use: Energy generated by local sources should be maximized.

There are two types of objective functions, i.e., to increase load factor for facility and to decrease cost of electricity produced. DSM program optimizes two of the following objective functions in Eqs. 12, 13, 14;

$$\text{Max L.F.} = \left[\left[\sum_{i=1}^{N} \sum_{j=1}^{J} P_{(i,j)} * t_j \right] \Big/ \sum_{j=1}^{J} t_j \right] \Big/ \sum_{i=1}^{N} P_{(i,k)} \qquad (12)$$

$$\text{Max L.F.} = \left[\left[\sum_{j=i}^{J} P_{(TO(j))} * t_j \right] \Big/ \sum_{j=1}^{J} t_j \right] \Big/ P_{TO(K)} \qquad (13)$$

$$\text{Min } C = \left[\sum_{i=1}^{N} \sum_{j=1}^{J} P_{(i,j)} * t_j * ce_{(i,j)} \right] + \left[\sum_{i=1}^{N} \sum_{j=1}^{J} P_{(i,j)} * cd_{(i,j)} \right] \qquad (14)$$

Objective functions for different DSM techniques are presented as follows;

8.1.1 Valley Filling

In this technique, off-peak loads are build up to improve economic efficiency of the building and to smooth load curve. Charging electric vehicle at night is an example of valley filling. In this case, utility is not required to produce more energy at day. Load during the day is decreased, while the load at night is increased which as a result smooths the load curve. Valley filling can be shown in Fig. 12;

Fig. 12 Valley filling

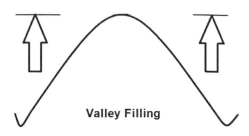

Valley Filling

Objective function is given in Eqs. 15 and 16 as follows;

$$\text{Max L.F.} = \left[\left[\sum_{i=1}^{N}\sum_{j=1}^{J}P_{(i,j)} * t_j\right] \Big/ \sum_{j=1}^{J}t_{(j)}\right] \Big/ \sum_{i=1}^{N}P_{(i,k)} \qquad (15)$$

$$\text{Max L.F.} = \left[\left[\sum_{j=1}^{J}P_{TO(j)} * t_j\right] \Big/ \sum_{j=1}^{J}t_{(j)}\right] \Big/ P_{TO(K)} \qquad (16)$$

8.1.2 Load Shifting

In load shifting, peak energy usage time is changed to increased energy generation time. Energy consumption remains unchanged, but peak load demand decreases. Cost of electricity decreases, while the load factor is improved. Load shifting is shown in Fig. 13.

Objective functions are given below in Eqs. 17 and 18;

$$\text{Max L.F.} = \left[\left[\sum_{j=1}^{J}P_{TO(j)} * t_j\right] \Big/ \sum_{j=1}^{J}t_{(j)}\right] \Big/ P_{TO(k)} \qquad (17)$$

$$\text{Min } C. = \left[\sum_{i=1}^{N}\sum_{j=1}^{J}P_{(i,j)} * t_j * ce_{i,j}\right] + \left[\sum_{i=1}^{N}\sum_{j=1}^{J}P_{(i,j)} * cd_{i,j}\right] \qquad (18)$$

8.1.3 Peak Clipping

In this technique, utility loads are decreased during peak load demand hours. The power consumption and load demand both are decreased, while the load factor is

Fig. 13 Load shifting

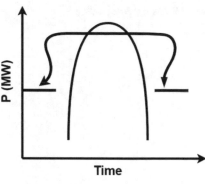

Fig. 14 Peak clipping

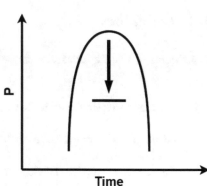

improved resulting in decrease in electricity cost. Peak clipping is shown in Fig. 14. Objective functions are given in Eq. 19;

$$\text{Max L.F.} = \left[\left[\sum_{j=1}^{J} P_{TO(j)} * t_j \right] / t_{(j)} \right] / P_{TO(k)} \tag{19}$$

8.1.4 Energy Conservation

In energy consumption method, aggregated power consumption and peak demand are minimized. Energy conservation is shown in Fig. 15. Objective functions formulated in Eq. 20;

$$\text{Min } C. = \left[\sum_{i=1}^{N} \sum_{j=1}^{J} P_{(i,j)} * t_j * ce_{(i,j)} \right] + \left[\sum_{i=1}^{N} \sum_{j=1}^{J} P_{(i,j)} * cd_{(i,j)} \right] \tag{20}$$

Fig. 15 Energy conservation

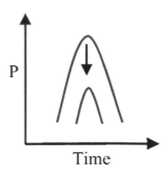

8.2   Constraints

Constraints of DSM optimization model are as follows [45];

8.2.1   Constraints on Electric Devices

1. Fixed electric device: In fixed electric devices, usage time and power consumption cannot be changed.
2. Shiftable electric device: Devices can be shifted in time without disturbing load profile.
3. Energy-based elastic electric devices: These devices must utilize a fixed amount of power within a fixed time.
4. Comfort-based elastic electric devices: It can control a physical variable which influence user's comfort [45].

8.2.2   Local Energy Generators

These generate power which can be produced locally or injected into the grid.

8.2.3   Energy Storage Systems

These devices can be charged/discharged while satisfying maximum rates and SOC constraints.

8.2.4   Energy Balance

It is an important restriction in power systems that there should be a balance between input and output energy.

8.2.5 Energy Market

1. Fixed tariff: Prices of electricity are not dependent on users.
2. Power-dependent tariff: Price of energy depends on users demand.
3. Reward tariff: Energy prices are the sum of fixed prices and rewards which customers can get if they adjust their demands properly.

9 Different Models

Different models are presented for DSM optimization in previous literature. Some of which are presented as follows [45];

1. Genetic algorithm
2. Differential evolution algorithm
3. Particle swarm optimization algorithm
4. Ant colony algorithms.

9.1 Genetic Algorithm

The concept of genetic algorithm (GA) originated from Darwin's theory of evolution which is survival of the fittest. GA is an optimization techniques which is inspired from concept of genes and chromosomes, represented as set of variables. Chromosomes corresponds to every solution for optimization problem while genes represent variables of the problem. If there are ten variables in problem, then GA will use ten genes. There are three major steps in GA technique: selection, crossover and mutation shown in Fig. 16.

The steps involved in GA are as follows;

1. **Start**: In this step, a random n chromosomes population is generated. As chromosomes represent solutions to problem, it means suitable solutions are generated.
2. **Fitness**: Every chromosome in population is tested for fitness. Only fit chromosomes are considered which passes a certain criteria.
3. **New population**: A new population is designed through following steps,

   (a) **Selection**: Two parent chromosomes are chosen according to fitness criteria.
   (b) **Crossover**: A new offspring is formed from crossover. With no crossover, offspring is same as the parent chromosome.
   (c) **Mutation**: New offspring is mutated with mutation probability at a specific position in chromosome.
   (d) **Accepting**: Now, new offspring is placed in population.

4. **Replace**: With this generated population, algorithm is run.

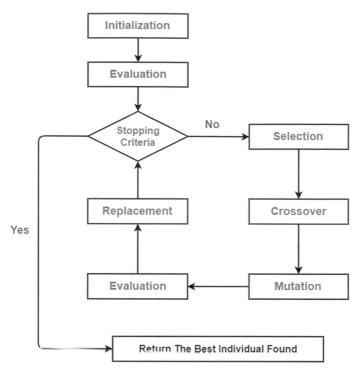

Fig. 16 Steps in GA

5. **Test**: Best solution is achieved, if end conditions are satisfied.
6. **Loop**: If end solutions are not achieved, Go to step 2

9.2 Differential Evolution Algorithm

Differential evolution algorithm is a stochastic optimization technique, developed in 1994 by Kenneth Price.

The steps are as follows given in Fig. 17; let us assume a function which consists of some real parameters D are to be optimized. The size of population is selected which should be at least 4.

- The extreme bounds (lower and upper) for every parameter is defined.
- For a given interval, the initial values of parameters are selected at random.
- Mutation, recombination and selection of N parameters are performed.
- The search space is expanded through mutation.
- Three vectors are selected at random for a given parameter.
- The weighted differences of two vectors are added to the third vector.
- The mutation factor F is a constant selected from an interval [0, 2].

Fig. 17 Differential
evolutionary algorithm

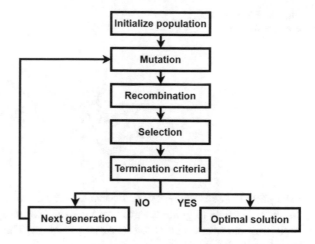

- Recombination is performed on successful solutions obtained from previous generations.
- From elements of donor and target vector, a trial vector is developed.
- In trial vector, the donor vector with a probability is entered.
- Trail vector is compared with target vector. The target vector with lowest function value is admitted to next generation.
- A stopping criteria are selected through which mutation, recombination and selection.

9.3 Particle Swarm Optimization (PSO) Algorithm

PSO is a stochastic optimization technique proposed by Dr. Eberhart and Dr. Kennedy in 1995 which is inspired by bird flocking and fish schooling. PSO is very similar to GA in a way that system starts with generating random populations and through updating generations for finding optimal solution. In PSO, particles being potential solutions fly through problem space by following current optimal particles. PSO is easy to implement as compared to GA.

As, PSO imitates bird flocking. Suppose there is a piece of food in a space. A group of birds is flying in that space but cannot find the food. So best way to search for the food is to follow that bird nearer to the food as shown in Fig. 18.

PSO starts with designing random particles where every particle represents a solution. Algorithm runs to find the best optimal solution though updating generations by iterations. Fitness function is designed to test every particle, and the value which originates from fitness functions is called as fitness function value. If this value is best one, then it is stored and called as best value, personal best (pbest). When the iterations stop, the best found fitness value is termed as global best (gbest). Hence,

Fig. 18 Block flocking
example for PSO

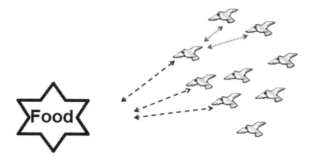

each particle keeps the record of two values pbest and gbest, which are responsible for every particle to guide toward best position. So the speed and position of every individual particle are based on its pbest and gbest. The next position of particle is found on the basis of;

- its current position found by an equation given in pseudocode
- its current velocity given by an equation in pseudocode
- the distance between its current position and pbest
- the difference between its current position and gbest.

The pseudocode of PSO is depicted in Fig. 19;

```
P= Particle_Initialization ();
For i=1 to it_max
        For each particle p in P do
            fp=f(p);
            If fp is better than f(pBest)
                    pBest = p;
            end
        end
        gBest=best p in P;
        For each particle p in P do
            v= v + c1*rand*(pBest - p) + c2*rand*(gBest - p);
            p=p + v;
        end
    end
```

Fig. 19 Pseudocode of PSO

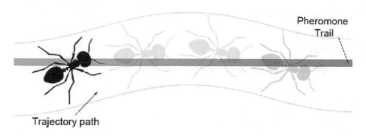

Fig. 20 Trajectory of ants

9.4 Ant Colony Algorithms ACA

Dorgio, in 1999, was the first one to propose this algorithm inspired by the process, in which ants find the optimal path being shortest to find food. While finding food, ants leave a trail by excreting a chemical named pheromone which serves as guide or method of communication for other ants to follow to find food. So the ants that choose shortest route will cover the distance at faster rate. Therefore, the ants will follow that path which has more pheromone creating a positive feedback. There are some ants working in parallel called as artificial ants that interact with each other through cumulative distribution function updated by weighting factors. These weighting factors are determined by the distance covered on the path chosen by ants analogous to pheromones. That is the procedure followed in ACA. This process is shown in Fig. 20. In ant colony optimization, for given optimization problem, software agents termed as artificial ants search for best solution. While applying ACA, the optimization of the given problem is converted into a problem of finding best path on graph. While moving on graph, artificial ants build many solutions. The process of building of solutions is stochastic in nature and affected by pheromone. Pseudocode of ACA is given below in Fig. 21.

10 Impact of DSM on Power Systems

The benefits provided by DSM are as follows

1. It maintains voltage stability and relieves transmission congestion.
2. It balances energy resources and mitigates the drawbacks posed by intermittency of renewable energy resources.
3. It increases utilization of renewable energy resources.
4. It improves reliability, quality, security and power factor of power systems.
5. It reduces running cost and improve efficiency of power systems.
6. Customer satisfaction is achieved, and most importantly, it is environmentally friendly.
7. Power losses are reduced after implementation of DSM.

Procedure of ACS Algorithm

Begin

    Initialize

    While stopping criterion not satisfied **do**

        Position each ant in a starting node

        Repeat

            For each ant **do**

                Choose next node by applying the state transition rule

                Apply step by step pheromone update

            End for

        Until every ant has built a solution

        Update best solution

        Apply offline pheromone update

    End While

End

Fig. 21 Ant colony algorithm

11 Obstacles in Implementing DSM Programs

Despite having advantages, there are some obstacles which affect the implementation of DSM program given as follows;

1. As, electricity prices structure, policies and regulations in implementing DSM are managed by the government, so these are affected by the political situation of the region.
2. Lack of funds for implementation of DSM programs.
3. Low awareness in customers can lead to hurdles in implementing DSM programs.
4. Energy-efficient appliances are costly than standard devices; hence, users prefer not to buy devices.
5. Lack of communication between utilities and customers.

12 Conclusion

In recent times, energy consumption is increasing due to increase in population and usage. The energy consumption pattern can change dramatically during any time frame. Usually, power systems are designed in such a way that if there comes a load demand higher than the normal routine, then power system will manage that increase in load. But, due to limited energy resources and increase in load requirement, power systems cannot maintain balance between energy generation and load demand. Power systems can be extended to avoid such situation, but due to limitation of space, resources and cost, this technique cannot be used for a long time. So, this chapter presents a comprehensive survey on a new technique on which many countries are working on called as demand side management, which manages the demand side to maintain balance between generation and demand. Ample articles have been written in the past to explain the concept of DSM. But, majority of those works concentrate on a certain aspect of this technique. In this chapter, demand side management as well as conventional energy management system is explained in detail. A detailed theoretical study with different programs and models has been presented in this chapter. The programs are differentiated into different categories with respect to their implementation and use. Architecture of optimal residential demand side management system with different types of loads is reviewed in detail. It is concluded that despite having challenges, DSM has been proved to be the most effective solution to power management problems. DSM is advantageous in terms of optimizing energy cost and consumption.

References

1. Jabir, H.J. Teh, J., Ishak, D., Abunima, H.: Impacts of demand-side management on electrical power systems: a review. Energies, **11**(5) (2018). https://doi.org/10.3390/en11051050
2. Fattahi Meyabadi, A.Â., Deihimi, M.H.: Reconsidering theoretical framework: a review of demand-side management. Renew. Sustain. Energ. Rev. **80**, 367–379 (2017). https://doi.org/10.1016/j.rser.2017.05.207
3. Karunanithi, K., Saravanan, S., Prabakar, B.R., Kannan, S., Thangaraj, C.: Integration of demand and supply side management strategies in generation expansion planning. Renew. Sustain. Energ. Rev. **73**, 966–982 (2017). https://doi.org/10.1016/j.rser.2017.01.017
4. Sahin, E.S., Bayram, I.S., Koc, M.: Demand side management opportunities, framework, and implications for sustainable development in resource-rich countries: case study qatar. J. Cleaner Prod. **241**, 118332 (2019). https://doi.org/10.1016/j.jclepro.2019.118332
5. Hussain, H.M., Javaid, N., Iqbal, S., Hasan, Q.U., Aurangzeb, K., Alhussein, M.: An efficient demand side management system with a new optimized home energy management controller in smart grid. Energies **11**(1) (2018). https://doi.org/10.3390/en11010190
6. Chuang, A.S., Gellings, C.W.: Demand-side integration in a restructured electric power industry. In: CIGRE Sess (2008). https://smartgrid.epri.com/doc/Demand-side%20Integration%20in%20a%20Restructured%20Electric%20Power%20Industry.pdf
7. Chuang, A., Gellings, C.: Demand-side integration for customer choice through variable service subscription. In: 2009 IEEE Power Energy Society General Meeting, pp. 1–7 (2009). https://doi.org/10.1109/PES.2009.5275910
8. De Ridder, F., Hommelberg, M., Peeters, E.: Four potential business cases for demand side integration. In: 2009 6th International Conference on the European Energy Market, pp. 1–6 (2009). https://doi.org/10.1109/EEM.2009.5207197
9. Silvestro, F., Bak-Jensen, B., Georgilakis, P., Baitch, A., Fan, M., Hatziargyriou, N., Pilo, F., Pisano, G., Petretto, G.: Demand side integration aspects in active distribution planning. In: 22nd International Conference and Exhibition on Electricity Distribution (CIRED 2013), pp. 1–4 (2013). https://doi.org/10.1049/cp.2013.1254
10. Ming, Z., Song, X., Mingjuan, M., Lingyun, L., Min, C., Yuejin, W.: Historical review of demand side management in china: management content, operation mode, results assessment and relative incentives. Renew. Sustain. Energ. Rev. **25**, 470–482 (2013). https://doi.org/10.1016/j.rser.2013.05.020

11. Murthy Balijepalli, V.S.K., Pradhan, V., Khaparde, S.A., Shereef, R.M.: Review of demand response under smart grid paradigm. In: ISGT2011-India, pp. 236–243 (2011). https://doi.org/10.1109/ISET-India.2011.6145388

12. Zehir, M.A., Batman, A., Bagriyanik, M.: Review and comparison of demand response options for more effective use of renewable energy at consumer level. Renew. Sustain. Energ. Rev. **56**, 631–642 (2016). https://doi.org/10.1016/j.rser.2015.11.082

13. Shan, K., Wang, S., Yan, C., Xiao, F.: Building demand response and control methods for smart grids: a review. Sci. Technol. Built Environ. **22**(6), 692–704 (2016). https://doi.org/10.1080/23744731.2016.1192878

14. Mazidi, M., Zakariazadeh, A., Jadid, S., Siano, P.: Integrated scheduling of renewable generation and demand response programs in a microgrid. Energ. Convers. Manage. **86**, 1118–1127 (2014). https://doi.org/10.1016/j.enconman.2014.06.078

15. Zhu, L., Yan, Z., Lee, W., Yang, X., Fu, Y., Cao, W.: Direct load control in microgrids to enhance the performance of integrated resources planning. IEEE Trans. Ind. Appl. **51**(5), 3553–3560 (2015). https://doi.org/10.1109/TIA.2015.2413960

16. Huang, J., Zuo, Q., Mu, F.: Automatic generation method of optimization scheme for orderly power utilization based on genetic algorithm. In: 2013 IEEE 11th International Conference on Dependable, Autonomic and Secure Computing, pp. 72–77 (2013). https://doi.org/10.1109/DASC.2013.40

17. Zhao, C., Wang, J., Watson, J., Guan, Y.: Multi-stage robust unit commitment considering wind and demand response uncertainties. IEEE Trans. Power Syst. **28**(3), 2708–2717 (2013). https://doi.org/10.1109/TPWRS.2013.2244231

18. Qian, L.P., Zhang, Y.J.A., Huang, J., Wu, Y.: Demand response management via real-time electricity price control in smart grids. IEEE J. Select. Areas in Commun. **31**(7), 1268–1280 (2013). https://doi.org/10.1109/JSAC.2013.130710

19. Kim, S., Giannakis, G.B.: Scalable and robust demand response with mixed-integer constraints. IEEE Trans. Smart Grid **4**(4), 2089–2099 (2013). https://doi.org/10.1109/TSG.2013.2257893

20. Falsafi, H., Zakariazadeh, A., Jadid, S.: The role of demand response in single and multi-objective wind-thermal generation scheduling: A stochastic programming. Energy **64**, 853–867 (2014). https://doi.org/10.1016/j.energy.2013.10.034

21. Alipour, M., Zare, K., Mohammadi-Ivatloo, B.: Short-term scheduling of combined heat and power generation units in the presence of demand response programs. Energy **71**, 289–301 (2014). https://doi.org/10.1016/j.energy.2014.04.059

22. Koliou, E., Eid, C., Chaves-Ávila, J.P., Hakvoort, R.A.: Demand response in liberalized electricity markets: analysis of aggregated load participation in the german balancing mechanism. Energy **71**, 245–254 (2014). https://doi.org/10.1016/j.energy.2014.04.067

23. Li, X.H., Hong, S.H.: User-expected price-based demand response algorithm for a home-to-grid system. Energy **64**, 437–449 (2014). https://doi.org/10.1016/j.energy.2013.11.049

24. Poudineh, R., Jamasb, T.: Distributed generation, storage, demand response and energy efficiency as alternatives to grid capacity enhancement. Energ Policy **67**, 222–231 (2014). https://doi.org/10.1016/j.enpol.2013.11.073

25. Ravindra, K., Iyer, P.: Decentralized demand-supply matching using community microgrids and consumer demand response: A scenario analysis. Energy **76**, 03 (2014). https://doi.org/10.1016/j.energy.2014.02.043

26. Zakariazadeh, A., Jadid, S., Siano, P.: Smart microgrid energy and reserve scheduling with demand response using stochastic optimization. Int. J. Electr. Power Energ. Syst. **63**, 523–533 (2014). https://doi.org/10.1016/j.ijepes.2014.06.037

27. Ahmad, A., Javaid, N., Qasim, U., Khan, Z.A.: Demand response: from classification to optimization techniques in smart grid. In: 2015 IEEE 29th International Conference on Advanced Information Networking and Applications Workshops, pp. 229–235 (2015). https://doi.org/10.1109/WAINA.2015.128

28. Xu, D., Li, P., Zhao, B.: Optimal scheduling of microgrid with consideration of demand response in smart grid. In: 2015 IEEE 12th International Conference on Networking, Sensing and Control, pp. 426–431 (2015). https://doi.org/10.1109/ICNSC.2015.7116075

29. Nguyen, D.T., Le, L.B.: Risk-constrained profit maximization for microgrid aggregators with demand response. IEEE Trans. Smart Grid **6**(1), 135–146 (2015). https://doi.org/10.1109/TSG. 2014.2346024

30. Ghazvini, M.A.F., Faria, P., Ramos, S., Morais, H., Vale, Z.: Incentive-based demand response programs designed by asset-light retail electricity providers for the day-ahead market. Energy **82**, 786–799 (2015). https://doi.org/10.1016/j.energy.2015.01.090

31. Dian ce Gao, Yongjun Sun, and Yuehong Lu. A robust demand response control of commercial buildings for smart grid under load prediction uncertainty. *Energy*, 93:275 – 283, 2015. https:// doi.org/10.1016/j.energy.2015.09.062

32. Faria, P., Vale, Z., Baptista, J.: Constrained consumption shifting management in the distributed energy resources scheduling considering demand response. Energ Convers. Manage. **93**, 309–320 (2015). https://doi.org/10.1016/j.enconman.2015.01.028

33. Neves, D., Pina, A., Silva, C.A.: Demand response modeling: a comparison between tools. Appl. Energ. **146**, 288–297 (2015). https://doi.org/10.1016/j.apenergy.2015.02.057

34. Richardson, D.B., Harvey, L.D.D.: Optimizing renewable energy, demand response and energy storage to replace conventional fuels in ontario, canada. Energy **93**, 1447–1455 (2015). https:// doi.org/10.1016/j.energy.2015.10.025

35. Pourmousavi, S.A., Nehrir, M.H., Sharma, R.K.: Multi-timescale power management for islanded microgrids including storage and demand response. IEEE Trans. Smart Grid **6**(3), 1185–1195 (2015). https://doi.org/10.1109/TSG.2014.2387068

36. Safamehr, H., Rahimi-Kian, A.: A cost-efficient and reliable energy management of a microgrid using intelligent demand-response program. Energy **91**, 283–293 (2015). https://doi.org/ 10.1016/j.energy.2015.08.051

37. Schreiber, M., Wainstein, M.E., Hochloff, P., Dargaville, R.: Flexible electricity tariffs: Power and energy price signals designed for a smarter grid. Energy **93**, 2568–2581 (2015). https:// doi.org/10.1016/j.energy.2015.10.067

38. Dong, J., Xue, G., Li, R.: Demand response in china: regulations, pilot projects and recommendations–a review. Renew. Sustain. Energ. Rev. **59**, 13–27 (2016). https://doi.org/ 10.1016/j.rser.2015.12.130

39. Feuerriegel, S., Neumann, D.: Integration scenarios of demand response into electricity markets: Load shifting, financial savings and policy implications. Energ. Policy **96**, 231–240 (2016). https://doi.org/10.1016/j.enpol.2016.05.050

40. Gils, H.C.: Economic potential for future demand response in germany–modeling approach and case study. Appl. Energ. **162**, 401–415 (2016). https://doi.org/10.1016/j.apenergy.2015. 10.083

41. Roh, H., Lee, J.: Residential demand response scheduling with multiclass appliances in the smart grid. IEEE Trans. Smart Grid **7**(1), 94–104 (2016). https://doi.org/10.1109/TSG.2015. 2445491

42. Leithon, J., Lim, T.J., Sun, S.: Battery-aided demand response strategy under continuous-time block pricing. IEEE Trans. Sign. Proc. **64**(2), 395–405 (2016). https://doi.org/10.1109/TSP. 2015.2483487

43. Nosratabadi, S.M., Hooshmand, R.-A., Gholipour, E.: Stochastic profit-based scheduling of industrial virtual power plant using the best demand response strategy. Appl. Energ. **164**, 590–606 (2016). https://doi.org/10.1016/j.apenergy.2015.12.024

44. Lima, D.A., Perez, R.C., Clemente, G.: A comprehensive analysis of the demand response program proposed in brazil based on the tariff flags mechanism. Electr. Power Syst. Res. **144**, 1–12 (2017). https://doi.org/10.1016/j.epsr.2016.10.051

45. Goel, L., Wu, Q., Wang, P.: Reliability enhancement and nodal price volatility reduction of restructured power systems with stochastic demand side load shift. In: 2007 IEEE Power Engineering Society General Meeting, pp. 1–8 (2007). https://doi.org/10.1109/PES.2007.385602

46. Haring, T.W., Mathieu, J.L., Andersson, G.: Comparing centralized and decentralized contract design enabling direct load control for reserves. IEEE Trans. Power Syst. **31**(3), 2044–2054 (2016). https://doi.org/10.1109/TPWRS.2015.2458302

47. Kim, Y., Norford, L.K., Kirtley, J.L.: Modeling and analysis of a variable speed heat pump for frequency regulation through direct load control. IEEE Trans. Power Syst. **30**(1), 397–408 (2015). https://doi.org/10.1109/TPWRS.2014.2319310
48. Kim, Y., Wang, J.: Power hardware-in-the-loop simulation study on frequency regulation through direct load control of thermal and electrical energy storage resources. IEEE Trans. Smart Grid **9**(4), 2786–2796 (2018). https://doi.org/10.1109/TSG.2016.2620176
49. Mortaji, H., Ow, S.H., Moghavvemi, M., Almurib, H.A.F.: Load shedding and smart-direct load control using internet of things in smart grid demand response management. IEEE Trans. Ind. Appl. **53**(6), 5155–5163 (2017). https://doi.org/10.1109/TIA.2017.2740832
50. Battegay, A., Hadj-Said, N., Roupioz, G., Lhote, F., Chambris, E., Boeda, D., Charge, L.: Impacts of direct load control on reinforcement costs in distribution networks. Electric Power Syst. Res. **120**, 70–79 (2015). https://doi.org/10.1016/j.epsr.2014.09.012
51. Stenner, K., Frederiks, E.R., Hobman, E.V., Cook, S.: Willingness to participate in direct load control: the role of consumer distrust. Applied Energy **189**, 76–88 (2017). https://doi.org/10.1016/j.apenergy.2016.10.099
52. Zhang, C., Xu, Y., Dong, Z.Y., Ma, J.: Robust operation of microgrids via two-stage coordinated energy storage and direct load control. IEEE Trans. Power Syst. **32**(4), 2858–2868 (2017). https://doi.org/10.1109/TPWRS.2016.2627583
53. Hobbs, B.F., Hu, M., Inon, J.G., Stoft, S.E., Bhavaraju, M.P.: A dynamic analysis of a demand curve-based capacity market proposal: The pjm reliability Pricing model. IEEE Trans. Power Syst. **22**(1), 3–14 (2007). https://doi.org/10.1109/TPWRS.2006.887954
54. Liu, Y.: Demand response and energy efficiency in the capacity resource procurement: Case studies of forward capacity markets in iso new england, pjm and great britain. Energy Policy **100**, 271–282 (2017). https://doi.org/10.1016/j.enpol.2016.10.029
55. Stavrakas, V., Flamos, A.: A modular high-resolution demand-side management model to quantify benefits of demand-flexibility in the residential sector. Energ. Convers. Manage. **205**, 112339 (2020). https://doi.org/10.1016/j.enconman.2019.112339
56. Roy, A., Auger, F., Dupriez-Robin, F., Bourguet, S., Tran, Q.T.: A multi-level demand-side management algorithm for offgrid multi-source systems. Energy **191**, 116536 (2020). https://doi.org/10.1016/j.energy.2019.116536
57. Afzal, M., Huang, Q., Amin, W., Umer, K., Raza, A., Naeem, M.: Blockchain enabled distributed demand side management in community energy system with smart homes. IEEE Access **8**, 37428–37439 (2020). https://doi.org/10.1109/ACCESS.2020.2975233
58. Sarker, E., Halder, P., Seyedmahmoudian, M., Jamei, E., Horan, B., Mekhilef, S., Stojcevski, A.: Progress on the demand side management in smart grid and optimization approaches. Int. J. Energ. Res. (2020). https://doi.org/10.1002/er.5631
59. Venizelou, V., Makrides, G., Efthymiou, V., Georghiou, G.E.: Methodology for deploying cost-optimum price-based demand side management for residential prosumers. Renew. Energ. **153**, 228–240 (2020). https://doi.org/10.1016/j.renene.2020.02.025
60. Morsali, R., Thirunavukkarasu, G.S., Seyedmahmoudian, M., Stojcevski, A., Kowalczyk, R.: A relaxed constrained decentralised demand side management system of a community-based residential microgrid with realistic appliance models. Appl. Energ. **277**, 115626 (2020). https://doi.org/10.1016/j.apenergy.2020.115626
61. Fangyuan, X., Chen, X., Zhang, M., Zhou, Y., Cai, Y., Zhou, Y., Tang, R., Wang, Y.: A sharing economy market system for private ev parking with consideration of demand side management. Energy **190**, 116321 (2020). https://doi.org/10.1016/j.energy.2019.116321
62. Adika, C.O., Wang, L.: Smart charging and appliance scheduling approaches to demand side management. Int. J. Electr. Power amd Energ. Syst. **57**, 232–240 (2014). https://doi.org/10.1016/j.ijepes.2013.12.004
63. Bradac, Z., Kaczmarczyk, V., Fiedler, P.: Optimal scheduling of domestic appliances via milp. Energies **8**(1), 217–232 (2015). https://doi.org/10.3390/en8010217
64. Jovanovic, R., Bousselham, A., Bayram, I.S.: Residential demand response scheduling with consideration of consumer preferences. Appl. Sci. **6**(1), 2016. https://doi.org/10.3390/app6010016

65. Gao, B., Liu, X., Zhang, W., Tang, Y.: Autonomous household energy management based on a double cooperative game approach in the smart grid. Energies **8**(7), 7326–7343 (2015). https://doi.org/10.3390/en8077326

66. Gao, B., Zhang, W., Tang, Y., Mingjin, H., Zhu, M.: Zhan, Huiyu: Game-theoretic energy management for residential users with dischargeable plug-in electric vehicles. Energies **7**(11), 7499–7518 (2014). https://doi.org/10.3390/en7117499

67. Vardakas, J.S., Zorba, N., Verikoukis, C.V.: Power demand control scenarios for smart grid applications with finite number of appliances. Appl. Energ. **162**, 83–98 (2016). https://doi.org/10.1016/j.apenergy.2015.10.008

68. Abushnaf, J., Rassau, A., Górnisiewicz, W.: Impact on electricity use of introducing time-of-use pricing to a multi-user home energy management system. Int Transactions on Electrical Energy Systems **26**(5), 993–1005 (2016). https://doi.org/10.1002/etep.2118

69. Elkazaz, Mahmoud H., Hoballah, Ayman, Azmy, Ahmed M.: Artificial intelligent-based optimization of automated home energy management systems. Int Transactions on Electrical Energy Systems **26**(9), 2038–2056 (2016). https://doi.org/10.1002/etep.2195

70. Wen, Z., O'Neill, D., Maei, H.: Optimal demand response using device-based reinforcement learning. IEEE Transactions on Smart Grid **6**(5), 2312–2324 (2015). https://doi.org/10.1109/TSG.2015.2396993

71. Chavali, P., Yang, P., Nehorai, A.: A distributed algorithm of appliance scheduling for home energy management system. IEEE Transactions on Smart Grid **5**(1), 282–290 (2014). https://doi.org/10.1109/TSG.2013.2291003

72. Rasheed, M.B., Javaid, N., Ahmad, A., Khan, Z.A.: Umar Qasim, and Nabil Ali Alrajeh. An efficient power scheduling scheme for residential load management in smart homes. Appl. Sci., **5**, 1134–1163 (2015). https://doi.org/10.3390/APP5041134

73. Rezaee Jordehi, A.: Optimisation of demand response in electric power systems, a review. Renew. Sustain. Energ. Rev. **103**, 308–319 (2019). https://doi.org/10.1016/j.rser.2018.12.054

74. Rinaldi, S., Pasetti, M., Sisinni, E., Bonafini, F., Ferrari, P., Rizzi, M., Flammini, A.: On the mobile communication requirements for the demand-side management of electric vehicles. Energies **11**(5), 2018. https://doi.org/10.3390/en11051220

75. Aalami, H.A., Moghaddam, M.P., Yousefi, G.R.: Evaluation of nonlinear models for time-based rates demand response programs. Int. J. Electrical Power Energ. Syst. **65**, 282–290. https://doi.org/10.1016/j.ijepes.2014.10.021

76. Faria, P., Vale, Z.: Demand response in electrical energy supply: An optimal real time pricing approach. Energy **36**(8), 5374–5384 (2011). https://doi.org/10.1016/j.energy.2011.06.049

77. Li, Y., Chang, Shanshan, L., Fu, Zhang, S.: A technology review on recovering waste heat from the condensers of large turbine units in china. Rene Sustain Energ Reviews **58**, 287–296 (2016). https://doi.org/10.1016/j.rser.2015.12.059

78. Tomofuji, D., Morimoto, Y., Sugiura, E., Ishii, T., Akisawa, A.: The prospects of the expanded diffusion of cogeneration to 2030 - study on new value in cogeneration. Applied Thermal Engineering **114**, 1403–1413 (2017). https://doi.org/10.1016/j.applthermaleng.2016.09.071

79. Chang, Tzu-Pu: Jin-Li, Hu: Total-factor energy productivity growth, technical progress, and efficiency change: An empirical study of china. Applied Energy **87**(10), 3262–3270 (2010). https://doi.org/10.1016/j.apenergy.2010.04.026

80. Cai, H., Shen, S., Lin, Q., Li, X., Xiao, H.: Predicting the energy consumption of residential buildings for regional electricity supply-side and demand-side management. IEEE Access **7**, 30386–30397 (2019). https://doi.org/10.1109/ACCESS.2019.2901257

81. Hamed Shakouri, G., Kazemi, A.: Multi-objective cost-load optimization for demand side management of a residential area in smart grids. Sustain. Cities. Soc. **32**, 171–180 (2017). https://doi.org/10.1016/j.scs.2017.03.018

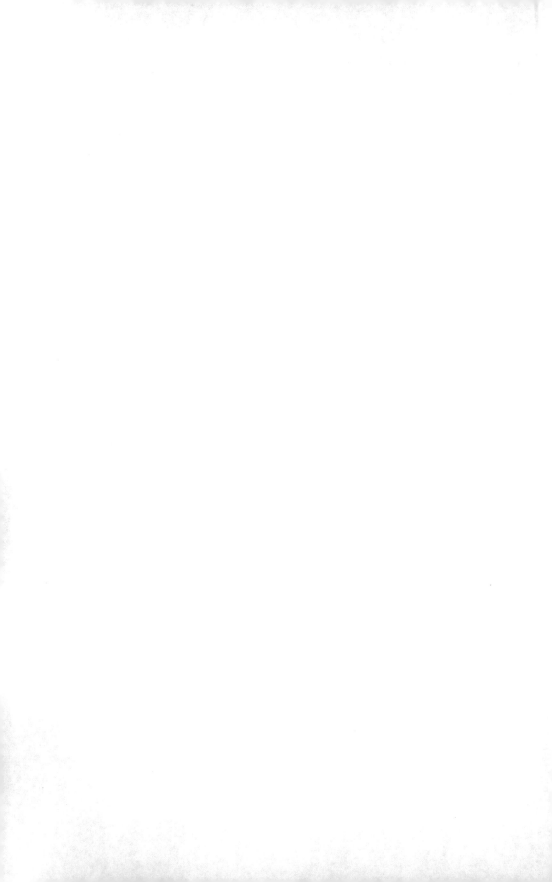

An Insight into Tool and Software Used in AI, Machine Learning and Data Analytics

Ruchi Mittal, Shefali Arora, Pragya Kuchhal, and M. P. S. Bhatia

Abstract Machine learning is a fantastic development on the off chance that you use it correctly. We can use machine learning models to demonstrate the importance of predictions on various projects. Acing machine learning tools would let you play with the information, train your models, find new systems, and make your computations efficiently. The pace of AI is overgrowing, and it is getting more noteworthy than some other time in late memory to perceive what choices you have for AI tools, libraries, stages, and so forward. Moreover, the need for investigation of critical information has opened various avenues in machine learning. Various open-source tools can be explored for performing analysis tasks as they are more renowned, straightforward, and executed orchestrated than the paid version. Many open-source tools do not require any coding and make sense of passing on the best results compared to paid structures. In this book chapter, we discuss the role of machine learning analytics in artificial intelligence. We survey the various kinds of open-source tools available on the Internet to take up projects in this field. Besides elucidating the application domains in which these analytics tools can be used, we also validate the results using a case study performed to detect fraudulent transactions. The chapter reviews data analytics tools, libraries, and software, what they are typically used for, what points of interest, and inconveniences they offer to choose from them based on his convenience.

R. Mittal (✉)
Department of Computer Science and Engineering, Ganga Institute of Technology
and Management, Jhajjar, Haryana, India
e-mail: ruchimittal138@gmail.com

S. Arora · M. P. S. Bhatia
Department of Computer Science, NSUT, Delhi, India
e-mail: arorashef@gmail.com

M. P. S. Bhatia
e-mail: bhatia.mps@gmail.com

P. Kuchhal
Department of Information Technology, NSUT, Delhi, India
e-mail: pragya.kuchhal@gmail.com

© The Author(s), under exclusive license to Springer Nature Singapore Pte Ltd. 2021
H. Malik et al. (eds.), *AI and Machine Learning Paradigms for Health Monitoring System*, Studies in Big Data 86,
https://doi.org/10.1007/978-981-33-4412-9_2

Keywords Machine learning · Artificial intelligence · Data analytics · Tools · Software's.

1 Introduction

1.1 Machine Learning

We have seen machine learning as a mainstream articulation as far back as relatively few years. The clarification behind this might be the high proportion of data made by applications, the extension of figuring power in the past scarcely any years, and the headway of better counts [2].

Machine learning has utilized anyplace from mechanizing regular assignments to offering short snippets of data, associations in each part attempt to profit by it. You may, beginning at now, be utilizing a gadget that uses it [27]. For instance, a wearable prosperity tracker like Fitbit, or a sharp home right hand like Google Home. Regardless, there are by and large more samples of ML being used.

1. **Forecast**—Machine learning can similarly be used in the desire systems. It is considering the complex model to enlist the probability of an issue. The structure should mastermind the available data in get-togethers.
2. **Picture recognition**—Machine learning can be used for face ID in an image as well. There is an alternate grouping for each person in a database of a couple of individuals.
3. **Speech Recognition**—It is the understanding of verbally communicated words into the substance. It is used in a voice look, and that is just a glimpse of something larger. Voice UIs join voice dialing, call coordinating, and machine control. In like manner, it can be used as an entire data area and the arranging of sorted out files.
4. **Clinical findings**—ML is trained to see harmful tissues.
5. **The financial business and exchanging**—associations use ML in distortion assessments and credit checks.

Machine learning (ML) is an order of a figuring that licenses programming applications to end up being more precise in anticipating results without being unequivocally redone. The crucial purpose behind machine learning is to amass measures that can get input data and use quantifiable assessment to envision a yield while invigorating yields as new data [19].

1.1.1 Types of Machine Learning

Machine learning can be characterized into three types [21].

1. Unsupervised Learning [20] The AI structures have unlabeled and uncategorized data in unsupervised learning. Likewise, the structure's estimations follow up on

the data without prior training. The yield is dependent upon the coded gauges. Presenting a structure to unsupervised learning is one technique for testing AI. It is of two types: Classification and Regression.

2. Supervised Learning [3] It has a limit that maps a commitment to yield subject to display information yield pairs. It concludes a limit from named training data involving many training models. In supervised learning, each model is a pair involving an information object (typically a vector) and ideal yield regard. A supervised learning figuring analyzes the training data and produces a concluded work, which can be used for arranging new models. A perfect circumstance will think about the figuring to precisely choose the class names for covered cases.

3. Reinforcement Learning [22] It is the training of machine learning models to make a course of action of decisions. The expert makes sense of how to achieve a target in an uncertain, possibly complex condition. In reinforcement learning, artificial intelligence faces a game-like situation. The PC uses experimentation to think about a response to the issue. To get the machine to do what the designer needs, artificial intelligence brings either rewards or disciplines for its exercises.

1.2 Artificial Intelligence [32]

Artificial intelligence (AI) is the limit of an electronic PC or PC-controlled robot to perform endeavors commonly associated with insightful animals. The term is applied to the assignment of making frameworks contributed with the norm of the academic strategy for individuals, for instance, the ability to reason, discover essentialness, summarize, or gain from earlier understanding. It is made from

- Thinking
- Learning
- Critical thinking
- Observation
- Etymological intelligence

1.3 Data Analytics

Data Analytics As the path toward separating raw data to find patterns and answer questions, data analytics' significance gets its large degree. Regardless, it fuses various methodologies with a broad scope of destinations [33]. The data analytics process has some essential parts that are required for any action. By uniting these fragments, a decisive data analytics action will part with a form of where you are, the spot you have been, and where you should go. All around, this technique begins with spellbinding analytics, and it is the route toward delineating evident patterns in data. Prominent analytics plans to address the request, "what happened?" This consistently incorporates evaluating standard markers, for instance, level of productivity. The pointers used will be different for each industry. Illuminating analytics does not choose estimates or prompt decisions. It revolves around summarizing data in a vast and informative way [33]. The accompanying essential bit of data analytics is progressed analytics. This bit of data science abuses impelled mechanical assemblies to isolate data, make gauges, and discover patterns. These instruments consolidate old-style estimations similarly to machine learning. Machine learning propels, for instance, neural frameworks, ordinary language getting ready, thought assessment, and more advanced analytics. This data gives new information from data. Advanced analytics addresses "envision a situation wherein?" questions. The accessibility of machine learning techniques, large datasets, and enduring enlisting power has enabled these systems' usage in various organizations. The collection of large datasets is instrumental in engaging these systems. Massive data analytics involves associations that draw significant closures from staggering and moved data sources, which is made possible by advances in equivalent getting ready and unassuming computational power [8].

1.3.1 Types of Data Analytics [25]

There are four fundamental sorts of data analytics: descriptive, demonstrative, prescient, and prescriptive analytics. Each type has a substitute goal and a prominent spot in the data examination process.

- Descriptive analytics helps answer inquiries regarding what occurred. These procedures sum up massive datasets to depict results to partners. By creating key execution markers (KPIs), these methodologies can help track victories or failures.
- Demonstrative analytics helps answer inquiries concerning why things occurred. These strategies supplement essential for engaging analytics. They take the discoveries from elucidating analytics and burrow further to discover the reason. The presentation pointers are additionally explored to find why they showed signs of improvement or more regrettable.
- Prescient analytics helps answer inquiries concerning what will occur later. These procedures utilize chronicled data to recognize inclines and decide whether they are probably going to repeat.
- Prescriptive analytics helps answer inquiries concerning what ought to be finished. By utilizing bits of knowledge from prescient analytics, data-driven choices can be made, which permits organizations to settle on educated decisions in the face regarding uncertainty.

Such data analytics give the knowledge that organizations need to settle on powerful and proficient choices.

2 Impact of Machine Learning, Artificial Intelligence, and Data Analytics [9]

Artificial intelligence (AI), machine learning, and data analytics are currently viewed as probably the most significant development. AI used to be a capricious thought from science fiction, but at this point it is transforming into a daily reality. Neural frameworks (imitating the technique of individual neurons in the brain) are preparing toward sending jumps in machine learning, called "machine learning."

Some express that AI is presenting another "cutting-edge change." Whereas the past Industrial Revolution outfitted physical and mechanical quality, this new disturbed will handle mental and mental limit. Sooner or later, PCs won't simply override physical work, yet likewise a profound practice. In any case, how accurately will this happen? Likewise, is it beforehand occurring? In Fig. 1, we show a connection between machine learning, artificial intelligence, and data analytics.

Here are 15 different ways artificial intelligence and machine learning will affect your regular daily existence.

- Smart Gaming [36]: Some of you may recollect 1997 when IBM's Deep Blue defeated Gary Kasparov in chess. Yet, on the off chance that you were not mature enough, at that point, you may recall when another PC program, Google Deep-Mind's AlphaGo, crushed Lee Sedol, the Go best on the planet, in 2016. Go is an old Chinese game, considerably harder for PCs to ace than chess. Yet, AlphaGo was explicitly trained to play Go, not by just dissecting the absolute best players'

Fig. 1 Co-relation between Machine Learning, Artificial Intelligence, and Data Analytics

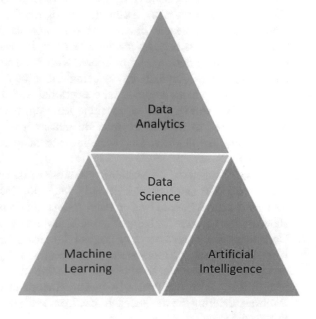

moves, yet by learning how to play the game better from rehearsing against itself many times.

- Self-Driving Cars and Automated Transportation [42] Taking everything into account, self-driving vehicles are presently a reality. These AI-fueled vehicles have even outflanked human-driven vehicles in security, as demonstrated by an examination with 55 Google vehicles that have turned over 1.3 million miles through. The course question has recently been handled a long time before. Google Maps, starting at now, sources zone information from your mobile phone. By taking a gander at the zone of a device beginning with one point in time, at that point onto the following, it can choose how rapidly the gadget is journeying. Put forward obviously, it can pick how direct traffic is reformist. It can solidify that information with scenes uncovered by customers to create the truck's picture at some irregular second. Aides can recommend the fastest course for you de-swinging on gridlocks, improvement work, or incidents among you and your objective.

- Cyborg Technology [12]: Our bodies and our brains have worked in constraints and shortcomings. As indicated by Oxford CS teacher Shimon Whiteson, innovation will improve to such a degree that we will have the option to enlarge a portion of our shortcomings and impediments with PCs along these lines upgrading vast numbers of our capacities. Be that as it may, wait before you begin imagining tragic universes of steel and tissue, consider for a second that a great many people strolling around are now "cyborgs" it might be said. What number of individuals do you realize who could endure the day without their trusty cell phone? As of now, we depend on these handheld PCs for correspondence, route, procuring information, getting essential news, and a large group of different exercises.

- Taking Over Dangerous Jobs [48] One of the riskiest occupations is bomb removal. Today, robots (or drones) are assuming control over these hazardous employments, among others. At present, most of these automatons require a human to control them. Be that as it may, as machine learning innovation improves later, these errands would be done totally by robots with AI. This innovation alone has just spared many lives. Another activity being redistributed to robots is welding. This sort of work produces commotion, exceptional warmth, and harmful substances found in the exhaust. Without machine learning, these robot welders would be pre-customized to weld in an area. Be that as it may, headways in PC vision and machine learning have empowered greater adaptability and more noteworthy exactness.

- Ecological Protection [18] Machines can store and access a more significant number of data than any individual could—including incredible insights. Utilizing enormous data, AI would be able today to distinguish patterns and use that data to show up at h answers for beforehand unsound issues. For instance, IBM's Green Horizon Project breaks down ecological data from many sensors and sources to item exact, developing climate and contamination gauges. It permits city organizers to run "imagine a scenario in which" situations and model approach to relieving natural effect. Also, that is merely starting. Energizing condition situated developments are entering the market each day, from self-altering keen indoor regulators to conveyed vitality matrices.

- Improved ElderCare [47] For some seniors, ordinary assignments can be a battle—many need to enlist outside assistance or depend on relatives. Senior consideration is a developing worry for some families. AI is at a phase where supplanting this need is not excessively far off, says Matthew Taylor, PC researcher at Washington State University. In-home robots could help old family members who would prefer not to leave their homes. That arrangement offers relatives greater adaptability in dealing with a friend or family member's consideration. These robots could assist seniors with regular errands and permit them to remain autonomous and to live in their homes for as far as might be feasible, improving their general prosperity.
- Developments in Banking [43] Consider what number of individuals have a ledger. Presently, on the head of that, consider the number of charge cards available for use. What number of worker hours would it take for representatives to filter through many exchanges that occur each day? When they saw an oddity, your ledger could be vacant, or your charge card maximized.

3 Current Trends in Machine Learning, AI, and Data Analytics [44]

Machine learning, data analytics, and artificial intelligence are not, now, the subject of science fiction. Instead, they are the central purposes behind billion-dollar organizations, such as self-administering driving vehicles, clinical determination, and aggression toward dread-based abuse. Taking everything into account, as far as stretching out as the employments of machine learning appears to be, there are examples to watch. These examples are critical in that they influence funds, society, and even the legal chief structure. Undoubtedly, various world bosses right now complement that the individual, state, or nation to control AI and machine learning will control the world.

1. Military independence [14] AI has shown up at a point that entirely free structures will, after a short time, control military ships and even bases. AI can measure the probability that pushing toward power is all around discarded or combative. Two or three ground vehicles arranged along these lines are controlled absolutely by AI to the degree that little human oversight is required. On these events, AI has filled human-made consciousness enough that an AI-controlled gatekeeper can recognize, assess, and even fire upon a peril with deadly force. The example here is one of the individuals getting more okay with machines choosing dangerous decisions.
2. Security in the home [17] AI-driven home-security frameworks are not exactly standard, yet they are on the ascent. Explicit parts, for example, smart locks, can speak with your cell phone. In any case, these frameworks are scheduled for substitution by observing structures that can see your home using video, identify danger, and advise specialists. Also, machine learning is anticipated to change home security and in-home individual security in that frameworks will have the

option to foresee a danger dependent on deciphering conduct, such as misuse or, in any event, hijacking. Machine learning has regularly been limited to numerical counts, factual investigation, and game-based execution. In any case, machine learning is currently ready to recognize certifiable items accurately. How these articles are deciphered relies upon the robot or software's utilization, yet vision-based machine learning can understand such things as individuals, felines, or terrain. Subsequently, sight-controlled AI is on the ascent required to affect home security, driving, and medicinal services.

3. Not any more secret elements A lot of what machine learning achieves gets mysterious at different purposes of the procedure. For example, the machine learning programs that grow superhuman thinking in other games make moves that people portray as outsiders. The explanations for the steps are not expected, and figuring out such choices are almost inconceivable. People are ordinarily in obscurity concerning seeing how AI works. For example, research is being led on developers' potential way to hardwire straightforwardness into machine learning. Moreover, machine learning is being coded in an approach to make the calculations more justifiable. At long last, simple endeavors are in progress to make machine learning reports on the execution procedure.

4. Removal Everybody realizes that occupations, including monotonous moves, are being made over by robots, shrewd or idiotic. Be that as it may, machine learning has additionally made specific desk callings defenseless against dislodging. For example, X-beam translation is something machine learning is making progress in, putting X-beam professionals' activity in the focus of AI relocation. Likewise, lawyers are relied upon to be uprooted by machine learning equipped for foreseeing the best pathways to winning a suit.

5. Internet of Things [45] Right now, gadgets that can interface with each other are considered keen. Nonetheless, this idea of intelligence is developing as machine learning is applied to the supposed web of things. For example, various organizations have created computerized guards that tune in on individuals through mobile phones, TVs, and speakers. Alexa and Siri are two such guards, and they are explicit to Amazon and Apple, separately. A broader character is coming as voice-based solicitation software that will be associated with the Internet of Things.

6. Cyborgs and general enlargement [12] On the ascent are gadgets that can screen our genetic data and react as needs are. For example, singular programmers are making gadgets associated with individuals, and these gadgets enlarge defective science by conveying insulin for individuals with diabetes. Be that as it may, AI is additionally being utilized to help widen individuals' discernment through expanded glasses. Increased cell phone applications are getting more rational, and machine learning brain PC interfaces permit people with quadriplegia to talk and cooperate with games. Even though the business is in its earliest stages, progress multiplies each year or something like that.

7. Adjusted AI fellowship [41] Machine learning is utilized by an assortment of retail organizations to make proposals to imminent clients. Be that as it may, machine learning is getting significantly more capable of serving the current needs of

individuals needing preoccupation or entertainment. For example, Netflix utilizes machine learning to comprehend what sort of shows individuals like. Making proposals for deals is a specific something. Making on-the-fly recommendations to current clients is very another because the plans are but rather a business device. They are methods for fulfillment. The machine learning that controlled this recommendation administration worked so well that it had the option to spare Netflix over 1,000,000,000 in lost income because of membership scratch-offs.

8. Natural language processing [28] It is on the ascent, and it has made extraordinary steps that permit machines to develop printed data dependent on arbitrary introductory information. One NLP can compose verses, stories, and news stories stunningly persuading. Upcoming advancement is scheduled to get conversational, permitting organizations to serve clients' specific requirements with inquiries regarding an organization's items or administrations.

9. Legislative issues and fake news [55] Profound fakes are on the ascent, and organizations and governments are supporting against the potential confounding effect such innovation will have on populaces. For example, machine learning has arrived at a point that it can tune in to sound data from somebody and afterward make nuanced speech designs that intently coordinate the genuine individual's sound and speech examples. Moreover, machine learning is getting more skilled at having the option to dissect many photos of a solitary individual. In the wake of breaking down the pictures, AI would then reproduce video-quality delineations of the individual. The aftereffect of these two innovations is something many refer to as a profound phony. Deep artificial sound and video will permit AI to develop bona fide messages from famous people, government pioneers, or even a healthy society. Also, the innovation is relied upon to be altogether persuading inside the following year.

4 Our Contribution

1. We review the various tools available in the domain of data analytics, machine learning and artificial intelligence as a whole. This study is one of its kind, which brings information about all the available software and technologies.

2. We identify the different domains in which we can utilize these tools to gain productive insights.

3. Our case study on detecting anomalies focuses on detecting fraudulent transactions done using credit cards, which validates the superiority of open-source machine learning tools in various such crucial domains centered around customers' security. The use of deep neural networks in a Python framework helps to achieve an accuracy of around 99.8 %.

5 Objective

AI and machine learning research objectives are thinking, data depiction, organizing, learning, natural language preparing, affirmation, and the ability to move and control objects. There are long-stretch goals in the general understanding division [40].

Approaches consolidate quantifiable systems, computational knowledge, and standard coding AI. We use various mechanical assemblies during the AI research related to looking and mathematical improvement, artificial neural frameworks, and procedures subject to estimations, probability, and financial viewpoints. Programming building draws in AI in the field of science, number juggling, brain science, phonetics, hypothesis, and so on [32].

The use of data analytics is extensive. Separating tremendous data can improve efficiency in different endeavors. Improving execution enables associations to prevail in an unyieldingly pitiless world. Data analytics is being used with extraordinary accomplishments in various fields [29]. Presumably, the soonest adopter is the financial part. Data analytics has a tremendous activity in the banking and finance organizations, used to promote floats and assess the possibility. FICO appraisals are an instance of data analytics that impacts everyone. These scores use various data centers around choosing advancing risk. Data analytics is additionally used to recognize and prevent coercion from improving viability and diminishing financial foundations. The utilization of data analytics goes past boosting benefits and ROI, be that as it may. Data analytics can give primary data to medicinal services (wellbeing informatics), wrongdoing counteraction, and ecological security. These utilizations of data analytics utilize these strategies to improve our reality. Even though measurements and data examination have consistently been utilized in logical exploration, progressed analytical methods and extensive data take numerous new bits of knowledge. These strategies can discover patterns in complex frameworks. Scientists are right now utilizing machine learning to ensure untamed life [15].

6 Software and Tools of Machine Learning, Artificial Intelligence, and Data Analytics

6.1 Data Analytics Tools [46]

1. **R Tool** [11]: R is the business's central analytics tool and used for estimations and data illustrating. It can control your data and present it in different manners. R consolidates and runs on a complete combination of stages, viz. UNIX, Windows, and macOS. It has more 11 K bundles and allows you to scrutinize the bundles by classes. R also offers tools to usually acquaint all packs agreeing with customer needs.

2. **Tableau Public** [7]:

   It is free programming that interfaces any data source, be it corporate Data Warehouse, Microsoft Excel, or online data. It makes data portrayals, guides, dashboards, etc. with regular reports on the web. They can, in like manner, be shared through online media or with the client. It allows the permission to download the record in different arrangements.

3. **Python** [52]

   Python is a scripting language that is definitely not hard to examine, create, keep up, and is open source. Guido van Rossum made it in the last aspect of the 1980s, supporting both commonsense and sorted out programming strategies. Python is not hard to learn as it is essentially equivalent to JavaScript, Ruby, and PHP. Also, Python has excellent AI libraries, viz. scikit-learn, Theano, TensorFlow, and Keras.

4. **Sas** [26]

   It is a programming language for data control and a pioneer in the assessment made by the SAS Institute in 1966 and later improved during the 1980s and 1990s. SAS is sufficiently available, reasonable, and can research data from any sources. It introduced an enormous game plan of push in 2011 for client information and various IT modules for web, web-based media, and publicizing examination to profile clients and potential outcomes. It can similarly anticipate their practices, administer, and update correspondences.

5. **Apache Spark** [49]

   It was made at University of California in 2009. It is a fast gigantic extension data planning engine and executes Hadoop packs' applications on numerous occasions quicker in memory and different events all the more rapidly on the plate. Streak depends on data science, and its thought makes data science simple. Spark is besides outstanding for data pipelines and AI models improvement. Gleam additionally unites a library—MLlib, which gives a one of a kind arrangement of machine assessments for dull being developed science methods like classification, regression, collaborative filtering, clustering, and so on.

6.2 Machine Learning Tools [54]

1. **Azure Machine Learning** [31] On the off chance that anyone doesn't have progressed programming aptitudes yet need to investigate AI, at that point, this instrument Azure machine learning is astounding. This cloud-based help gives tooling to conveying prescient models as investigative arrangements. It can likewise be utilized to test mama chine learning models, run calculations, and make recommender frameworks, to give some examples. It needs the exhibition and unintuitive UI (User Interface), particularly with regards to composing code.

2. **Deeplearning4J** [23] DeepLearning4J sees itself as an open-source, circulated deep learning library for the Java Virtual Machine (JVM). It's fitting for preparing appropriated deep learning organizations and can handle monster data without

losing its pace. It can likewise incorporate with Hadoop and Spark and can execute the AI calculations. Then again, Java isn't uncommonly notable for AI, so DL4J can't rely upon creating codebases as different libraries can. Improvement costs will probably be higher. Moreover, because it's worked with Java, we should make certain classes all alone to include lattices together, rather than Python, in which we don't need to make a point-by-point classes.

3. **IBM Watson** [16] IBM Watson is a "question answering machine." It utilizes scientific forces and computerized reasoning to impersonate human-like abilities to respond to questions, preferably. It can help you make mind-boggling business bits of knowledge and settle on educated choices dependent on informed decisions. IBM likewise ensures that your data is guaranteed with elite security and encryption limits and that they won't share your data aside from on the off chance that you express that they can. It is just accessible in English, it doesn't handle organized data straightforwardly, and exchanging and coordinating accompany significant expenses.

4. **Scikit-Learn** [39] Scikit-learn is an open-source AI system for Python that helps data mining, data investigation, and data perception. It helps order, relapse, grouping, dimensionality decrease, model choice, and preprocessing, to give some examples. It depends on NumPy, SciPy, and Matplotlib. Using Python, it works quicker than R and has fantastic execution. In any case, there is no appropriated variant accessible, and it isn't ideal for more significant datasets.

5. **TensorFlow** [1] At first, created by Google's Machine Intelligence research division to direct profound learning neural organizations and AI research, TensorFlow is a semi open-source library that grants designers the to perform mathematical computations. Human-made intelligence engineers can utilize the TensorFlow library to construct and train neural organizations in design acknowledgment. It is written in Python and C++, two fantastic and popular programming vernaculars, and thinks about circulated preparing. It doesn't contain various pre-prepared models, and there's no assistance for outside datasets, as Caffe.

6.3 Artificial Intelligence Tools [6]

1. **Knime** [30] Knime is an open-source AI instrument that relies upon Graphical User Interface (GUI). The best thing about Knime is it doesn't need any information on programming. One can at a present profit from the offices gave by Knime. It is usually used for significant data purposes, for instance, data manipulation and data mining, and so on. Furthermore, it measures data by making different work processes and afterward executes them. It goes with vaults that are loaded with other hubs. These hubs are then brought into the Knime entry. Lastly, the work process of hubs is made and executed.

2. **Weka** [50] It is likewise open-source programming. It tends to be gotten through a GUI and very easy to use. I t is utilized in exploration and instructing. Alongside this, Weka lets you access other AI instruments too, for instance, R, scikit-learn, and so forth.

3. **Pytorch** [38] Pytorch is a deep learning system. It is incredibly quick similarly, as versatile to use because Pytorch has a proper order over the GPU. It is one of the most significant AI devices since it is used in the essential parts of ML, which incorporates fabricating deep neural organizations and tensor computations. Pytorch is wholly founded on Python. Alongside this, it is the ideal alternative for NumPy.

4. **Google Cloud AutoML** [4] The aim of this tool is to make AI open to everybody. It additionally gives the models which are pre-prepared to the customers to outline different administrations. For test pl, text acknowledgment, discourse acknowledgment, and so on. Google Cloud AutoML is well known among associations/organizations. As the organization needs to apply human-made brainpower in each business area anyway, they experience been defying difficulties in doing so because talented AI individuals are absent in the market.

5. **Jupyter Notebook** [37] It is one of the most comprehensively used AI devices among all. It is quick handling just as a significant stage. Also, it upholds three dialects, viz. Julia, R, Python. Accordingly, the name of Jupyter is framed by the mix of these three programming dialects. This Notebook permits the client to store and offer the live code as a scratchpad. One can likewise get to it through a GUI, for example, WinPython pilot, Boa Constrictor guide, etc.

7 Application Domain of Machine Learning, Artificial Intelligence, and Data Analytics

Analytics and prediction have found its way in almost every sector today. Some of the popular domains where machine learning is gaining a lot of popularity are:

1. **Marketing**: An algorithm built from customers would be an asset for marketing products. Thus, machine learning tools are being extensively used in this domain in the industries [34]. In the early 2000s, we would generally search for an item on the online store. These days, with the help of ML tools, customers get recommendations and suggestions of products based on their recent searches, which has not only profited companies but has also made shopping a lot easier and fun for customers. A case of this is finding the correct motion pictures on Netflix. A few films are proposed to clients dependent on their past watches. ML apparatuses give an exact expectation conditional on responses of clients to these motion pictures. As the dataset develops, this innovation is getting more astute and more astute each day [51]. With the developing headway in AI, soon, it might be workable for customers on the web to purchase items by snapping a photograph.

2. **Banking and Finance**: Machine learning and artificial intelligence are overgrowing in this domain. Many banks have opted for tools that can predict credit card fraud, anomalies, and customer support [13]. A case of this is HDFC bank, which has built up an AI-based chatbot called Electronic Virtual Assistant (EVA) to address more than 3 million client queries [24]. EVA can gather information from a considerable number of sources and give straightforward answers in under 0.4 seconds. The utilization of analytics for misrepresentation anticipation can be utilized to upgrade security over a few business areas, including retail and account. Associations depend on these apparatuses, which examine the behavior of exchanges. Numerous organizations, like MasterCard and RBS WorldPay, are relying on these procedures.

   Numerous analytics devices on PCs are being utilized to decide future patterns in the market. Exchanging relies upon the capacity to foresee the future precisely. These tools can help observe past patterns and predict if these would repeat in the future. Thus, financial organizations are turning toward these tools to improve their profit ratios. Many trade data is stored in systems along with the prices. Therefore, these systems are reservoirs of information and can be used to make much analysis. For instance, it might confirm that current economic situations resemble the conditions fourteen days back and anticipate how offer costs will be changing a couple of moments down the line [35].

3. **Agriculture**: There would be a need to produce 50% more food in the coming days than what we have today. Analytics tools can help farmers to get more land and resources based on the predictions. These predictions can be made based on climate change, food security issues, and population growth. Many organizations are relying on artificial intelligence and machine learning to find efficient ways to do this [2]. Such sort of investigation can likewise assist with sparing yields from unsafe weeds. Blue River Technology has built up a robot called See and Spray, which utilizes PC vision innovations to screen and decisively shower weedicide on cotton plants. Aside from this, a Berlin-based rural tech fire up called PEAT has built up an application called Plantix finds any sorts of supplement insufficiencies in the dirt through imaging, which can help in discovering arrangements like soil rebuilding. It is said that such instruments can assist with obtaining an exactness of over 95

4. **Health Care**: A lot of doctors and medical centers are relying on ML tools to help patients all throughout the world. For instance, an association called Cambio Health Care built up a clinical choice emotionally supportive network for stroke anticipation. Numerous automated frameworks investigate patients' boundaries, for example, pulse, temperature, and so on. This can help specialists to screen patients distantly and break down their conditions [53]. Another such model is Coala life, which builds up an apparatus to distinguish cardiovascular issues in patients. Numerous devices in this domain are being created to deal with patients in mature age homes and nursing focuses. Along these lines, the consideration of AI and ML in human services is ending up being a shelter for the clinical world.

5. **Research**: Plagiarism in research work is checked with the help of software like Turnitin, which is used to analyze students' writing. ML and analytics can be applied in this domain to develop plagiarism detectors. Historically, plagiarism detection relies on checking a massive database of references. ML tools can help to locate sources that are not included in the database, such as old sources that are not digitized or sources in a foreign language [10].

6. **Commuting**: Decreasing commute times is a significant issue in the present period, and a solitary outing can include different transportation methods. An individual may get late because of development, mishaps, street maintenance, climate conditions, etc. Utilizing area data from cell phones, Google Maps can use ML and analytics to break down traffic speed anytime. These guides can join announced traffic occurrences or development exercises. Hence, Maps can diminish commutes by proposing the quickest courses to and from work [5]. While taking a ride utilizing Uber or Ola, these apparatuses can be utilized to decide the ride's cost, limit the wait time, coordinate a traveler with others to offer administrations like carpool, and so on.

7. **Social networking**: Many social networking apps like Facebook also use ML and AI-based tools to personalize our news feed [46]. We can also see ads that are relevant to our interest. In the first quarter of 2016, Facebook and Google made sure about a sum of 85% of the online promotion showcase—unequivocally due to profoundly focused on notices. In 2016, Facebook reported the utilization of DeepText, a book understanding motor to understand the substance of a few thousand posts for each second, spreading over more than 20 dialects. In this manner, it is utilized in the courier to identify the plan of a client. DeepText is likewise utilized to computerize spam's expulsion, helping famous available figures sort through the vast number of remarks on their presents on observing those generally pertinent, recognizing available to be purchased posts naturally, and removing essential data identify and surface substance in which you may be intrigued. Stages like Pinterest utilizes AI-based apparatuses to recognize objects from pictures naturally. Different employments of these instruments are spam counteraction, adaptation, email advertising, and so forth.

8 Case Study Data Analytics Using Python

We apply analytics on the detection of anomalies in transactions performed using credit cards. With the help of deep neural networks, we can detect any differences in the transaction's behavior and single it out. These points are known as outliers, data points that do not conform to the expected behavior. The different types of anomalies are discussed below:

8.1 Types of Anomalies

Anomaly detection is known as identifying rare items or observations that raise suspicions by differing from the rest of the data. Anomalies can be broadly categorized as: Point anomalies in which a single instance of data is an outlier if it is far from the other data points. Credit card fraud detection is an example of such an anomaly.

- Contextual anomalies: These kinds of anomalies are specific to time series problems and own some context. Many business use cases have outliers based on this anomaly.
- Collective anomalies: These anomalies refer to a set of data points that help in collective analysis of anomalies present in a system. For example, if a user is trying to copy data from a remote machine, it would be considered an anomaly.

8.2 Techniques Used for Anomaly Detection

8.2.1 Statistical Methods

Many statistical methods can be used to identify irregularities in the data. These include mean, median, quantiles, and other parameters; an anomalous data point would deviate by a specific standard deviation from the actual mean value. We can also make use of a rolling window to compute the average of data instances. Moving averages can help in distinguishing between short-term and long-term variations. The drawbacks of using these techniques for anomaly detection are:

- If the data being used is noisy, there would be no clear boundary between the normal and abnormal points. Thus, the calculation will not be precise.
- A threshold calculated using a moving average may not be applicable in situations where the definition of abnormal data points changes with time.

8.2.2 Machine Learning-Based Approaches

Analytics tools based on machine learning can help in the effective detection of anomalies present within the data. Some of these techniques are:

1. **Density-Based Anomaly Detection**: It is based on the K-nearest neighbors' algorithm. It is considered that regular data points occur within a neighborhood, and the abnormal points are farther away. Further, the data points near each other can be evaluated using the Euclidean score or a similar measure, depending on the data type. Some of these measures are Euclidean, Manhattan, Minkowski, or Hamming distance.

2. **Clustering-Based Anomaly Detection**: It works on the assumption that similar data points belong to similar clusters, which can be determined based on distance from centroids. K-means is a widely used clustering method, which is used to create k similar clusters out of data points. All other data points which are away from these groups are termed as anomalies.
3. **Support Vector Machine-Based Anomaly Detection**: A support vector machine is another useful technique for detecting anomalies. It learns boundaries between normal and abnormal data points to learn from patterns. Thus, it can predict any abnormalities in the transactions.
4. **Neural Network-Based Anomaly Detection**: Multilayer perceptrons are used in various systems such as intrusion detection systems for finding abnormal behavior or anomalies. The number of hidden layers would help to extract features from the data and learn from them using weights and biases on the inputs; the output obtained is subjected to an activation function. Such as ReLU or Tanh for the creation of nonlinear boundaries between the two classes—standard data points and abnormal data points.

8.2.3 Anomaly Detection Using Multilayer Perceptrons

In this case study, we detect the presence of anomalies in data comprising of credit card transactions. The multilayer perceptron or neural network is capable of learning anomalies from labeled data and can predict anomalies or fraudulent transactions in the future based on the learning. The dataset has been taken from Kaggle, and it comprises transactions made by European citizens in September 2013. This data consists of 492 frauds out of 284,807 transactions. Python has been used for the analysis. The statistical parameters of the fraudulent transactions are as follows (Table 1):

We further train a multilayer perceptron to learn from these anomalies and detect the presence of fraudulent transactions after evaluating the test data instances. The parameters of the multilayer perceptron are as follows (Table 2):

It is observed that the multilayer perceptron can detect anomalies or fraudulent transactions with an accuracy of 99.8%. Thus, fraudulent transactions can be easily captured with the use of analytics in machine learning.

Table 1 Statistical parameters of the fraudulent transactions

Fraudulent transactions	Value
Count	492
Mean	122.211
Standard deviation	256.683

Table 2 Parameters of the multilayer perceptron

Hyperparameter	Value
Hidden layers	5
Optimizer	lbfgs
Activation function	ReLu
Learning rate	0.00001

9   Conclusion and Future Work

This chapter reviews the various machine learning approaches and the open-source analytics tools that we can use in multiple application domains. The chapter gives insight into the usefulness of these tools and how they can help us obtain superior results compared to traditional tools used for analysis. Our case study on the detection of anomalies focuses on detecting fraudulent transactions done using credit cards, which validates the superiority of open-source machine learning tools in various such crucial domains centering around the security of customers. The use of deep neural networks in a Python framework helps achieve an accuracy of around 99.8 %. We also list their pros and cons compared to paid tools and traditional software used for data analysis. In the future, we would use analytics tools on more real-life applications.

References

1. Abadi, M., et al.: Tensorflow: a system for large-scale machine learning. In: 12th fUSENIXg Symposium on Operating Systems Design and Implementation (fOSDIg 16), pp. 265–283 (2016)
2. Alpaydin, E.: Introduction to Machine Learning. MIT Press (2020)
3. Apache Spark. In: Retrieved January 17 (2018), p. 2018
4. Basştanlar, Y., Özuysal, M.: Introduction to machine learning. In: miRNomics: microRNA Biology and Computational Analysis (2014)
5. Borkowski, A.A., et al.: Google Auto ML versus Apple Create ML for Histopathologic Cancer Diagnosis; Which Algorithms Are Better? arXiv preprint arXiv:1903.08057 (2019)
6. Caballé, N.C., et al.: Machine learning applied to diagnosis of human diseases: a systematic review. Appl. Sci. **10**(15), 5135 (2020)
7. Datig, I., Whiting, P.: Telling your library story: tableau public for data visualization. In: Library Hi Tech News (2018)
8. Dimiduk, D.M., Holm, E.A., Niezgoda, S.R.: Perspectives on the impact of machine learning, deep learning, and artificial intelligence on materials, processes, and structures engineering. In: Integrating Materials and Manufacturing Innovation, vol. 7, issue 3, pp. 157–172 (2018)
9. Dyckhoff., A.L.: Implications for learning analytics tools: a meta-analysis of applied research questions. Int. J. Comput. Information Syst. Industrial Manage. Appl. **3**(1), 594–601 (2011)
10. Gardener, M., Beginning, R.: The Statistical Programming Language. John Wiley & Sons (2012)

11. Garry, T., Harwood, T.: Cyborgs as frontline service employees: a research agenda. J. Service Theor. Pract. (2019)
12. Giebe, C., Hammerström, L., Zwerenz, D.: Big Data & Analytics as a sustainable Customer Loyalty Instrument in Banking and Finance (2019)
13. Gupta, R., et al.: Machine learning models for secure data analytics: a taxonomy and threat model. Comput. Commun. **153**, 406–440 (2020)
14. Hashimoto, D.A., et al.: Artificial intelligence in surgery: promises and perils. Anna. Surg. **268**(1), 70 (2018)
15. Helder Coelho and Tiago Thompsen Primo: Exploratory apprenticeship in the digital age with AI tools. Progress Artif. Intell. **6**(1), 17–25 (2017)
16. High, R.: The Era of Cognitive Systems: An Inside Look at IBM Watson and How it Works. IBM Corporation, Redbooks, pp. 1–16 (2012)
17. Holzinger, A., et al.: Current advances, trends and challenges of machine learning and knowledge extraction: from machine learning to explainable AI. In: International Cross-Domain Conference for Machine Learning and Knowledge Extraction. Springer, Heidelberg, pp. 1–8 (2018)
18. Huntingford, C., et al.: Machine learning and artificial intelligence to aid climate change research and preparedness. Environ. Res. Lett. **14**(12), 124007 (2019)
19. Joe Qin, S., Chiang, L.H.: Advances and opportunities in machine learning for process data analytics. In: Computers & Chemical Engineering, vol. 126, pp. 465–473 (2019)
20. Kodratoff, Y.: Introduction to Machine Learning. Elsevier (2014)
21. Kotsiantis, S.B., Zaharakis, I., Pintelas, P.: Supervised machine learning: a review of classification techniques. In: Emerging Artificial Intelligence Applications in Computer Engineering **160**(1), 3–24 (2007)
22. Kubat, M.: An Introduction to Machine Learning. Springer (2017)
23. Lagoudakis, M.G., Parr, R.: Reinforcement learning as classification: Leveraging modern classifiers. In: Proceedings of the 20th International Conference on Machine Learning (ICML-03), pp. 424–431 (2003)
24. Lang, S., et al.: Wekadeeplearning4j: a deep learning package for weka based on deeplearning4j. Knowl.-Based Syst. **178**, 48–50 (2019)
25. Leite, R.A., et al.: Eva: visual analytics to identify fraudulent events. IEEE Trans. Vis. Comput. Graphics **24**(1), 330–339 (2017)
26. Levy, Y., Ramim, M.: [Chais] A study of online exams procrastination using data analytics techniques. Interdisc. J. E-Learn. Learn. Objects **8**(1), 97–113 (2012)
27. Li, A.: Handbook of SAS®DATA Step Programming. CRC Press (2013)
28. Lison, P.: An Introduction to Machine Learning. Language Technology Group (LTG) 1.35 (2015)
29. Lupu, M.: Information Retrieval, Machine Learning, and Natural Language Processing for Intellectual Property Information (2017)
30. Martis, R.J., et al.: Recent Advances in Big Data Analytics, Internet of Things and Machine Learning (2018)
31. Massaro, A., et al.: ESB platform integrating KNIME data mining tool oriented on Industry 4.0 based on artificial neural network predictive maintenance. In. J. Artif. Intell. Appl. (IJAIA) **9**(3), 1–17 (2018)
32. Milad, A.: Using an azure machine learning approach for flexible pavement maintenance. In: 16th IEEE International Colloquium on Signal Processing & Its Applications (CSPA). IEEE, pp. 146–150 (2020)
33. Mitchell, R.S., Michalski, J.G., Carbonell, T.M.: An Artificial Intelligence Approach. Springer, Heidelberg (2013)
34. Moreira, J.: André Carlos Ponce de Leon Ferreira, and Tomáš̌s Horváth. A General Introduction to Data Analytics. Wiley Online Library (2019)
35. Mou, X.: Artificial Intelligence: Investment Trends and Selected Industry Uses. International Finance Corporation, pp. 1–8 (2019)

36. Nabrzyski, J., et al.: Agriculture data for all-integrated tools for agriculture data integration, analytics, and sharing. In: 2014 IEEE International Congress on Big Data. IEEE, pp. 774–775 (2014)
37. Nayak, A., Dutta, K.: Impacts of machine learning and artificial intelligence on mankind. In: 2017 International Conference on Intelligent Computing and Control (I2C2). IEEE, pp. 1–3 (2017)
38. O'Hara, K.J., Blank, D., Marshall, J.: Computational Notebooks for AI Education (2015)
39. Paszke, A., et al.: Pytorch: an imperative style, high-performance deep learning library. In: Advances in Neural Information Processing Systems, pp. 8026–8037 (2019)
40. Pedregosa, F., et al.: Scikit-learn: machine learning in python. J. Mach. Learn. Res. **12**, 2825–2830 (2011)
41. Riaz, I.B.R., et al.: Gender Differences in Faculty Rank and Leadership Positions Among Hematologists and Oncologists in the United States. In: JCO Oncology Practice (2020), OP-19
42. Rigas, E.S., Ramchurn, S.D., Bassiliades, N.: Managing electric vehicles in the smart grid using artificial intelligence: a survey. IEEE Trans. Intell. Transp. Syst. **16**(4), 1619–1635 (2014)
43. Sabharwal, C.L.: The rise of machine learning and robo-advisors in banking. IDRBT J. Banking Technology, 28 (2018)
44. Saiyeda, A., Mir, M.A.: Cloud computing for deep learning analytics: a survey of current trends and challenges. Int. J. Adv. Res. Comput. Sci. **8**(2) (2017)
45. Samanpour, A.R., Ruegenberg, A., Ahlers, R.: The future of machine learning and predictive analytics. In: Digital Marketplaces Unleashed. Springer, Heidelberg, pp. 297–309 (2018)
46. Sapountzi, A., Psannis, K.E.: Social networking data analysis tools & challenges. Future Generation Comput. Syst. **86**, 893–913 (2018)
47. Schure, M.B., Odden, M., Turner Goins, R.: The association of resilience with mental and physical health among older American Indians: the native elder care study. In: American Indian and Alaska Native Mental Health Research (Online), vol. 20, issue 2, p. 27 (2013)
48. Siau, K., Wang, W.: Building trust in artificial intelligence, machine learning, and robotics. Cutter Bus. Technol. J. **31**(2), 47–53 (2018)
49. Srivastava, S.: Weka: a tool for data preprocessing, classification, ensemble, clustering and association rule mining. Int. J. Comput. Appl. **88**(10) (2014)
50. Thomas Davenport and Jeanne Harris. Competing on analytics: Updated, with a new introduction: The new science of winning. Harvard Business Press (2017)
51. Van Esch, P., Stewart Black, J., Ferolie, J.: Marketing AI recruitment: the next phase in job application and selection. Comput. Human Behav. **90**, 215–222 (2019)
52. Van Rossum, G., et al.: Python programming language. In: USENIX Annual Technical Conference, vol. 41, p. 36 (2007)
53. Yang, H., Lee, E.K.: Healthcare Analytics: From Data to Knowledge to Healthcare Improvement. John Wiley & Sons (2016)
54. Yuan, J., et al.: A survey of visual analytics techniques for machine learning. arXiv preprint arXiv:2008.09632 (2020)
55. Zellers, R., et al.: Defending against neural fake news. In: Advances in Neural Information Processing Systems, pp. 9054–9065 (2019)

Security Enhancement and Monitoring for Data Sensing Networks Using a Novel Asymmetric Mirror-Key Data Encryption Method

Linoy A. Tharakan, Sherly Daniel, and R. Dhanasekaran

Abstract Today, the world is moving to fully enable Internet technologies and gadgets. Devices become smarter and intelligent, and the data exchanges between the devices become exponentially increased and more private data in being transmitted through the Internet. By the use of the Internet and other digital technology such as mobile gadgets, social media networks, the Internet of Things (IoT), and personalized services, enormous quantities of data are open and continuously gathering, processing, evaluating, and using massive data on different networks like the cloud through individuals and organizations, and the term Big data is named for such a massive data manipulation. Then, it becomes a big challenge to data scientists to secure the data which is transmitted through the various medium. Historically, data is secured using cryptographically, and number of techniques is globally accepted. This chapter proposes a semi-asymmetric mirror dual encryption approach. Here, the encrypted key is appended along with the data, but even the intruder collects the data or the key, then they cannot hack the key or the data because of the mirroring cryptographic technique. This method is safer because it does not transfer the actual data, or the actual key for encryption. The key generated through a mirroring algorithm at the receiver side only. So this technique is secured than other symmetric key encryption because it is neither transmitting the actual data nor the encryption actual key as in conventional methods. The key is generated through a noble algorithm at the receiver side only.

Keywords Big data · Cryptography · Data security · Encryption · The mirror key · WSN

L. A. Tharakan
Mar Thoma Institute of Information Technology, Kollam, Kerala, India
e-mail: lino.net4u@gmail.com

S. Daniel
Mar Thoma College of Science and Technology, Kollam, Kerala, India
e-mail: sherlino@gmail.com

R. Dhanasekaran (✉)
ECE, Saveetha School of Engineering, SIMATS, Chennai, India
e-mail: dhanasckaranr.sse@saveetha.com

1 Introduction

People incline toward to socialize, and for this, they communicate with one another and wish their communications to be secure. Secure communication is once two parties are passing information which they do not need any third party to encourage to get it intruding or spying the content. For this, information needs to be sent in an exceedingly kind that is not prone to interference. The science of using mathematics to make the data unreadable and rearrange to the original form on demand is called secret writing. The encryption is utilized to store or transmit delicate data over an unreliable systems, so that, it cannot be capturing by any interlopers. Data from various sources are now become too heavy and countless, and that data needs to be securely handled [1–26]. The huge data from various sensors and gadgets, and other devices are flowing to and from across the network and that data is called Big data [25, 26]. Securing that data is the primary role of system, and encryption and decryption then become an inevitable component of Big data.

1.1 Big Data

Big data, a typical term recently, is referring to a good range of very large and diverse data sets that face severe privacy and security concerns. Attributable to the properties of Big data, like the speed, data volume with large cloud architecture services, and therefore, the Internet of Things (IoT), conventional systems for security and confidentiality are ineffective and being unable to function unable to handle the vigorous burst of information in a very really diverse Big data environment. Security risk mitigation plays an enormous role in the Big data infrastructures worldwide with Big data analytics being popularly used among companies and the government for deciding. Common security methods have struggled to attain contemporary scalability, interoperability, and flexibility [1].

By the use of the Internet and other digital technology such as mobile gadgets, social media networks, the Internet of Things (IoT) and personalized services, enormous quantities of data are open and continuously gathering, processing, evaluating, and using massive data on different networks like the cloud through individuals and organizations, and the term Big Data is named for such a massive data manipulation.

Before the term Big data was used to mention large quantities of data on the Internet, three widely used measurements characterizing huge databases and data warehouses were the 3Vs, namely volume, velocity, and variety. Now along with the mentioned V's, valence and vulnerability dimensions have been associated with Big data to represent privacy and security challenges. Although Big data may be huge, if the links between the data objects are not really formed, we will have clusters or regions of fragmented data whose inter dependencies might not be fully known neither adapted. Any links could be created when info gets acquired since they get transmitted [2]. However, finding indirect links among elements be far challenging, and they contribute value to the business. These interdependencies lead in different realm, namely valence of Big data. The shortcomings owing to privacy and security issues, and the lack of specifications are correlated to Big data systems, processes, and governance. Recently identified vulnerabilities of security and confidentiality of Big data has received extensive interest to look into the vulnerability dimension of Big data.

1.2 Big Data Security

Services such as cloud storage and services are being used extensively to cope with the Big data world increasing data access from the Internet. Massive availability of data and therefore companies gain a lot of knowledge about data mining that can help in their smart business decision making. Although Big data can provide companies and consumers in their daily operations with many value-added opportunities, it also creates security challenges. The hackers and intruders are extremely motivated to execute various tools to crack the cloud security because of the companies and business services moved their working platform to the Internet and intelligent digital technologies. Rich information could be gathered on the individual's preferences, desire, activity, and action habits, and these interesting and useful data could have been exposed. Throughout the life cycle of Big data, adequate security and privacy must also be implemented [1, 2].

Usually, the security and privacy of any data strengthened using the cipher key generation approach. The chapter proposed here gives a novel approach to improve the security with a minimum processes power and the memory usage without sharing the secret key as in the case of private key encryption. The proposed algorithm in the chapter gives a dynamic key generation using the random key generator approach, but the key which generated will not send to the receiver side as in its actual form which makes this system more unique.

2 Data Security Concerns

The collection of data includes multiple data sources from the Internet, cloud, social, and IoT networks. While large sensing data streams have new encryption systems, attacks from the phase of data procurement are possible Therefore, in order to allow data mining itself metadata on these data sources, as the data root, the method used for dissemination and intermediate calculation can be registered.

Hence, metadata approximate those records sources consisting of the records origin, the procedure used for dissemination, and any intermediate calculations that can be recorded that allows you to facilitate mining of the statistics on the time of records streaming itself [3].

2.1 Insecure Computation

The intruders and hackers use software tools together and transfer confidential data from the remote cloud. Aside from the critical data loss, these sorts of unreliable computing also tamper the data and cause inaccurate prediction or data analytical results. This leads a crucial bottleneck of removing the property of using parallel programming language on Big data solution and result in Denial of Services (DoS).

2.2 Input Validation and Filtering

Big data gather data from a number of sources, so validation of the information is very necessary and compulsory. It includes determining what form of data is untrusted and what the untrusted sources of data are. This additionally needs to filter rogue or malicious information from them. Signature-based filtering of data frequently has drawbacks consisting of being not able to locate rogue, or malicious records with any behavioral dimension. When a significant volume of malicious data is introduced into the dataset, tremendous control is exerted on the result generated.

2.3 Insecure Data Storage

The Big data is processed at number of nodes, authentication, authorization, and security of data on those nodes is an intimidating process. When every approach offers real-time data protection, this may not be the case useful, because real-time data protection can have impacts on efficiency. Safe communication between various nodes, middleware's, and end users is disabled by default, so explicit triggering is necessary.

3 Cryptography

3.1 The Basic Terms Used in Cryptography

- **Data confidentiality**—The aim of confidentiality is to create sure that only those nodes or user can understand what information are exchanged while two or more parties are involved in communication. Encryption is employed to supply confidentiality.
- **Data integrity**—This ensures that data not been altered, added, damaged, or lost in an unauthorized or accidental manner [3, 4] while transmitted. A robust

mathematical function is applied to the message being transmitted to impart the data integrity.

- **Non-repudiation**—This happens when denial by any of the nodes associated in communication.
- **Plain text**—The node or user who desires to transfer with the other will send a message that is called plain text.
- **Cipher text**—The message that cannot be readable by anyone is also known as the encrypted data. Actual message is converted to a non-readable format before transmission.
- **Encryption**—Process of converting the readable message into unreadable format is called encryption. The encryption technique is used to send confidential messages through an untrusted medium. For encryption, the system needs two programming functions—an encryption algorithm and a key.
- **Decryption**—The process of converting cipher text into plain text is called decryption. The decryption function used in the cryptography at the receiver side to obtain the original message from non-readable message. The decryption process requires two things—a decryption algorithm used at the receiver side and unique key to open the cipher message.
- **Key**—Key's unique combination of special symbols or a gaggle of numeric data or an alphanumeric text. Selection of key in cryptography makes the system more secure because the security of encryption algorithm depends directly thereon.

4 Classification of Cryptography Algorithms

4.1 Symmetric Cryptography

There is only one key in this cryptography both for encryption and decryption, and it is also called secret key cryptography [5, 6]. This method worked according to: (1) the message is encrypted with the key and that key has been sent to the recipient to decrypt cipher text. (2) The recipient uses the same key to decipher the cipher text and can retrieve plain text. Figure 1 demonstrates the block diagram for the symmetric key encryption [5].

Both the sender and the recipient must know the same key in symmetric key cryptography to use the technique. In this method, the stream cipher and the block cipher are two typical patterns. The stream ciphers produce a sequence of bits that are used as a key called a key stream, and the encryption is achieved by merging the key stream with the plain text. Typically, this is achieved with the Exclusive-OR (XOR) function at bit wise. The stream cipher is synchronous if the key stream does not depend on plain text and cipher text, and if it relies on data and its encryption, the stream cipher synchronizes itself. A block cipher transforms a fixed-length plaint text block into a cipher-text block [6–8].

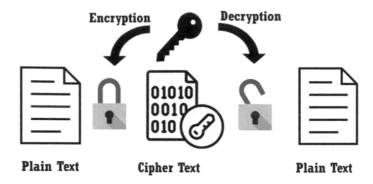

Fig. 1 Symmetric encryption

4.2 Asymmetric Cryptography (Public Key Cryptography)

This method produces two types of keys: one to encrypt plain text, and one to decode cipher text, and without one or the other, it does not function. It is named asymmetric encryption when a pair of keys are used: the first is the public key that the owner will release to whomever he chooses, and another is the private key and is identified only by the owner [9–11]. The most popular public key algorithm is the Rivest–Shamir–Aleman (RSA) algorithm used for key sharing, digital signatures or small data block encryption [14, 20, 21]. It uses a random size key and a variable lengths encryption block. Figure 2 illustrates the block diagram of the asymmetric key to encryption.

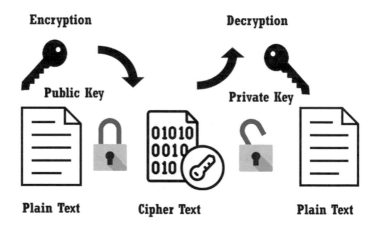

Fig. 2 Asymmetric key encryption

5   Literature Review

In papers [11, 13, 15], Huffman suggested a method which would create a tree T in a hastily manner corresponding to the optimal code. Huffman tree construction starts with a series of C leaves and executes C-$1''$ merging operations to construct the final tree. Here, we assume that C is a set of n symbols that each symbol is an entity with only a given frequency $f[c]$. A priority queue, Q, is keyed on f and used to determine the two least frequent objects to merge between. The merger of two variables leads to a new entity whose frequency is the sum of the frequencies of the two combined entities. Huffman's average run time on a set of n characters is $O\ (n \log n)$. The key benefits of this algorithm are, (1) Simple to apply and achieves lossless image compression (2) Allows best, efficient code. It also has diverse drawbacks. Huffman algorithm is relatively slow [12]. It depends on data model which is purely statistical. Decryption is challenging because of the different lengths of code. Huffman's tree sometimes becomes an overhead.

Arithmetic coding is an effective technique of encoding used in lossless data compression [15–17] which uses a fraction to represent the whole source message, rather than a code word to describe a text symbol. Now, this encoder splits the actual interval through sub-intervals, each representing a fraction of the current interval proportional to the symbol's probability in the current context, and figures out the interval corresponding to the actual symbol as the interval in the next step, using symbol probability to encode the text.

The key benefits of this coding are (1) It is almost optimal. (2) It can code very large occurrences in only a fraction of a bit. (3) It is quick, and the simulation distinguishes from the coding. (4) It significantly decreases file size (5) and facility to adapt [19]. The term adaptation refers to change of the frequency tables during data processing. Handful drawbacks to arithmetic coding are (1) To start decoding the symbols, full codeword must be received, and even if there is an incorrect bit in the codeword, the entire message may get incorrect. (2) The amount that may be encoded is reduced in length, thereby restricting the number of symbols to be encoded within a codeword.

The Lempel Ziv Welch Coding (LZW) is another lossless data compression algorithm. This algorithm is easy to implement relative to other algorithms and achieves high performance in practical systems. Either arithmetic encoding or Huffman coding is defined as a statistical model, i.e., an alphabet and the probability distribution of a source while LZW is focused on a dictionary model [18, 22]. This "dictionary" LZW uses encoding algorithm, which encodes data by referring to a dictionary rather than tabulating counts of characters and constructing trees. To encrypt a substring, only a single code number is applied to the output file that corresponds to the substring index in the dictionary. While it can be extended to various file formats, this algorithm is mainly used to compress text files. The dictionary initially contains 256 single-character entries (e.g., ASCII codes).

The longest sequence of the source text is defined for each line and is then represented in the current dictionary by the indices. These result in a new entry if the existing dictionary does not find such a match or if a match is found in the dictionary where the same section is used in the future. Initially, this algorithm begins with a 28 character dictionary (in the case of 8 bits) and uses them as the set of "ordinary" characters. 8 bits are read at one time (e.g., not, 'r', etc.), and the data is encoded as the number in the dictionary which represents its index. When reading, once a substring is found, it reads the new digit and connects it to the current string to create a new substring, and when a new substring is found (say 'tr'), it is added to the dictionary.

While revisiting the next substring, this is represented with a single digit. Monochrome images or repeated data greatly raise the file size, and LZW is the best strategy to minimize the size of those files. The key benefit is that (1) It is easy to install and one of the powerful lossless algorithms. (2) No need to transfer the string table to the code for decompression, using the input stream as data will reconstruct the table as it was during compression. The biggest drawback is the string table that is difficult to handle, and the amount of storage needed cannot be calculated.

The other most commonly employed algorithm is data encryption protocol (DES) [23]. This algorithm is intended to provide a consistent procedure for protecting strategically sensitive and unclassified information. The DES algorithm uses data key 56 bit and data block 64 bit. This technique calculates 16 rounds of iteration. The major disadvantage of DES [20] is the use of the 56 bit key size. It has already been proved vulnerable to attacks through brute force attack and other crypto-analytic approaches.

Blowfish is an 8-round block cipher with a block size of 64 bits and a key length of 32–448 bits. Blowfish algorithm serves as a substitution for DES [23, 24]. This algorithm is even simpler than other algorithms, and the key quality is excellent. This algorithm is only useful for applications where the function remains fundamentally the same. Through comparing this algorithm, it takes less time to implement, achieves high throughput, and speeds efficiency nearly four times higher than the advanced encryption standard (AES) and two times higher than DES. AES and DES are more energy intensive than blowfish.

6 The Proposed Encryption Method

6.1 Sender Side

This method uses a semi-asymmetric mirror-key dual encryption approach. Here, the encrypted "mirror-key" is appended along with the data, but even the intruder collects the data or the key, then they cannot hack the real-key or the data because of the mirroring cryptographic technique.

This technique is more secure because it is neither transmitting the actual data nor the encryption actual key. The key is generated through a mirroring algorithm at the receiver side only. On the transmitter side, it is by calculating the frequency of each symbol occurring in the data collected by the sensor and arrange the frequencies of letters in ascending order. Take two least frequent symbols and calculate the sum, until we generate a single digit key as adjacent sum generator (ASG). Encrypt the stream of data using the generated ASG. Figure 3 shows the block diagram of the proposed encryption/decryption algorithm.

Using a random generator, function generates a 4 bit mirror key. Then, divide the ASG with that mirror key generated, so that the actual encryption key will be masked. By division, the system will generate a 4 bit quotient and remainder. Separate the quotient and remainder (QR). Convert the QR data to gray code as named the dual encrypted key (DEK). Append the encrypted data with DEK. Transmit the encrypted data. Figure 3 shows the data flow diagram of the proposed algorithm at transmitter side.

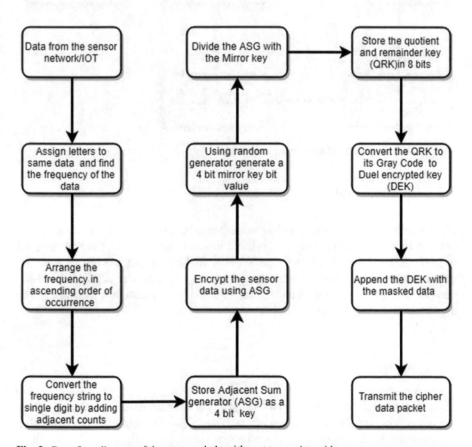

Fig. 3 Data flow diagram of the proposed algorithm at transmitter side

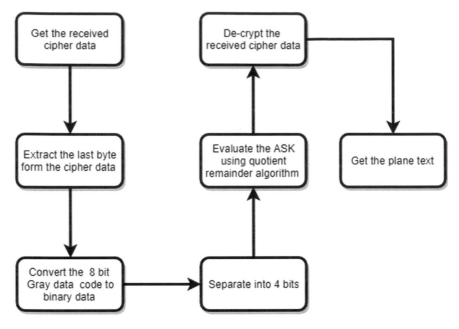

Fig. 4 Data flow diagram of receiver side algorithm

6.2 *Receiver Side*

The algorithm at the receiver end is not exactly in reverse. Here, as the obtained encrypted data stops on the server, the last 8 bits are first collected. Convert the 8 bit of gray code to binary where the device gets two 4 bits. From that binary data, the quotient–remainder (Q–R) function generates the adjacent sum key (ASK) which used to decrypt the received data stream. Figure 4 shows data flow diagram of the algorithm at the receiver end.

7 Analysis

The proposed algorithm's performance analysis is calculated using the three popular cryptographic algorithms, such as AES, DES, and blowfish which demonstrates the measurement bench marking report with respect to proposed algorithm. The smallest set of data used for checking the algorithm is the 100 bytes, and the maximum set of data used here is the 1000 bytes. The analysis is conducted on a 2.5 GH, PC I3 with Windows 7 operating system. Three metrics of execution are measured encryption time, use of the central processing unit (CPU) and memory usage. The time for encryption is defined as the time it takes for an encryption process to build a plain text cipher. Encryption time is used to estimate an encryption algorithm's performance. It reveals how fast encryption is. The encryption throughput is calculated as the complete plain text in encoded bytes divided by the time taken for encryption. Figures 5 and 6 give a graphical representation of the CPU execution and memory

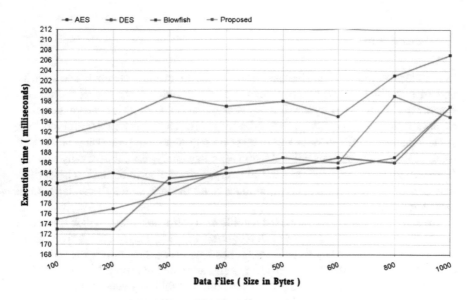

Fig. 5 CPU execution time analysis

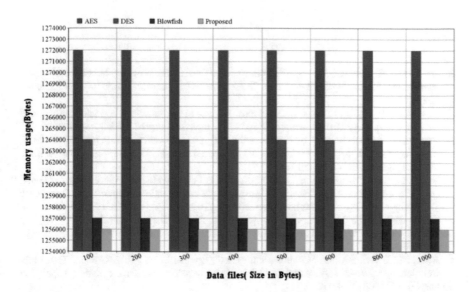

Fig. 6 Memory usage in bytes

utilization results. CPU execution time that a CPU is submitted to the given computation period is identical. The more CPU utilization is utilized in the encryption cycle, the higher is the heap of CPU. The test is conducted to determine the effect of the increasing information size and the phase for measurement of cryptography.

8 Conclusion

In any electronic communication scenario, data is the primary element. The security and privacy of the data is primarily taken into consideration for any data transmission sensor. The advantage of symmetric key encryption is that it has less processing time but less secure also, and the key has to be sent between the transmitter and receiver. An asymmetric public–private key encryption requires more processing power and more complex. But in conventional symmetric key encryption, it uses only one key (a hidden key) for both encryption and decryption of electronic data. The entities that interact by symmetric encryption must share the key, so that it can be used in decryption.

Here, in this chapter, we proposed a noble encryption algorithm where the actual key or the encrypted key is not transferring between transmitter and receiver rather than sending a mirror key (false-key). It has less processing power needed when compared with any other asymmetric key generation and recovery. Moreover, it has dual level security similar to the private key and the public key encryption approach. So it gives better performance in securing the transmitted data.

References

1. Lv, Z., Ota, K., Lloret, J., Xiang, W., Bellavista, P.: Complexity problems handled by big data technology. Complexity **2019**, 7, Article ID 9090528 (2019). https://doi.org/10.1155/2019/909 0528
2. Zhang, X., Wang, S., Cong, G., Cuzzocrea, A.: Social big data: mining, applications, and beyond. Complexity **2019**, 2, Article ID 2059075. https://doi.org/10.1155/2019/2059075
3. Kumari, S.: A research paper on cryptography encryption and compression techniques. Int. J. Eng. Comput. Sci. **4**(4), 20915–20919 (2017). Accessed on 11/09/2020 at https://www.ijecs. in/index.php/ijecs/article/download/3630/3378/
4. Tharakan, L.A., Dhanasekaran, R.: Security enabled energy efficient middleware for WSN. In: IEEE International Conference on Advanced Communications, Control and Computing Technologies (2015). https://doi.org/https://doi.org/10.1109/ICACCCT.2014.7019201
5. Liestyowati, D.: Public key cryptography. J. Phys. IOP Publishing Conf. Ser. **1477**, 052062 (2020). Accessed on 11/09/2020 at https://iopscience.iop.org/article/10.1088/1742-6596/1477/ 5/052062/pdf
6. Joshi, M.R., Avinash, R.: Network security with cryptography. Int. J. Comput. Sci. Mob. Comput. **4**(1), 201–204. Accessed on 11/09/2020 at https://www.ijcsmc.com/docs/papers/Jan uary2015/V4I1201544.pdf
7. Tharakan, L.A., Dhanasekaran, R.: Energy aware data compression in wireless sensor network using an advanced RLE method—matrix RLE (M-RLE). Int. J. Appl. Eng. Res. **10**(17) (2015).

ISSN 0973-4562. Accessed on 11/09/2020 at https://www.researchgate.net/publication/296 680223_Energy_Aware_Node_Deployment_in_Wireless_Sensor_Network_with_Straight_Line_Topology

8. Chaudhary, S., Joshi, N.K.: Secured blended approach for cryptographic algorithm in cloud computing. Int. J. Pure Appl. Math. **118**(20), 297–304 (2018). Accessed on 11/09/2020 at https://acadpubl.eu/jsi/2018-118-20/articles/20a/40.pdf

9. Stoyanov, B., Nedzhibov, G.: Symmetric key encryption based on rotation-translation equation. Symmetry **12**, 73 (2020). Accessed on 11/09/2020 at https://www.mdpi.com/2073-8994/12/1/73/pdf

10. Pradeep, K.V., Vijayakumar, V., Subramaniyaswamy, V.: An efficient framework for sharing a file in a secure manner using asymmetric key distribution management in cloud environment. J. Comput. Netw. Commun. **2019**, 8, Article ID 9852472 (2019). https://doi.org/10.1155/2019/9852472

11. Saha, R., Geetha, G., Kumar, G., Kim, T.-H.: RK-AES: an improved version of AES using a new key generation process with random keys. Secur. Commun. Netw. **2018**, 11, Article ID 9802475 (2018). https://doi.org/10.1155/2018/9802475

12. Abood, O.G., Guirguis, S.K.: A survey on cryptography algorithms. Int. J. Adv. Res. Comput. Sci. Softw. Eng. **6**(2) (2016). https://doi.org/10.29322/IJSRP.8.7.2018.p7978

13. Kumar, S., Jayadevappa, Bhopale, S.D., Naik, R.R.: Implementation of Huffman image compression and decompression algorithm. Int. J. Innov. Res. Electr. Electron. Instrum. Control Eng. **2**(4) (2014). Accessed on 11/09/2020 at https://ijireeice.com/wp-content/uploads/2013/03/IJIREEICE1E-s-sharankumar-IMPLEMENTATION-OF-HUFFMAN.pdf

14. Tharakan, L.A., Dhanasekaran, R.: Security enhancement of WSN data using symmetric data encryption through tabulation method of boolean function reduction. In: IJCA Proceedings on International Conference on Emerging Trends in Technology and Applied Sciences (2015). Accessed on 11/09/2020 at https://www.ijcaonline.org/proceedings/icettas2015/number3/22386-2586

15. Sharma, M.: Compression using Huffman coding. IJCSNS Int. J. Comput. Sci. Netw. Secur. **10**(5) (2010). Accessed on 11/09/2020 at https://paper.ijcsns.org/07_book/201005/20100520.pdf

16. Usman, M., Shoukat, I.A., Malik, M.S.A., Abid, M., Hasan, M.M., Khalid, Z.: A comprehensive comparison of symmetric cryptographic algorithms by using multiple types of parameters. Int. J. Comput. Sci. Netw. Secur. **18**(12) (2018). Accessed on 11/09/2020 at https://paper.ijcsns.org/07_book/201812/20181218.pdf

17. Bansal, S., Jagdev, G.:Comparative analysis and implementation of cryptographic algorithms in cloud computing. Int. J. Res. Stud. Comput. Sci. Eng. **5**(1), 17–25 (2018). Accessed on 11/09/2020 at https://www.arcjournals.org/pdfs/ijrscse/v5-i1/3.pdf

18. Hasan, Md.R.: Data compression using Huffman based LZW encoding technique. Int. J. Sci. Res. Publ. **8**(7) (2018). Accessed on 11/09/2020 at https://www.ijser.org/ResearchPaperPublishing_November2011.aspx

19. Panda, M.: Text and image encryption decryption using symmetric key algorithms on different platforms. Int. J. Sci. Technol. Res. **8**(09) (2019). Accessed on 11/09/2020 at https://www.ijstr.org/final-print/sep2019/Text-And-Image-Encryption-Decryption-Using-Symmetric-Key-Algorithms-On-Different-Platforms.pdf

20. Wahid, M.N.A., Ali, A., Esparham, B., Marwan, M.: A comparison of cryptographic algorithms: DES, 3DES, AES, RSA and blowfish for guessing attacks prevention. J. Comput. Sci. Appl. Inf. Technol. (2018). ISSN Online: 2474-9257. Accessed on 11/09/2020 at https://symbiosisonlinepublishing.com/computer-science-technology/computerscience-information-technology32.pdf

21. Narasingapuram, P.B., Ponnavaikko, M.: DNA cryptography based user level security for cloud computing and applications. Int. J. Recent Technol. Eng. (IJRTE) **8**(5) (2020). ISSN: 2277-3878. Accessed on 11/09/2020 at https://www.ijrte.org/wp-content/uploads/papers/v8i5/B2845078219.pdf

22. Gahan, A.V., Devanagavi, G.D.: A empirical study of security issues in encryption techniques. Int. J. Appl. Eng. Res. **14**(5), 1049–1061 (2019). ISSN 0973-4562. Accessed on 11/09/2020 at https://www.ripublication.com/ijaer19/ijaerv14n5_02.pdf
23. Sivakumar, R., Balakumar, B., Arivu Pandeeswaran, V.: A study of encryption algorithms (DES, 3DES and AES) for information security. Int. Res. J. Eng. Technol. (IRJET) **05**(04 Apr 2018). Accessed on 11/09/2020 at https://www.irjet.net/archives/V5/i4/IRJET-V5I4919.pdf
24. Senthilkumar, Mathivanan: Analysis of data compression techniques using Huffman coding and arithmetic coding. Int. J. Adv. Res. Comput. Sci. Softw. Eng. **6**(5) (2016). Accessed on 11/09/2020 at https://ijarcsse.com/Before_August_2017/docs/papers/Volume_6/5_May2016/V6I5-0357.pdf
25. Iqbal, A., et al.: Big-data analytics based energy analysis and monitoring for multi-story hospital buildings: case study. In: Springer Nature Book: Soft Computing in Condition Monitoring and Diagnostics of Electrical and Mechanical Systems, pp. 325–343 (2019). https://doi.org/10.1007/978-981-15-1532-3_14
26. Iqbal, A., et al.: Data driven intelligent model for sales prices prediction and monitoring of a building. In: Springer Nature Book: Soft Computing in Condition Monitoring and Diagnostics of Electrical and Mechanical Systems, pp. 407–421 (2019). https://doi.org/10.1007/978-981-15-1532-3_18

Introduction to Cuckoo Search and Its Paradigms: A Bibliographic Survey and Recommendations

Wahid Ali, Mohd Shariq Khan, Mashhood Hasan,
Mohammad Ehtisham Khan, Muhammad Abdul Qyyum,
Mohammad Obaid Qamar, and Moonyong Lee

Abstract Metaheuristic algorithms are found to be more effective and helpful in working out on complex problems (e.g., optimization and mining, etc.). This chapter presents a survey with a brief overview of the cuckoo algorithm, its latest developments, as well as recommendation for the applications in various disciplines. The presented survey analyzes the algorithm search insight, its Lévy flight strategy, and search mechanism efficiency. It was found that despite being capable of solving various complex and multimodal problems researcher further improves cuckoo search algorithm performance. The chapter presents the cuckoo search algorithm, and explains the variants and hybrids of the cuckoo algorithm. Further, the chapter unveils various complex problems of science and engineering where the algorithm can be applied successfully with better convergence and global optimization results.

W. Ali (✉) · M. E. Khan
Department of Chemical Engineering Technology, College of Applied Industrial Technology (CAIT), Jazan University, Jazan 45971, Kingdom of Saudi Arabia
e-mail: wahid8petro@gmail.com; wzali@jazanu.edu.sa

M. E. Khan
e-mail: mekhan@jazanu.edu.sa

M. S. Khan
Department of Chemical Engineering, Dhofar University, Salalah 211, Oman
e-mail: mskhan@du.edu.om

M. Hasan
Department of Electrical Power Engineering Technology, College of Applied Industrial Technology (CAIT), Jazan University, Jazan 45971, Kingdom of Saudi Arabia
e-mail: mirmashhood2010@gmail.com

M. A. Qyyum · M. Lee
School of Chemical Engineering, Yeungnam University, Gyeongsan 712-749, South Korea
e-mail: maqyyum@gmail.com

M. Lee
e-mail: mynlee@ynu.ac.kr

M. O. Qamar
Department of Civil Engineering, Yeungnam University, Gyeongsan 712-749, South Korea
e-mail: obaid.qamar@zhcet.ac.in

H. Malik et al. (eds.), *AI and Machine Learning Paradigms for Health Monitoring System*, Studies in Big Data 86,
https://doi.org/10.1007/978-981-33-4412-9_4

Keywords Cuckoo search · Metaheuristic algorithm · Optimization · Variants · Hybrids · Applications · Survey

1 Overview and Analysis

1.1 Optimization and Cuckoo Search Concept

The essence of any algorithm is to fulfill the purpose of exploring optimal solutions by utilizing a system of evolving agents [1]. The system of obtaining a solution arises by iterations, governed by the rules of the set, leading to self-organizing states [2]. As soon the self-organized states are achieved, it indicates that the system converges, and a global solution is discovered. The iterations required for an optimal search for a given accuracy helps in describing the performance of any algorithm. Hence, an efficient optimizing algorithm mimics the evolution of a self-organizing system. However, the increasing size of the problem due to high dimensional complexity and the objectives with the interacting constraints made a typically nonlinear, non-convex optimization problem [3]. Hence, an efficient algorithm must use less computation with fewer iterations [1].

Nowadays, there are diverse optimization algorithms with a range of important applications. Among the modern algorithms, metaheuristics are becoming more familiar contributing to a new subdivision called metaheuristic optimization. These metaheuristic algorithms such as ant colony (AC), particle swarm optimization (PSO), and cuckoo search algorithm (CSA) are nature-inspired [4, 5]. Further, these algorithms can be categorized as trajectory-based and population-based [6]. Trajectory-based algorithms, for example, Simulated Annealing (SA) algorithm, mainly work by using only one agent to find the optimal solution; however, in population-based algorithms (e.g., PSO), multiple agents work, search, and communicate with each other in a decentralized manner. These agents usually move in two phases, namely exploration and exploitation. Most swarm intelligence-based algorithms are a set of population-based, bio-inspired optimization techniques. These features exploit collective behavior within a swarm and, therefore, make the overall functionality of the algorithm much richer than the simple sum of individual tasks [3, 7]. In this chapter, a metaheuristic population-based Cuckoo Search (CS) algorithm for the various class and areas of optimization problem has been undertaken. The chapter beside the CS concept is featured with the Lévy flight focuses on its implementation and its use. Many recently used variants and hybrids CS algorithm with their application in the diverse discipline have been described. Further, the chapter illustrated the popularity and applicability of CSA not only in science and engineering rather in other disciples such as economics, data mining et cetera in the CSA analysis, section.

1.2 Cuckoo Breeding and Search Concept

Cuckoos are a family of fascinating birds known because of their beautiful sound and unique reproductive strategy. Cuckoo species such as Guira and Ani lay their eggs in a host nest (crow), moreover, to increase the chance of hatching, they also move out the host eggs from the nest. Another Cuckoo species Tapera, however, uses the parasitism method. These species play their cards at the place where the host has just given their eggs. Tapera cuckoo species have precise timing of laying, and their eggs normally hatch quicker. Soon after hatching, the foreign chick (cuckoo) moves the host bird eggs from the host nest. This act of cuckoo reduces the chance of abandonment of their eggs and thus increases the breeding and feeding share of cuckoo chick [5, 8]. Based on this concept Yang and Deb in 2009 [9] developed an algorithm known as the CS algorithm that obligates the same concept of brood parasitism. Figure 1 presents a cuckoo search approach for better understanding and representation. The algorithm is inspired by the reproduction strategy of the cuckoo birds and fall into the class of metaheuristics. CS algorithm search uses the feature of Lévy flights to utilize the population-based swarm intelligence and to improve the performance [9, 10]. A brief about the Lévy flight mechanism is explained in the following subsection.

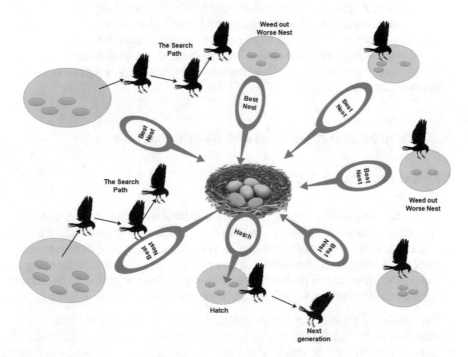

Fig. 1 Cuckoo search strategy for migration and brood parasitism

1.3 Lévy Flights Strategy

Lévy flights follow the class of non-Gaussian random processes. Paul Pierre studied that in Lévy walk stationary increments are distributed according to stable distributions. The properties of the stable distribution can be represented by the following noteworthy attributes of stable distributions [11]:

- Stability
- Generalized central limit theorem
- Power law asymptotics (Heavy tails):

$$f(|x| \rightarrow \infty) \approx \frac{\Gamma(\alpha\phi)\sin\left(\frac{\pi\phi}{2}\right)}{\pi}|x|^{(-1-\phi)} \tag{1}$$

where $\phi(1 \leq \phi \leq 2)$ is the external Lévy noise index. It is believed that Lévy's stats represent a model for the description of many natural phenomena. These natural phenomena from a general point of view may include biological, physical, chemical, and economic systems. In summary, Lévy flights are a type of random walk in which the step-length has a heavy tail's type probability distribution. These heavy-tailed distributions are those probability distributions that have heavier tails than the exponential distribution [12]. Actually, Lévy flights are like Markov processes where the step-size general distributions satisfy the power–law condition. Further, the walk distance from the origin reaches to a stable distribution owing to the generalized central limit theorem after a large number of steps. Details theory about the Lévy-flight, random-walk, and Markov processes can be obtained from the Yang study [13].

2 Cuckoo Search Algorithm and Implementation

2.1 Cuckoo Search Algorithm

Since the natural/physical systems are complex, their modeling gives a complex mathematical model. It is difficult to code them exactly in a computer algorithm. The simplification of these natural complex systems is an essential part of their successful execution [14]. Therefore, the cuckoo search behavior of laying and hatching eggs is required to simplify for developing the algorithm. The simplified assumptions (idealized rules) to develop the CS algorithm are presented as follows [5, 9]:

- Each cuckoo lay one egg at a time, and put it in a randomly selected nest,
- Excellent nests with high-quality eggs will be passed on to future generations,
- The available number of host nests is fixed, and the egg laid is spotted by the host allowed by a chance $p_a \in (0, 1)$. In this case, the trapped bird can either eliminate the egg or simply vacate the old nest and build a new one.

Further, we can use the simple postulate that each egg in a nest considers as a solution (or each nest has only one egg), and each cuckoo can give one egg only (i.e., one solution) with the objective to use the new and better solutions by replacing a local (bad results).

In the CSA, the algorithm utilizes a proportionate combining of a local walk with the global explorative walk. These random walks are controlled by a switching parameter represented by p_a. The local random walk can be represented by the following equation:

$$x_i^{t+1} = x_i^t + \alpha s \otimes H(p_\alpha - \varepsilon) \otimes \left(x_j^t - x_k^t\right), \tag{2}$$

where x_j^t and x_k^t are two separate solutions selected by random permutation. Further, $H(u)$ is a Heaviside function, ε is chosen from a uniform distribution, and s is the step size.

When generating new solutions x^{t+1} for, *say cuckoo i*, the global explorative random walk is performed by Lévy random walk. The above equation folded with the Lévy random walk can be represented as:

$$x_i^{t+1} = x_i^t + \alpha \otimes \text{Lévy } (\lambda). \tag{3}$$

Lévy flights basically provide a random walk in which the random steps are taken from a Lévy distribution for large steps. The Lévy (λ) distribution can be represented as:

$$\text{Lévy } (\lambda) \sim u = t^{-\lambda}, \quad (1 < \lambda \le 3); \tag{4}$$

The distribution shown above has both, infinite variance and infinite mean. Moreover, the consecutive steps/jumps in the cuckoo process basically form a random walk governed by power-law step-length distribution with a heavy tail (see Sect. 1.3) [5]. The dynamic switching parameters used in the CSA are described in Table 1.

2.2 Implementation of Algorithm

The objective to be optimized based on the problem layout, and the fitness of a solution is simply proportional to the value of the objective function. For CSA implementation, the above-mentioned rules are summarized in compact pseudocode as shown in Fig. 2a and the corresponding flowchart of the CS algorithm is represented in Fig. 2b [15]. Moreover, the detailed pseudocode for CSA can be obtained from Civicioglu and Besdok's study [16].

It is reported that CSA can be controlled by a few important tuning parameters compared to other available nature-inspired algorithms [15]. This is one of the most favorable advantages of using the CS algorithm and encourages the user from diverse areas. The tuning parameters of CSA are given in Table 2 with their commonly used

Table 1 Switching parameters used in the CSA

Parameter	Description
x_i^t and x_k^t	Randomly selected current positions
x_i^{t+1}	Next position
$\alpha > 0$	Step size scaling factor
s	Step size
$\otimes$	Product of two vectors
H	Heavy-side function
$p_a \in [0, 1]$	Switching parameter (help to switch between local random and global random walks)
ε	A number drawn from the uniform distribution
$L(\lambda) \sim u$	Lévy distribution

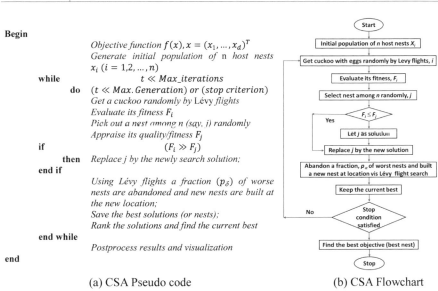

Begin

Objective function $f(x), x = (x_1, \ldots, x_d)^T$
Generate initial population of n host nests
x_i ($i = 1, 2, \ldots, n$)

while $t \ll Max\_iterations$
     do   ($t \ll Max. Generation$) or ($stop\ criterion$)
       Get a cuckoo randomly by Lévy flights
       Evaluate its fitness F_i
       Pick out a nest among n (say, i) randomly
       Appraise its quality/fitness F_j

if $(F_i \gg F_j)$
     then   *Replace j by the newly search solution;*
end if

Using Lévy flights a fraction (p_δ) of worse nests are abandoned and new nests are built at the new location;
Save the best solutions (or nests);
Rank the solutions and find the current best

end while

Postprocess results and visualization

end

(a) CSA Pseudo code

(b) CSA Flowchart

Fig. 2 Pseudocode and flowchart of the CSA [15]

Table 2 Parameters of the CSA [15]

Parameter	Symbol	Range	Commonly used
Nest	N	[15, 50]	$N = 15$
Fraction	p_α	[0, 1]	$p_\alpha = 0.25$
Step size	α	$\alpha \gg 0$	$\alpha = 1$

values [15]. However, the MATLAB codes for a single [17] and multi-objective problem [18] for the CSA are available on MATLAB official webpage.

3 Cuckoo Search Algorithm Variants, Hybrids and Applications

3.1 Variants Algorithm

CSA is the latest swarm-based algorithm, proposed by Yang in 2009, in comparison with the firefly (2008), bee colony (2005), PSO (1995), and AC (1992) algorithms [15], as it is being claimed by developers that CSA can deal with diverse problems naturally and efficiently [19]. However, premature convergence and high computational time of CSA further encouraged the researchers to attempt to improve CSA efficiency, in terms of convergence time its premature convergence in a high-dimensional and multi-modal environment, and fewer iterations [7] and to obtain a better solution [19, 20], to fulfill the requirement of a better optimization algorithm. Hence to improve CSA, researchers had developed many variants to grapple with the nature of the search space and to improve the results in a diverse field of optimization problems [15].

The researcher had developed various CSA variants by tuning the control parameters only without any modification in the original CSA. These slight changes correspond to small modifications since the operating mechanism of the algorithm remains unchanged. The major category of the CS variants and years of development are summed up in Table 3.

3.2 Hybrids of Algorithm

Since many complex optimization problems are difficult to handle by pure CSA and sometimes CSA variants are also incapable of achieving the purpose in complex optimization system. Further, the CSA variants were obtained by just a slight alteration in the algorithm parameters; hence, it requires big modifications that alter the searching mechanism of the algorithm [37, 38]. As mentioned above (see Sect. 3.1), the major problem usually associated with the CS algorithm is the convergence to a suboptimal solution. This problem arises when an algorithm is not able to keep the diversity in the solutions with the number of iteration or the solution searched in the search domain [20]. As against creating or developing the variants of CS researchers made a strategy to strengthen the results of algorithms by using the hybridization methodology. The hybridization can be performed by adopting and incorporating other available algorithms or any suitable mathematical alterations to reduce the likelihood of premature convergence. These hybridization strategies involve deep changes in the original and

Table 3 Variants of cuckoo search [19]

Multi-objective cuckoo search	A novel complex-valued	Quantum-based CSA
Emotional chaotic CS	Gaussian-based disturbance CSA	CS based Levenberg–Marquardt
Parallelized	Discrete	Modified
Modified adaptive	CSA-based on Gauss distribution	Discrete binary
Neural based		

Famously used variants of CS algorithm	Year	References
Novel CSA under adaptive parameter control	2019	[21, 22]
Adaptive CSA	2018	[23]
Hybrid self-adaptive CS	2016	[24]
CSA-based on frog leaping and chaos theory	2015	[25]
Discrete CS for travelling salesman problem	2014	[26]
Neural-based CS	2013	[27]
CSA-based Levenberg–Marquardt (LM)	2013	[28]
Multi-objective CSA	2013	[28]
Discrete binary CS	2012	[29]
Discrete CS	2012	[30]
Emotional chaotic cuckoo	2012	[31]
Parallelized CS	2012	[32]
Modified CS	2012	[33]
Modified adaptive CS	2012	[34]
CS-based on Gaussian disturbance	2011	[35]
Quantum inspired CS	2011	[36]

basic form of the CS algorithm's search components such as initialization procedure, function evaluation, moving function, rather in every possible state [19]. However, it is also true that these hybrid algorithms may have their own disadvantages that they may normally require more computational time than the original [20].

The main suggestions and study work for hybridization of CSA obtained from the survey are based on the complying main features (i) matheuristics, in which math model are combined with metaheuristic algorithms [39], (ii) hybrid heuristics, the combination with various metahcuristic methodologies [40], (iii) simheuristics, that facilitates both simulation and metaheuristics [41], and (iv) the hybridization with the combination among machine learning and metaheuristics [42]. The short detail of the hybridized CS algorithms developed are mentioned in Table 4 however, the interested reader may go through literature/research presented by García et al. [43].

In summary, the study on the various aspects of variants and hybrids cannot be individually discussed, as it is beyond the scope of this chapter; however, the

Table 4 Hybrid cuckoo search available in the literature

Name	Year	References
Intelligent hybrid CS/β-hill climbing algorithm	2020	[20]
Hybrid k-means CSA	2020	[43]
Hybrid CS and differential evolution	2019	[47]
Hybrid ant colony/CSA	2018	[48]
Hybrid CS with Nelder–Mead method	2016	[8]
Hybrid CS/harmony (global harmony) search algorithm	2016	[49]
Hybrid PSO/CS	2015	[50]
Hybrid CS/improved shuffled frog leaping algorithm	2014, 2019, 2020	[51–53]
Hybrid CS/GA	2012	[54]

application parts and type of problems solved using such diverse CSA may leave the area for separate literature review. Apart of this, some examples are given in [44–46].

3.3 Applications

CS algorithm including its variants and hybrids has been applied in many disciplines with promising efficiency. Considering, for instance, in the engineering design applications, medical field, image processing, decision making, data mining, etc., it is evident by many researchers that CS has superior performance over other algorithms in many real-world applications [20, 55–57]. Significant portions of the published study have concrete proofs that dignify the performance of CSA. Table 5 shows a summary of the application in various areas of CSA.

Table 5 Application of kind of CSA across the various field of discipline

S. No.	Application area	References/Publications
1	Benchmarking functions for optimization	[20]
2	Area of medical application	[58]
3	Data clustering and data mining	[59]
4	Image processing	[60]
5	Economic load dispatch	[61]
6	Engineering design applications	[62]
7	Energy and power	[63]
8	Decision making and scheduling optimization	[64]
9	Neural network/Artificial intelligence	[65]
10	Data mining applications	[66]

4 Analysis of Algorithm

The analysis of the structural model of the CSA, it is analogously grounded on a simplified mathematical set of equations of lineage genesis behavior of cuckoos, since it is possible to create the model of the nature of the living birds (i.e., cuckoo), motion, and search for the host nest or food. To make possible the movement of the bird, few analytical random-walk methods are available. These random-walk methods usually use Brownian-walk or Lèvy-flight (walk), or both strategies. P. Civicioglu and his colleague in their study found that the Lèvy-walk strategy could discover more new locations than the Brownian-walk strategy. Hence, developers make it possible by using the Lèvy-walk strategy in CSA. This strategy makes the CSA more useful that can find more resources and conspicuously decrease the search time [16]. McCulloch's algorithm has been used in CSA to generate random solutions in specified domains of distributions for most commodious nest [67]. Further, the overall structure of CSA is substantially like the evolutionary algorithms that comprise of two basic search stages. First stage predicates all possible nest in which the best solution is screen out, i.e., the system be led by an elite strategy. Through this stage, speedy access for a better solution can be achieved, located between a nest and the nest having the best result. Second stage forces every nest to evolve randomly toward a different nest in a fast manner. It explores a nest which gives a better solution that may exist among two nests. All these search techniques allow the CS algorithm to establish powerful stability to explore between global and local regions of search space.

Because of all these capabilities and the beautiful nature of the bird, Pinar and Erkan verified that CS has been succeeded in solving various benchmark optimization problems. They compared CSA optimization results with three renowned algorithms, i.e., PSO, differential evolution (DE), and artificial bee colony (ABC) by utilizing statistical tests [16]. X. S. Yang also found evidence that CS is an excellent combination of DE, PSO, and SA in one algorithm and without a doubt, providing an efficient and global convergence [19]. Some other studies also reported that CSA is potentially better and efficient than PSO and GA [6, 9]. Xin-She also claims that DE, SA, and PSO are peculiar classes of the CS algorithm [6]. Hence, the reason why an estimate of CSA popularity can be made by the number of publications in various filed and areas of application. Figure 3 shows the number of publications from 2009 to 2016 on CSA [15].

5 Conclusion

The chapter describes the basic need for the optimization of complex problems. As expected, the multi-agent metaheuristic algorithms are most prone to find the best possible optimal solution, and it may be called as global optimum. In this chapter, the basics of CSA with Lévy flights random-walk strategy is presented beside the

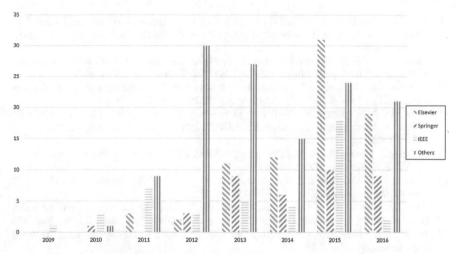

Fig. 3 CSA-based publications by Elsevier, Springer, IEEE, and others, per annum (2009–2016) [15] (Figure rights included with the files)

new developments in the same algorithm. Since CSA is simple in implementation with a few tuning parameters, however, there are many important issues with CS, and based on the theoretical analysis, many researchers created many variants and hybrids and claimed that the cuckoo algorithm has the superior solving capability. It can also be there may still more room to improve the CSA. Furthermore, many applications of CSA based on the variants and hybrids were highlighted (see Sect. 3) in the various areas and discipline which focus on large and real-world applications.

References

1. Ahmed, A.M., Rashid, T.A., Saeed, S.A.M.: Cat swarm optimization algorithm: a survey and performance evaluation. Comput. Intell. Neurosci. **2020**, 4854895 (2020). https://doi.org/10.1155/2020/4854895https://doi.org/10.1155/2020/4854895
2. Yang, X.-S.: Swarm intelligence based algorithms: a critical analysis. Evol. Intell.**7**(1), 17–28 (2014). https://doi.org/10.1007/s12065-013-0102-2
3. Aghaei, J., et al.: Optimal robust unit commitment of CHP plants in electricity markets using information gap decision theory. IEEE Trans. Smart Grid**8**(5), 2296–2304 (2017). https://doi.org/10.1109/TSG.2016.2521685
4. Yang, X.S.: Nature-Inspired Metaheuristic Algorithms. Luniver Press (2008)
5. Yang, X.-S., Deb, S.: Engineering optimisation by cuckoo search. Int. J. Math. Model. Numer. Optim.**1**(4), 14 (2010)
6. Yang, X.-S.: Nature Inspired Optimization Algorithms. Illustrated, Reprint. Elsevier Science, Amsterdam (2016)
7. Huang, Z., Gao, Z., Qi, L., Duan, H.: A heterogeneous evolving cuckoo search algorithm for solving large-scale combined heat and power economic dispatch problems. IEEE Access**7**, 111287–111301 (2019). https://doi.org/10.1109/ACCESS.2019.2933980

8. Ali, A.F., Tawhid, M.A.: A hybrid cuckoo search algorithm with Nelder Mead method for solving global optimization problems. SpringerPlus**5**(1), 473 (2016). https://doi.org/10.1186/s40064-016-2064-1

9. Yang, X.-S., Deb, S.: Cuckoo search via Levy flights. In: Proceedings of the World Congress on Nature and Biologically Inspired Computing (NaBIC 2009), p. 7, Dec 2009

10. Pavlyukevich, I.: Lévy flights, non-local search and simulated annealing. J. Comput. Phys.**226**(2), 1830–1844 (2007). https://doi.org/10.1016/j.jcp.2007.06.008

11. Chechkin, A.V., Metzler, R., Klafter, J., Gonchar, V.Y.: Introduction to the theory of Lévy flights. In: Anomalous Transport, pp. 129–162, 23 July 2008. https://doi.org/10.1002/978352 7622979.ch5

12. Asmussen, S. (ed.): Steady-State Properties of GI/G/1 BT—Applied Probability and Queues, pp. 266–301. Springer, New York (2003)

13. Yang, X.: Random walk and Markov chain. In: Engineering Optimization, pp. 153–170, 21 June 2010. https://doi.org/10.1002/9780470640425.ch10

14. Ali, W., Qyyum, M.A., Khan, M.S., Duong, P.L.T., Lee, M.: Knowledge-inspired operational reliability for optimal LNG production at the offshore site. Appl. Therm. Eng. **150**, 19–29 (2019). https://doi.org/10.1016/j.applthermaleng.2018.12.165https://doi.org/10.1016/j. applthermaleng.2018.12.165

15. Shehab, M., Khader, A.T., Al-Betar, M.A.: A survey on applications and variants of the cuckoo search algorithm. Appl. Soft Comput. **61**, 1041–1059 (2017). https://doi.org/10.1016/j.asoc. 2017.02.034https://doi.org/10.1016/j.asoc.2017.02.034

16. Civicioglu, P., Besdok, E.: Comparative analysis of the cuckoo search algorithm BT. In: Yang, X.-S. (ed.) Cuckoo Search and Firefly Algorithm: Theory and Applications, pp. 85–113. Springer International Publishing, Cham (2014)

17. Yang, X.-S.: Cuckoo Search (CS) Algorithm Matlab Code. Matlab official page (2020)

18. Yang, X.-S.: Multiobjective Cuckoo Search (MOCS). Matlab official page (2020)

19. Yang, X. S.: Cuckoo Search and Firefly Algorithm: Theory and Applications. Springer International Publishing, Berlin (2013)

20. Abed-Alguni, B.H., Alkhateeb, F.: Intelligent hybrid cuckoo search and β-hill climbing algorithm. J. King Saud Univ. Comput. Inf. Sci.**32**(2), 159–173 (2020). https://doi.org/10.1016/j. jksuci.2018.05.003

21. Wei, J., Yu, Y.: A novel cuckoo search algorithm under adaptive parameter control for global numerical optimization (7) (2019). https://doi.org/10.1007/s00500-019-04245-3

22. Abdullahi, H., Onumanyi, A.J., Zubair, S., Abu-Mahfouz, A.M., Hancke, G.P.: A cuckoo search optimization-based forward consecutive mean excision model for threshold adaptation in cognitive radio. Soft Comput.**24**(13), 9683–9704 (2020). https://doi.org/10.1007/s00500-019-04481-7

23. Mareli, M., Twala, B.: An adaptive Cuckoo search algorithm for optimisation. Appl. Comput. Inform. **14**(2), 107–115 (2018). https://doi.org/10.1016/j.aci.2017.09.001https://doi.org/10. 1016/j.aci.2017.09.001

24. Mlakar, U., Fister, I., Fister, I.: Hybrid self-adaptive cuckoo search for global optimization. Swarm Evol. Comput. **29**, 47–72 (2016). https://doi.org/10.1016/j.swevo.2016.03.001https:// doi.org/10.1016/j.swevo.2016.03.001

25. Liu, X., Fu, M.: Cuckoo search algorithm based on frog leaping local search and chaos theory. Appl. Math. Comput. **266**, 1083–1092 (2015). https://doi.org/10.1016/j.amc.2015. 06.041https://doi.org/10.1016/j.amc.2015.06.041

26. Ouaarab, A., Ahiod, B., Yang, X.S.: Discrete cuckoo search algorithm for the travelling salesman problem. Neural Comput. Appl. **24**(7), 1659–1669 (2014). https://doi.org/10.1007/ s00521-013-1402-2https://doi.org/10.1007/s00521-013-1402-2

27. Khan, K., Sahai, A.: Neural-based cuckoo search of employee health and safety (HS). Int. J. Intell. Syst. Appl. **5**, 76–83 (2013)

28. Nawi, N.M., Khan, A., Rehman, M.Z.: A New cuckoo search based Levenberg-Marquardt (CSLM) algorithm. Comput. Sci. Appl. ICCSA **2013**, 438–451 (2013). https://doi.org/10.1007/ 978-3-642-39637-3_35https://doi.org/10.1007/978-3-642-39637-3_35

29. Gherboudj, A., Layeb, A., Chikhi, S.: Solving 0–1 knapsack problems by a discrete binary version of cuckoo search algorithm. IJBIC **4**, 229–236 (2012). https://doi.org/10.1504/IJBIC. 2012.048063https://doi.org/10.1504/IJBIC.2012.048063
30. Jati, G.K., Manurung, H.M., Suyanto: Discrete cuckoo search for traveling salesman problem. In: 2012 7th International Conference on Computing and Convergence Technology (ICCCT), pp. 993–997 (2012). https://doi.org/10.1007/s00521-013-1402-2
31. Lin, J.-H., Lee, I.-H.: Emotional chaotic cuckoo search for the reconstruction of chaotic dynamics (2012)
32. Subotic, M., Tuba, M., Bacanin, N., Simian, D.: Parallelized cuckoo search algorithm for unconstrained optimization. In: Proceedings of the 5th WSEAS Congress on Applied Computing Conference, and Proceedings of the 1st International Conference on Biologically Inspired Computation, pp. 151–156 (2012)
33. Tuba, M., Subotic, M., Stanarevic, N.: Modified cuckoo search algorithm for unconstrained optimization problems. In: Proceedings of the 5th European Conference on European Computing Conference, pp. 263–268 (2011)
34. Zhang, Y., Wang, L., Wu, Q.: Modified adaptive cuckoo search (MACS) algorithm and formal description for global optimisation. Int. J. Comput. Appl. Technol.**44**(2), 73–79 (2012). https://www.doi.org/10.1504/IJCAT.2012.048675
35. Wang Fan, W.Y., Xing-Shi, H.: The cuckoo search algorithm based on gaussian disturbance. J. Xi'an Polytech. Univ.**4** (2011)
36. Layeb, A.: A novel quantum inspired cuckoo search for knapsack problems. IJBIC **3**, 297–305 (2011). https://doi.org/10.1504/IJBIC.2011.042260https://doi.org/10.1504/IJBIC. 2011.042260
37. Crawford, B., Soto, R., Astorga, G., García, J.,Castro, C., Paredes, F.: Putting continuous metaheuristics to work in binary search spaces. Complexity**2017**, 8404231 (2017). https://doi. org/10.1155/2017/8404231
38. Calvet, L., de Armas, J., Masip, D., Juan, A.A.: Learnheuristics: hybridizing metaheuristics with machine learning for optimization with dynamic inputs. Open Math. **15**(1), 261–280 (2017). https://doi.org/10.1515/math-2017-0029https://doi.org/10.1515/math-2017-0029
39. Caserta, M., Voß, S.: Metaheuristics: intelligent problem solving BT—matheuristics: hybridizing metaheuristics and mathematical programming. In: Maniezzo, V., Stützle, T., Voß, S. (eds.) Mathheuristics Hybridizing Metaheuristics and Mathematical Programming, pp. 1–38. Springer, Boston (2010)
40. Talbi, E.-G.: Combining metaheuristics with mathematical programming, constraint programming and machine learning. Ann. Oper. Res.**240**(1), 171–215 (2016). https://doi.org/10.1007/ s10479-015-2034-y
41. Juan, A.A., Faulin, J., Grasman, S.E., Rabe, M., Figueira, G.: A review of simheuristics: extending metaheuristics to deal with stochastic combinatorial optimization problems. Oper. Res. Perspect. **2**, 62–72 (2015). https://doi.org/10.1016/j.orp.2015.03.001https://doi.org/10. 1016/j.orp.2015.03.001
42. Sayed, G.I., Tharwat, A., Hassanien, A.E.: Chaotic dragonfly algorithm: an improved metaheuristic algorithm for feature selection. Appl. Intell.**49**(1), 188–205 (2019). https://www.doi. org/10.1007/s10489-018-1261-8
43. García, J., Yepes, J., Martí, V.: A hybrid k-means cuckoo search algorithm applied to the counterfort retaining walls problem. Mathematics**8**(4), 555 (2020). https://doi.org/10.3390/ math8040555
44. Iqbal, A., et al.: Metaheurestic algorithm based hybrid model for identification of building sale prices. In: Springer Nature Book: Metaheuristic and Evolutionary Computation: Algorithms and Applications. Studies in Computational Intelligence (2020). https://doi.org/10.1007/978-981-15-7571-6_32
45. Faiz Minai, A., et al.: Metaheuristics paradigms for renewable energy systems: advances in optimization algorithms. In: Springer Nature Book: Metaheuristic and Evolutionary Computation: Algorithms and Applications. Studies in Computational Intelligence (2020). https://doi. org/10.1007/978-981-15-7571-6_2

46. Yadav, A.K., et al.: Optimization of tilt angle for intercepting maximum solar radiation for power generation. In: Springer Nature Book: Optimization of Power System Problems (Methods, Algorithms and MATLAB Codes), pp. 203–232 (2020). https://doi.org/10.1007/978-3-030-34050-6_9

47. Chi, R., Su, Y., Qu, Z., Chi, X.: A hybridization of cuckoo search and differential evolution for the logistics distribution center location problem. Math. Probl. Eng.**2019**, 7051248 (2019). https://doi.org/10.1155/2019/7051248

48. Zhang, Y., et al.: A hybrid ant colony and cuckoo search algorithm for route optimization of heating engineering. Energies**11**(10) (2018). https://doi.org/10.3390/en11102675

49. Feng, Y., Wang, G.G., Gao, X.Z.: A novel hybrid cuckoo search algorithm with global harmony search for 0–1 Knapsack problems. Int. J. Comput. Intell. Syst. **9**(6), 1174–1190 (2016). https://doi.org/10.1080/18756891.2016.1256577https://doi.org/10.1080/18756891.2016.1256577

50. Wang, L., Zhong, Y., Yin, Y.: A hybrid cooperative cuckoo search algorithm with particle swarm optimisation. Int. J. Comput. Sci. Math.**6**(1), 18–29 (2015). https://doi.org/10.1504/IJCSM.2015.067537

51. Feng, Y., Wang, G.-G., Feng, Q., Zhao, X.-J.: An effective hybrid cuckoo search algorithm with improved shuffled frog leaping algorithm for 0-1 knapsack problems. Comput. Intell. Neurosci.**2014**, 857254 (2014). https://doi.org/10.1155/2014/857254

52. Li, J., Li, Y., Tian, S., Xia, J.: An improved cuckoo search algorithm with self-adaptive knowledge learning. Neural Comput. Appl.**32**(16), 11967–11997 (2020). https://doi.org/10.1007/s00521-019-04178-w

53. Shao, S.: An improved cuckoo search-based adaptive band selection for hyperspectral image classification. Eur. J. Remote Sens.**53**(1), 211–218 (2020). https://doi.org/10.1080/22797254.2020.1796526

54. Ghodrati, A., Lotfi, S.: A hybrid CS/GA algorithm for global optimization, pp. 397–404 (2012)

55. Gandomi, A.H., Yang, X.S., Alavi, A.H.: Cuckoo search algorithm: a metaheuristic approach to solve structural optimization problems. Eng. Comput. **29**(1), 17–35 (2013). https://doi.org/10.1007/s00366-011-0241-yhttps://doi.org/10.1007/s00366-011-0241-y

56. Pandian Vasant, V.N.D., Weber, G.-W.: Handbook of Research on Modern Optimization Algorithms and Applications in Engineering and Economics. IGI Global (2016)

57. Yang, X.-S.: Cuckoo search and firefly algorithm: overview and analysis BT. In: Yang, X.-S. (ed.) Cuckoo Search and Firefly Algorithm: Theory and Applications, pp. 1–26. Springer International Publishing, Cham (2014)

58. Bustamam, A., Nurazmi, V. Y., Lestari, D.: Applications of cuckoo search optimization algorithm for analyzing protein-protein interaction through Markov clustering on HIV. AIP Conf. Proc.**2023**(1), 20232 (2018). https://doi.org/10.1063/1.5064229

59. Abbas, A.K., Sadeq, A.T.: Database clustering using intelligent techniques. Al-Nahrain J. Sci. **17**(3), 195–203 (2018)

60. Peng, K., Chen, Z., Huang, L., Wu, X.: Application of cuckoo search algorithm for texture recognition based on water areas. In: Proceedings SPIE, vol. 10806, Aug 2018. https://doi.org/10.1117/12.2503078

61. Yasin, Z.M., Aziz, N.F.A., Salim, N.A., Wahab, N.A., Rahmat, N.A.: Optimal economic load dispatch using multiobjective cuckoo search algorithm. Indonesian J. Electr. Eng. Comput. Sci. **12**, 168–174 (2018)

62. Kaveh, A., Bakhshpoori, T.: An efficient multi-objective cuckoo search algorithm for design optimization 1, Jan 2016. https://doi.org/10.12989/ACD.2016.1.1.087

63. Devabalaji, K.R., Yuvaraj, T., Ravi, K.: An efficient method for solving the optimal sitting and sizing problem of capacitor banks based on cuckoo search algorithm. Ain Shams Eng. J. **9**(4), 589–597 (2018). https://doi.org/10.1016/j.asej.2016.04.005https://doi.org/10.1016/j.asej.2016.04.005

64. García, J., Altimiras, F., Peña, A., Astorga, G., Peredo, O.: A binary cuckoo search big data algorithm applied to large-scale crew scheduling problems. Complexity **2018**, 8395193 (2018). https://doi.org/10.1155/2018/8395193https://doi.org/10.1155/2018/8395193

65. Cristin, R., Kumar, B.S., Priya, C., Karthick, K.: Deep neural network based rider-cuckoo search algorithm for plant disease detection. Artif. Intell. Rev. (2020). https://doi.org/10.1007/s10462-020-09813-https://doi.org/10.1007/s10462-020-09813-w
66. Abdualrhman, M.A.A., Padma. M.C.: CS-IBC: cuckoo search based incremental binary classifier for data streams. J. King Saud Univ. Comput. Inf. Sci.**31**(3), 367–377 (2019). https://doi.org/10.1016/j.jksuci.2017.05.008
67. Soneji, H., Sanghvi, R.C.: Towards the improvement of cuckoo search algorithm. In: 2012 World Congress on Information and Communication Technologies, Oct 2012, pp. 878–883. https://doi.org/10.1109/WICT.2012.6409199

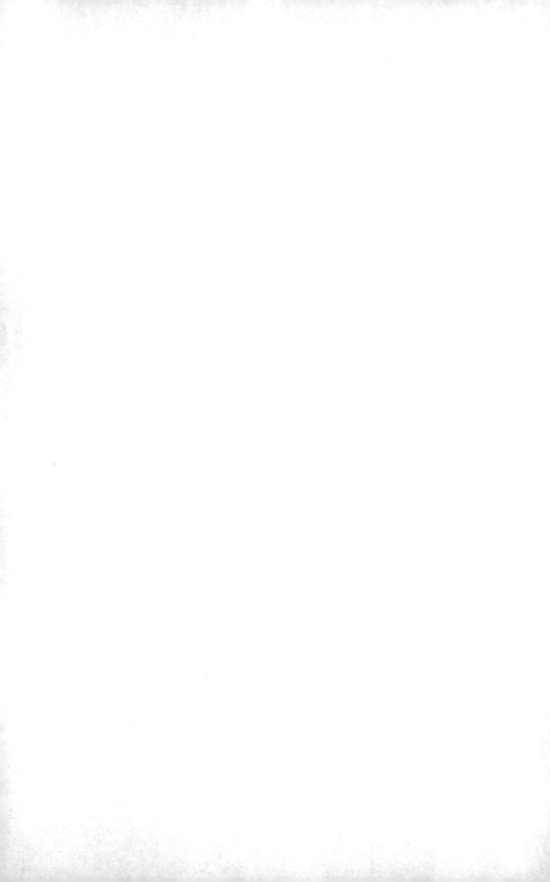

Routing Protocols for Internet of Vehicles: A Review

Farhana Ajaz, Mohd. Naseem, Gulfam Ahamad, Qamar Rayees Khan, Sparsh Sharma, and Ehtesham Abbasi

Abstract As the rapid invention and innovation has been performed in the automobile sectors, the modern vehicles are supposed to perform communication through heterogeneous technologies. In this process, the modern vehicles should be able to commutate tremendous amount of data and information within their neighborhood. To incorporate these requirements of modern vehicles, the conventional VANET are emerging to the Internet of Vehicles (IoV). In this chapter, we intend to contribute in review of routing protocols of the IoV. We will classify different type of routing protocols based on different parameters (information based, topology based, position based, delay based, target network). We will also discuss the challenges of routing protocols and future direction. This chapter ought to guide and motivate researchers of IoV to develop efficient routing protocols.

Keywords Broadcast · Multicast · Unicast · Routing · Internet of vehicles

1 Introduction

In VANET, all the autonomous vehicles are connected in an adhoc network in which each vehicle serves as node, and the adhoc network in this particular coverage area is called VANET. The VANET is especially adapted in autonomous vehicles where a vehicle can have breaking controls or can change lanes, turning, etc. Nowadays,

F. Ajaz · Mohd. Naseem (✉) · G. Ahamad · Q. R. Khan
Department of Computer Sciences, Baba Ghulam Shah Badshah University, Rajouri, Jammu & Kashmir 185234, India
e-mail: mohdnaseemshakeel@gmail.com

S. Sharma
Department of Computer Engineering, College of Engineering and Technology, Baba Ghulam Shah Badshah University, Rajouri, Jammu & Kashmir 185234, India

E. Abbasi
Green Economics Institute, Reading, UK

Sustainable Urban Development, Kellogg College University of Oxford, Oxford, UK

© The Author(s), under exclusive license to Springer Nature Singapore Pte Ltd. 2021   95
H. Malik et al. (eds.), *AI and Machine Learning Paradigms for Health Monitoring System*, Studies in Big Data 86,
https://doi.org/10.1007/978-981-33-4412-9_5

transportation has extended in limits as the quantity of individuals that use these vehicles keep on growing. The recent report has shown a tremendous hike in the number of vehicles worldwide which is marginally greater than 1000 million [1] and assumed to reach 2000 million by the year 2035 [2]. Every year, there are approximately 8 million road accidents. 1.2 million people die because of these accidents, and more than 70 lakh people get injuries. Fatalities and traffic congestion occur because of the hike in quantity of the vehicles. As vehicles increase, a need for management of these vehicles arises for avoiding accidents and road menace. So, IoV came into existence. IoV is a moving network made up of Internet of Things (IoT)-enabled vehicles using modern electronics and integrated information. As shown in Fig. 1, IoV keeps all the smart vehicles connected where each vehicle serves as a node. The vehicle could be sensor platform, collecting data (information) from driver, utilizing it for secure route (navigation), controlling pollution, managing the traffic. Using IoV, drivers can find out the traffic plans of the road and can fix their driving routes accordingly, thus avoiding traffic jams and accidents. Electronics used in IoV include sensors, GPS, entertainment system, brakes, and throttles. Internet of vehicles is an advancement of vehicle-to-vehicle (V2V) communication. The biggest challenge in IoV is to store and process big data. Cloud computing and mobile cloud play an important role in handling big data [3–5].

The rest of the chapter is systematized as follow. General characteristics of IoV are discussed in Sect. 2, whereas Sect. 3 overviews the challenges of IoV. Section 4

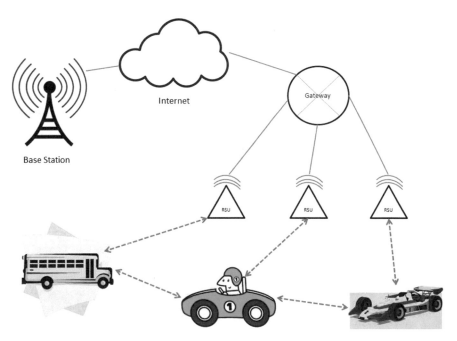

Fig. 1 Typical example of internet of vehicles

presents state-of-the-art of routing protocols. Lastly, in Sect. 5, conclusions are drawn.

2 Characteristics

Some of the characteristics of IoV are as follows:

- **Information collection**: The data is gathered by making use of various sensors (pollution checking sensors, cameras, road sensors, etc.) that gives drivers sufficient information to react to the environment changes in an adequate and efficient way [6].
- **Highly mobile**: Vehicular networks have highly mobile nodes, related to speed of cars, so a node can add and abscond in a small span of time, thus leads to repeated change in topology [6].
- **Type of information transported**: The messages are transported according to the degree of involvement in the triggered event. The message can be sent from a single initiator to a single target (unicasting) or sending messages from a single initiator to a particular cluster by using multiple hop communication (multicasting) or vehicles can also send messages to all other vehicles by broadcasting [7].
- **Handling big data**: Huge amount of data is generated because large numbers of vehicles are connected, so IoV uses cloud computing for processing and storing of the big data.
- **Internet facility**: IoV has a unique characteristic of having access to Internet. The vehicles that are connected can take benefit from this huge network [6].

3 Challenges

There are lots of challenges while proposing anything in IoV. Some of the challenges are as follows:

- Economical techniques must be used by the researchers such as IP addressing over digital maps [6].
- Future research of the researchers must focus on the highway and rural areas.
- Design the routing protocols that are scalable.
- Routing protocols must consider the bandwidth constraints [7, 8].
- Researchers must consider the density of network that is inadequately balanced [9].
- Using efficient means to truncate and trim a network's fragmentation problem [6].

4 Routing Protocols

Design of the efficient routing protocol is biggest challenge in IoV. In literature, several routing protocols have been proposed. These routing protocols can be categorized according to Fig. 2.

4.1 Information-Based Routing Protocol

It distributes the routing information by either sending the smaller incremental updates or sending the entire dumps infrequently.

4.2 Topology-Based Routing Protocol

In this category, some of the routing protocols are as follows:

4.2.1 DSDV

It depends on Bellman Ford calculation. DSDV uses table-driven routing. In routing table, all entries have sequence number; these sequence numbers are even in presence of link, odd otherwise. It uses sequence number in routing tables for loop freeness. A node will update its table if it receives its updated route to the destination. The information of routing is disseminated between nodes by sending tinier incremental updates more repeatedly and sending full dumps infrequently [10].

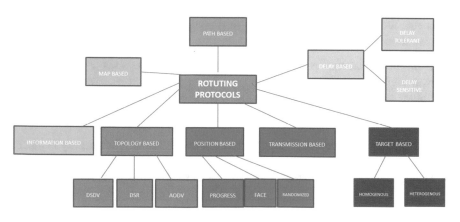

Fig. 2 Routing protocols in IoV

4.2.2 DSR

It is type of protocol that follows reactive routing. The first phase is route discovery in which node discovers route by producing a RREQ message that is overflowed in network. As RREQ message propagates through the network, packet header of RREQ which has list of the hops is added incrementally to packet header of RREQ. Once the RREQ reaches destination, RREP is directed back along inverse path. Source node will cache (store) route to destination. In future, if source wants to send packet to the same destination, it will get route from the cache. If any link is broken, information is broadcasted to make them update their cached route. RERR message is sent to transmitting node and process repeats. Contrast to AODV, DSR is the form in which how the information about the route is kept. Within AODV, the route information is accumulated in the middling nodes, while route information of DSR is accumulated in source and in header of the transferred packets [11].

4.2.3 AODV

It is a reactive routing protocol where on demand routes are formed as and when required. Route discovery in DSR and AODV is same. Until the connection is required, the network remains silent. Once a node wants to search a route to some target, it broadcasts route request message (RREQ) that other nodes receive it, progresses it, and keeps track of node from where they got it. When the target node comes across the RREQ, it responds in a way that it sends the RREP packet to the requesting node through a temporary (path) route. Source then starts using the path. If there is a failure in the link, route error packet (RERR) is sent back to the transmitting node. One of main disadvantages of DSR is that routing information gets stored in header of data packet which is to be transmitted. If the network size grows, the length of the route path also increases, and thus, the data packet's header increases, so most of the bandwidth will be consumed by the route path. It is hence not the efficient utilization of network bandwidth. AODV is reactive, and it does not require routing table. So, additional traffic is not required for managing routing tables, but it takes more time for establishing routes as compared to DSDV [12].

4.3 Position-Based Routing Protocol

Another approach of routing is position based that makes use of the location of the node to find next hop. This is called geo-routing also. One the most reliable routing protocol for vehicular networks is position-based routing protocol (PBR), it is because of the actuality that nodes (vehicles) can get the information about the position from onboard GPS receivers and obtain the information of the road layout from the on boarded digital map. This position-based routing (PBR) eliminates some of limitation of the topology-based protocols such as maintaining routes. One of the most familiar techniques that exploit location information for routing packets is known as greedy approach [13–16].

Using this approach, the neighboring node which is nearest to target node is eligible for advancing the data packet into network. Geographic protocols are divided into three types of classes. First is face-based. Second is progress-based, and the third is randomized-based.

4.3.1 Progress-Based

In this protocol, packet is forwarded to node that is making most progress toward the destination by the node that is currently holding the packet.

4.3.2 Randomized-Based Approach

The node that currently holds the data packet sends it by randomly choosing the next node or by using probability of distribution from a set of the candidate nodes [6].

4.3.3 Face-Based

Face-based approach makes use of the algorithm which is known as face [13], and it forwards the packets that are between the faces and always guarantee packet delivery in 2D network. In three-dimensional (3D) space, geographical routing is very difficult than the routing of two-dimensional (2D) topologies. The approach that is known as greedy forwarding in 3D reaches more local minima than in case of 2D. More ever many 2D position-based routing protocols cannot be extended to 3D. Durocher et al. stress on impossibility of the routing protocols to assure delivery in the 3D adhoc networks [14].

4.3.4 Greedy Perimeter Stateless Routing (GPSR)

It is given by H. T. Kung and Brad Karp, and it makes uses of the position of the neighboring nodes, position of the target node, and its current position for making decisions about forwarding the packets. It is effective protocol for mobile wireless networks. It makes the packet forwarding decisions by exploiting the position of the nodes. It makes use of the greedy forwarding nodes that are making most progress toward the destination [13].

4.3.5 Greedy Perimeter Coordinator Routing (GPCR)

GPCR is proposed by Christian Lochert et al. Main goal of this protocol is improving the performance of GPSR. There are two parts in GPCR, the first is restricted greedy forwarding procedure and the second is repairing strategy. It is completely based on junctions and real-world street topology. In order to determine the next hop, all the packets are first forwarded to a junction node. Local maximum problem cannot be completely solved by this protocol in a way that while forwarding packet, it may arrive at a situation where its distance to the target is closer than neighbor's distance to the target [14].

4.3.6 Intersection-Based Geographic Routing Protocol IGRP

This protocol was given for solving QOS problems in VANETs in non-rural or metropolitan scenarios [15]. Genetic algorithm is used to identify best solutions in order to satisfy the constraints of QOS on the performance metrics of backbone building routes established on adjacent and intermediate intersections of road toward Internet gateway.

4.4 Delay Routing Protocols

DRP is categorized into delay-sensitive protocol and delay-Tolerant protocol.

4.4.1 Delay-Sensitive Protocol

They cannot tolerate delay and requires transmitting the road's information rapidly. Delay-sensitive protocols need exchange of the packets as soon as possible. DSP should reduce probability of bottleneck of the routing packets and maintain low latency with high delivery ratio [16].

4.4.2 Delay-Tolerant Protocol

DTP use a carry forward mechanism. They can manage the failures during carry forward mechanism [17]. It deals with cases of occasional connectivity problems. Their representative is geospray. It improves the probability of delivering packets and also reduces the delay in delivering packets. One of the limitations of DTN routing protocol is that it limits the network transmission while achieving high degree of network coverage.

4.5   Target Network Routing Protocols

Under this category, there are two types of networks: homogeneous network and heterogeneous network.

4.5.1   Homogeneous Network

It refers to type of access technology which a vehicle could use. The classical routing protocol in VANETs targets on transmitting the packet over short distances using wireless technologies, like "Wireless Access in Vehicular Environment" [18, 19].

4.5.2   Heterogeneous Network

This divergent nature of IoV includes various radio access technologies [18]. IoV is more complex than VANET's because IoV comprises of various distinct radio access technologies; hence, it forms heterogeneous network. However, one of the big problems that occur in heterogeneous networks including IoV's is handoff [20].

4.6   Path-Based Routing

Zhao and Cao have presented the vehicle-assisted data delivery protocol (VADD). VADD uses carry forward mechanism in order to route the data from sender to the target. The problem of frequent disconnections and high mobility are dealt using this protocol. VADD is not that efficient when dealing with sparsely connected networks. VADD minimizes delay by choosing the highly dense path where the density of network is high. VADD calculates best path that has lowest data delivery delay [21].

5   Conclusion

IoV is mainly concerned with communicating information among roadside units, humans, and vehicles. As the number of vehicles increase, a need for management of these vehicles arises for avoiding accidents and road menace. So, IoV came into existence. IoV is the communication between vehicles over a network. The vehicle could be sensor platform, collecting data (information) from driver and utilizing it for safe route, controlling pollution, and managing the traffic. In this chapter, we have analyzed characteristics and challenges of IoV. In addition to this, we have also categorized the different types of routing protocols. Under each category, various routing protocols have been discussed in detail.

References

1. Organisation Internationale des Constructeurs d'Automobiles (OICA): Number of Passenger Cars and Commercial Vehicles in Use Worldwide from 2006 to 2014 in (1,000 Units) (2014)
2. Voelcker J: It's Official: We Now Have One Billion Vehicles on the Planet, Aug 2011
3. Dhaliwal, J.K., Naseem, M., Lawaye, A.A., Abbasi, E.H.: Fibonacci Series Based Virtual Machine Selection for Load Balancing in Cloud Computing
4. Mahto, T., et al.: Traffic signal control to optimize run time for energy saving: a smart city paradigm. In: Springer Nature Book: Metaheuristic and Evolutionary Computation: Algorithms and Applications. Studies in Computational Intelligence (2020). https://doi.org/10.1007/978-981-15-7571-6_21.
5. Iqbal, A., et al.: Big-data analytics based energy analysis and monitoring for multi-story hospital buildings: case study. In: Springer Nature Book: Soft Computing in Condition Monitoring and Diagnostics of Electrical and Mechanical Systems, pp. 325–343 (2019). https://doi.org/10.1007/978-981-15-1532-3_14
6. Cheng, J.J., et al.:Routing in internet of vehicles: a review. IEEE Trans. Intell. Transp. Syst. **16**(5), 2339–2352 (2015)
7. Naseem, M., Kumar, C.: Congestion-aware Fibonacci sequence based multipath load balancing routing protocol for MANETs. Wireless Pers. Commun. **84**(4), 2955–2974 (2015)
8. Naseem, M., Kumar, C.:Distributed bandwidth guarantee using multi-path routing protocol in mobile ad hoc network. In: 2014 International Conference on Science Engineering and Management Research (ICSEMR). IEEE (2014)
9. Naseem, M., Kumar, C.: Queue-based multiple path load balancing routing protocol for MANETs. Int. J. Commun. Syst. **30**(6), e3141 (2017a)
10. Naseem, M., Kumar, C.:EDSDV: Efficient DSDV routing protocol for MANET. In: 2013 IEEE International Conference on Computational Intelligence and Computing Research. IEEE (2013)
11. Johnson, D.B., Maltz, D.A., Broch, J.: DSR: the dynamic source routing protocol for multi-hop wireless ad hoc networks. Ad Hoc Netw. **5**(1), 139–172 (2001)
12. Perkins, C.E., Royer, E.M.:Ad-hoc on-demand distance vector routing. In: Proceedings WMCSA'99. Second IEEE Workshop on Mobile Computing Systems and Applications. IEEE (1999)
13. Karp, B., Kung, H.T.: GPSR: greedy perimeter stateless routing for wireless networks. In: Proceedings of the 6th Annual International Conference on Mobile Computing and Networking, New York, NY, USA, pp. 243–254 (2000)
14. Contreras-Castillo, J., Zeadally, S., Guerrero-Ibañez, J.A.:Internet of vehicles: architecture, protocols, and security. IEEE Internet Things J **5**(5), 3701–3709 (2017)
15. Maihofer, C.: A survey of geocast routing protocols. IEEE Commun. Surv. Tutorials **6**(2), 32–42, 2nd Quart. (2004)
16. Bose, P., Morin, P., Stojmenovic, I., Urrutia, J.: Routing with guaranteed delivery in ad hoc wireless networks. In: Proceedings of the ACM DIAL M Workshop, pp. 48–55 (1999)
17. Naseem, M., Kumar, C.: QSLB: queue size based single path load balancing routing protocol for MANETs. Int. J. Ad Hoc Ubiquitous Comput. **24**(1–2), 90–100 (2017b)
18. Lochert, C., et al.: A routing strategy for vehicular ad hoc networks in city environments. In: Proceedings of the IEEE Intelligent Vehicles Symposium, pp. 156–161 (2003)
19. Sharma, S., Kaul, A.: A survey on intrusion detection systems and honeypot based proactive security mechanisms in VANETs and VANET cloud. Veh. Commun. **12**, 138–164 (2018)
20. Sharma, S., Kaul, A.: VANETs cloud: architecture, applications, challenges, and issues.Arch. Comput. Methods Eng. 1–22
21. Xiang, Y., Liu, Z., Liu, R., Sun, W., Wang, W.: GeoSVR: a map-based stateless VANET routing. Ad Hoc Netw. **11**(7), 2125–2135 (2013)

Introduction to Particle Swarm Optimization and Its Paradigms: A Bibliographic Survey

Mohd Shariq Khan, Wahid Ali, Muhammad Abdul Qyyum, Khursheed B. Ansari, and Moonyong Lee

Abstract Particle swarm optimization (PSO) belongs to evolutionary computation algorithms that are inspired by the swarming motion of living organisms. PSO has a humble beginning where it was only able to solve the single-objective continuous optimization problems. Since then through numerous refinements and contribution voiding weakness and combining elements of other methods proposing modifications, hybridizations, velocity update rules, and population topologies, PSO has matured with immense scope of real-world applications. Though swarm stagnation and dynamic environment are still identified as significant challenges nevertheless, continued interest in PSO shows no sign of slowing. More than ten thousand contributions in the IEEE database alone after 25 years of the first appearance is a strong indicator that the mentioned challenges will come to pass. This chapter enlists and discusses in brief the major developments in PSO along with the area of successful application in a concise form.

Keywords Particle swarm optimization · Stochastic · Swarm movement · Single multi-objective · Continuous · Discrete

M. S. Khan (✉)
Department of Chemical Engineering, Dhofar University, Salalah 211, Oman
e-mail: mskhan@du.edu.om

W. Ali
Department of Chemical Engineering Technology, College of Applied Industrial Technology (CAIT), Jazan University, Jazan 45971, Kingdom of Saudi Arabia
e-mail: wzali@jazanu.edu.sa

M. A. Qyyum · M. Lee
School of Chemical Engineering, Yeungnam University, Gyeongsan 712-749, Republic of Korea
e-mail: maqyyum@yu.ac.kr

M. Lee
e-mail: mynlee@ynu.ac.kr

K. B. Ansari
Department of Chemical Engineering, Zakir Husain College of Engineering and Technology, Aligarh Muslim University, 202001 Aligarh, India
e-mail: ansarikh5@gmail.com

© The Author(s), under exclusive license to Springer Nature Singapore Pte Ltd. 2021   105
H. Malik et al. (eds.), *AI and Machine Learning Paradigms for Health Monitoring System*, Studies in Big Data 86,
https://doi.org/10.1007/978-981-33-4412-9_6

1   Introduction

Optimization is an important stage in any design where the best possible solution relative to a given set of prioritized criteria is achieved. These criteria comprise several maximizing factors like strength, reliability, productivity, longevity, efficiency, and utilization [1] or minimization factors such as losses, manpower, cost, waste, time consumed, and material/resources used. Now, based on the number of variables involved and problem complexity, two main strategies, deterministic and stochastic, were evolved with time to solve the optimization problems [2]. If the problem is untractable NP-hard, deterministic approaches may early converge to any sub-optimal solution [3] besides being CPU-intensive, and their dependence on a good starting point is also a challenge. Stochastic approaches evolved to overcome those challenges by sampling the search space without exploring it exhaustively and show robustness in convergence and fully exploit increasingly available parallel computing power to navigate highly nonlinear problems with a multitude of available variables [4]. The working structure of the PSO is represented in Fig. 1 [5–7].

Evolutionary computation (EC) belongs to stochastic approach that is inspired by the biological evolution [8]. There are many variants of EC and the few that find most applications are genetic algorithms (GA) [9], differential evolution [10], ant colony optimization [11], and particle swarm optimization (PSO) [12]. Among these, GA [13–15] and PSO [16, 17] have been widely applied and researched, and it is safe to say that PSO was evolved to rectify the challenges faced in GA mainly many tuning

Particle velocity update $V_{i+1} = wV_i + c_1r_1(pBest_i - X_i) + c_2r_2(gBest_i - X_i)$
Particle position update $X_{i+1} = X_i + V_{i+1}$

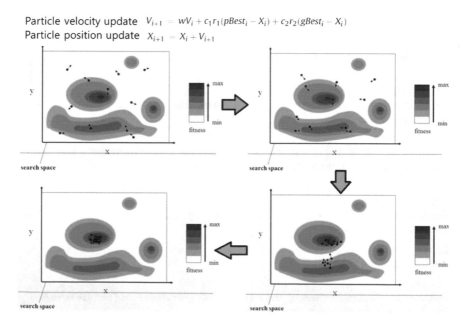

Fig. 1 Graphical representation of PSO

parameters and higher function evaluations and inherently discrete in handling design variables [18]. Better performance of PSO over GA in terms of function evaluation [19] and inherently continuous in terms of design variable handling is reported [18].

1.1 PSO Inspiration, Concept, and Major Developments

PSO was introduced by Kennedy and Eberhart in 1995 [12] and inspired by the social interaction in a flock of birds that bring the best for both flock and bird. The social behavior of a bird flock was studied and simulated to answer the flowing three questions:

- How a large population of birds (or organisms) gracefully flocking and changing directions suddenly, regrouping, and scattering without colliding with each other?
- Are there any benefits to this swarming behavior to the individual bird in a group?
- Is it possible for humans to display social behaviors similar to swarming like other organisms?

After asking these three fundamental questions about swarming behavior, Kennedy and Eberhart [12] concluded that the swarming birds can only keep in mind the inter-individual distances while keeping pace to avoid the collision. This makes individual bird behavior as a decentralized local process. The answer to the second question yields that the birds can profit from the discoveries of others and share their discoveries for instance food, evading predators, adjusting to the environment with the swarm. Thus, information sharing produces evolutionary advantages to the individual and the swarm. Humans show swarming behavior at a more abstract level where they adjust their attitudes to avoid confrontation and comply with societal standards. After learning, the swarming behavior of birds the Kennedy and Eberhart concluded that individuals in a population tend to gravitate from their current state toward their best found or the state that those with whom they are in contact found best. Since 1995, a lot of improvement has been made in PSO, and it is impossible to summarize all here; however, the major development related to PSO is enumerated in Table 1. IEEE database was explored to access the activity of PSO in conferences and journal publications, and the trends are illustrated in Fig. 2.

2 PSO Algorithm

PSO works by employing the swarming motion of a population of agents distributed randomly that spread across the search space of N dimensions (R^N). These dimensions comprise of real number every agent is described by a N component vector whose real number elements represent value or attributes. The agents swarm toward the global best and adapt by returning to previously successful regions.

Table 1 Major contributions on PSO: Thesis, books, and review

Authors	Publication
Ph.D. Thesis	
Changhe Li	Swarm optimization in stationary and dynamic environments [20]
Pedersen, M. E. H.	Tuning & simplifying heuristical optimization[21]
Bai, Q.	An analysis of particle swarm optimizers[22]
Schoeman, I. L.	Niching in particle swarm optimization[23]
Liang, J.	Novel PSO with hybrid, dynamic & adaptive neighborhood structures[24]
Helwig, S.	Particle swarms for constrained optimization[25]
Dasheng, L.	Multi-objective PSO: Algorithms and applications[26]
Omran, M. G.	PSO methods for pattern recognition and image processing[27]
Birattari, M.	The problem of tuning metaheuristics[28]
Schmit B. I.	Convergence analysis for particle swarm optimization [29]
Talukder, S.	Mathematical modeling and applications of particle swarm optimization [30]
Vis, J. K.	Particle swarm optimizer for finding robust optima [31]
Major Reviews & Books	
Kennedy et al.	Particle swarm optimization [12]
Parsopoulos et al.	Particle swarm optimization and intelligence: advances and applications [32]
Mikki et al.	Particle swarm optimization: A physics-based approach [33]
James Kennedy	Chapter 6, Swarm intelligence in handbook of nature-inspired and innovative computing: integrating classical models with emerging technologies [34]
Clerc, M.	Particle swarm optimization [35]
Poli, R.	Analysis of the publications on the applications of particle swarm optimization [36]
Poli et al.	Particle swarm optimization An overview [37]
Banks et al.	A review of particle swarm optimization. Part I: background and development [38]
Banks et al.	A review of particle swarm optimization. Part II: hybridisation, combinatorial, multicriteria and constrained optimization, and indicative applications [39]

There are three stages in the PSO algorithm (illustrated in Fig. 3) first is *swarm initialization* where a velocity vector is generated for each agent in search space of N dimensions (R^N) [18]. For swarming motion (or iterations), each agent matches the velocity of the neighbor. Randomness is added in the velocity of each agent to allow for exploratory behavior. In the second stage, *swarm updates* its current fitness by comparing its position to the global best position (G_{best}). This is possible only if each agent remembers its best-ever fitness (P_{best}) and exchanges this information

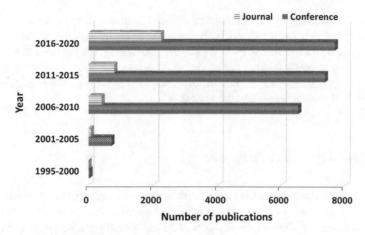

Fig. 2 PSO publication in the IEEE database till 2020

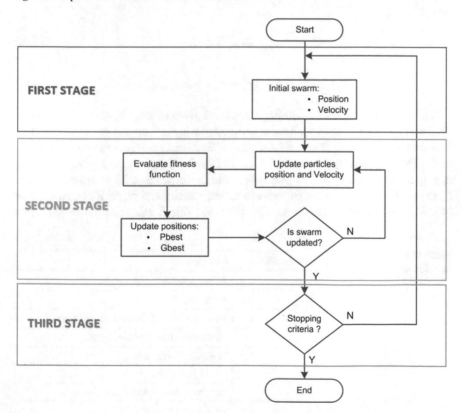

Fig. 3 Basic PSO algorithm

with other swarm members whereby everyone compares their position and adjust their velocities to converge toward the global best (G_{best}). In the second stage, two weighting factors to control local and global exploration were introduced by Shi and Eberhart [40] to better control the global exploration and local exploitation. In the third stage, agents check for the maximum change in best fitness, if it became smaller than specified, *swarm lands* on global best.

2.1 PSO Algorithm Structure

The basic PSO algorithm proposed by Kennedy and Eberhart [12] consists of two key properties position and velocity. Once the swarm of agents is initialized across the search space R^n, their randomly generated individual position ($x_0^i \in D$ in R^n for $i = 1, ..., p$.) and velocity are updated ($0 < v_0^i < v_0^{max}$ for $i = 1, ..., p$.) through Eqs. 1 and 2.

$$x_{k+1}^i = x_k^i + v_{k+1}^i \tag{1}$$

$$v_{k+1}^i = v_k^i + c_1 r_1 (p_k^i - x_k^i) + c_1 r_1 (p_k^g - x_k^i) \tag{2}$$

The description of the individual parameter is given in Table 2. After initialization, PSO evaluate the fitness of each agent and store the best ever agent position p_k^i and the best swarm position p_k^g. The last two terms of Eq. 2 represent two competing features of the PSO algorithm, i.e., the exploration of the local and whole region; hence, the choice of parameter c_1 and c_2 play a key role in the process. The parameter c_1 and c_2 are positive constants set by users to provide social and cognitive learning rates [40, 41] also known as acceleration coefficients [42]. Proper selection of the values

Table 2 PSO parameter descriptions

Parameters	Descriptions
x_k^i	Agent position
v_k^i	Agent velocity
p_k^i	Best remembered individual agent position
p_k^g	Best remembered swarm position
c_1	Cognitive parameter
c_2	Social parameter
r_1, r_2	Random number between 0 and 1
w	Inertia weight factor
$w^{(0)}$	Initial value of w
$w^{(t_{max})}$	Final value of w
C	Construction factor

of c_1 and c_2 have a substantial influence on the convergence success. The normal working range of c_1 is found to be between 1.5 and 2, while for c_2 is 2–2.5 [18]. The first term in Eq. 2 drives the rate of exploration, and one of the early modifications of PSO involves the introduction of an inertia weight factor w as given Eq. 3.

$$v_{k+1}^i = wv_k^i + c_1r_1(p_k^i - x_k^i) + c_1r_1(p_k^g - x_k^i) \tag{3}$$

This introduction of w gives satisfaction in the convergence where large values promote global exploration and smaller effectively evaluate the local region; Chatterje and Siarry [43] propose inertial value between $0 < w < 1$. The static value of the inertia factor w provides challenges when the search narrows down toward optimum. To overcome this challenge, gradually decreasing value of w as the optimization proceeds were proposed [44] given in Eq. 4

$$w^t = w^{(0)} - w^{(t_{max})} \frac{(t_{max} - t)}{t_{max}} + w^{(t_{max})} \tag{4}$$

Another method that modified the value of the inertia factor is based on the relative improvement in the fitness value that is approximate to the optimum value [16]. A higher value of inertia factor in the beginning also makes the agents' velocity fly past the potential solution; thus, a velocity clamping parameter was introduced. Constriction coefficient (C) (see Eq. 5) as a multiplier of velocity equation controls the nature of the exploration process, which depends on Φ, if $\Phi \geq 4$ and $k \in [0, 1]$, then Clerc and Kennedy [45] demonstrate guaranteed swarm converge.

$$C = \frac{2k}{|2 - \Phi - \sqrt{\Phi(\Phi - 4)}|} \tag{5}$$

The value of k control exploration for small k fast local convergence is achieved, and for large k, the search space is explored thoroughly. Consequently, the velocity (Eq. 3) is adjusted to incorporate the constriction factor as a special case of inertia weight variant as Eq. 6.

$$v_{k+1}^i = C[v_k^i + c_1r_1(p_k^i - x_k^i) + c_1r_1(p_k^g - x_k^i)] \tag{6}$$

2.2 Pseudocode

The pseudocode given by Kennedy and Eberhart [12] for real number version is given below:

```
set population size
for i =1 to i = max                        // initialize agents' positions and velocities, compute fitness
        for d =1 to dimensions
                x_{i,d} = Rnd(x_{min}, x_{max})
                v_{i,d} = Rnd(-v_{max}, v_{min})
next i
loop
        for i =1 to i = max                // compare best position of each agent with its best so far
                if G(x_i) > G(p_i) then    // G( ) evaluates fitness
                        for d =1 to dimensions
                                p_{i,d} = x_{i,d}    // p_{i,d} is best so far
                        next d
                end if
                g = j                      // g is index of best performer in the neighborhood
                for j = indices of neighbors
                        if G(p_i) > G(p_g) then g = j
                next j
                for d =1 to dimensions // compute velocity and new position
                        v_{k+1}^i = C[v_k^i + c_1 r_1(p_k^i − x_k^i) + c_1 r_1(p_k^g − x_k^i)]
                        v_k^i = (−v_{max} + v_{min})
                        x_{k+1}^i = x_k^i + v_k^i
                next d
        next i
stopping criterion
end
```

Several efforts were made to share the PSO codes in different programming languages and disseminate the development related to different variants of PSO, in terms of toolboxes and visualization materials. These efforts were made public through dedicated public Web sites; their details are given in Table 3.

3   PSO Variants, Hybrids, and Modifications

Since its first occurrence, numerous PSO variants appeared in the literature addressing different aspects of PSO often refining and voiding weakness and combining elements of other methods proposing modifications, hybridizations, velocity update rules, population topologies, etc., and these variants are keep growing rapidly. Berthold [29] classifies PSO variants based on neighborhood topologies, constraints and bound handling, and movement equation. Macro [46] classify PSO variants based on neighborhood topologies, enhanced diversity, velocity update rules,

Table 3 Public materials related to PSO

Web site	Source URL
Scholarpedia	www.scholarpedia.org/article/Particle_swarm_optimization
Swarmintelligence	www.swarmintelligence.org/index.php
MathWorks	www.mathworks.com/matlabcentral/fileexchange/7506-particle-swarm-optimization-toolbox
PSO Toolbox	psotoolbox.sourceforge.net/
Scilab	https://forge.scilab.org/index.php/p/pso-toolbox/
swMATH	https://cran.r-project.org/web/packages/hydroPSO/index.html
Softwareheritage	https://archive.softwareheritage.org/browse/origin/?origin_url=https://github.com/cran/hydroPSO
PSO Resources	https://bee22.com/resources/

components using other approaches, and discrete optimization problems. Dorigo et al. [47] described discrete PSO, constriction coefficient, bare-bone PSO, and fully informed PSO as some of the "most important developments" in PSO variants. Selleri et al., [48] proposed three PSO variants by introducing more than one swarm and keeping those swarms apart from each other using social distancing rules and making best performing swarm not repelled by other swarms. Finding all the variants of PSO and writing about them is a monumental work, so this section describes in brief two main variants of PSO in Sects. 3.1 and 3.2. Table 4 compiles the breakthroughs in PSO variants with a short comment.

3.1 Barebones PSO

After proposing the PSO first time in 1995 [44], Kennedy revised the PSO to a new variant called barebones PSO (bbPSO) [49] in 2003. This modification was made after analyzing the converge characteristic of original PSO in which each particle only has position vector bbPSO that eliminates the need for velocity vector, and thus the inertial, social, and cognitive parameters are no longer needed. In bbPSO, new position is updated by the Gaussian sampling given by Eq. 7

$$x_{k+1}^i = N\left(\frac{g_{best} + p_{best_i}}{2}, \left| g_{best} - p_{best_i} \right|\right) \tag{7}$$

where N indicates a Gaussian distribution with mean as $\frac{(g_{best} + p_{best_i})}{2}$ and the standard deviation $\left| g_{best} - p_{best_i} \right|$.

Table 4 Breakthrough in PSO variants

PSO variant	Unique characteristic
BBMOPSO	Bare-bone multi-objective PSO [42]
Meta PSO	Varied from PSO in using more than a single swarm [48]
Modified Meta PSO	Keeping meta PSO swarm apart from each other to "widening global search" [48]
SMMPSO	Best performing swarm in modified meta PSO not repelled by other swarms [48]
bbPSO	Barebone PSO strips traditional features of the PSO [49]
BPSO	Binary PSO, Maximum likelihood estimate MLE-BPSO, entropic PSO [50]
DPSO	Discrete PSO: solve the problem associated with discrete-valued space [50]
QPSO	Quantum PSO, quadratic programming & Gaussian chaotic mutation operators [51]
hydoPSO	PSO variant with focus on optimizing environmental models [52, 53]
ScPSO	Scout PSO: Scout bee phase added to the end of PSO eliminating regeneration[54]
C-PSO	Clubs-PSO: Socializing clubs for agents to learn and increase convergence [55]
FPSO	Fuzzy PSO: Charisma is defined for more than one agent in each neighborhood [56]
TVPSO	PSO with time-varying acceleration coefficients (TVAC) [57]
OPSO	Opposition PSO: Dynamic Cauchy mutation on the best particle to fast convergence [58]
PSOAG	Age group PSO: Population diversity through separating particles on their age group [59]
APSO	Adaptive PSO: Inactive particles taken off to maintain swarm social attribution [60]
AugPSO	Augmented PSO: Increase convergence & diversity by boundary-shifting agents [61]
PSO-GA	Genetic-PSO: Introduce dying probability for the agents [62]
ANN-GA-PSO	Artificial neural-network optimization using a hybrid genetic algorithm and PSO [63]
MOPSO	Multi-objective PSO: Integrating elements of ant colony and PSO [64]
PSO-SA	Simulated annealing PSO used for dynamics power flow problems [65]
BPSO	Biogeography-based PSO: Uses the geographical distribution of biological organisms [66]
IMPSO-PS	Improved multi-objective PSO preferential strategy [67]

(continued)

Table 4 (continued)

PSO variant	Unique characteristic
PF-PSO	Particle filter PSO: Particle degeneracy improved by resampling operation [68]
TBSLB-PSO	Task-based load balancing PSO for overloaded virtual machine [69]
ELPSO	Enhanced leader PSO: Diversity enhancing mechanism [70]
UPSO	Unified PSO, combine global, and local search [71]
FIPSO	Fully Informed PSO, modified velocity [72]
CLPSO	Comprehensive learning PSO [73]
NSPSO	Neighbors of particles search PSO [74]
CPSO	Cooperative PSO: Employ multiple swarms to optimize different components [75]

3.2 Binary PSO

PSO was initially developed in 1995 for continuous problems and cannot handle discrete problems; hence, to answer the problem associated with discrete-valued space, Kennedy and Eberhart in the year 1997 proposed a discrete binary version of PSO [50], where each particle represents its position through binary values of 0 or 1. Binary PSO (BPSO) mainly differs from the original continuous PSO version in defining velocities in terms of probabilities that restrict the velocity to the range of [0,1]. The normalized velocity function in BPSO is a sigmoid function defined using Eq. 8, and the new position of the particle is obtained using Eq. 9. Parameters and memory were found to be the main problems associated with BPSO.

$$v'_{ij}(k) = \text{sig}(v_{ij}(t)) = \frac{1}{1 + e^{-v_{ij}(t)}} \tag{8}$$

$$x_{ij}(k+1) = \begin{cases} 1 & \text{if } r_{ij} < \text{sig}(v_{ij}(k+1)) \\ 0 & \text{otherwise} \end{cases} \tag{9}$$

4 PSO Applications

PSO has been effectively deployed to address a wide range of applications and surprisingly show promise where other methods yield unsatisfactory results. So far, PSO is virtually applied to every discipline that deals with optimization problems. If a problem is converted to optimization one, PSO through its numerable variants can be applied to solve it. Its first application was reported along with the algorithm itself and was in the field of neural-network training [12]. Initially, PSO was only able to solve single-objective unconstrained problems, but it was evolved to solve constrained multi-objective problems and the problems with dynamically changing landscape as well. Few selected areas where PSO has been successfully applied ranging from pattern recognition, multi-objective optimization, system design, signal processing, decision making, biological system modeling, classification, robotics, games, and many more.

Zhang et al. [42] through their excellent annotated review paper classified the applications of PSO in ten different working areas. They also identified symbolic regression, floor planning, supply chain management, weapon targets as the potential areas where PSO if applied can show promising results. Poli et al. [36] in the year 2008 through 650 publications identified 23 application areas, and since then, the applications of PSO have seen exponential growth (see Fig. 2), and in the IEEE database alone, there are more than 8000 conferences and 2000+ journal papers addressing mostly PSO applications. It is virtually impossible to discuss even in brief all the applications of PSO; thus through Table 5 (selected and not exhaustive, application area list), authors would like to give an impression about PSO penetration, its multifaceted working areas, and success of PSO in solving real-world problems.

5   Concluding Remarks

This chapter introduces the reader to the major developments related to PSO and its successful applications area provides useful links (Table 3) for accessing the open-source PSO toolboxes. Further the chapter discusses the originally proposed PSO and how through numerous contributions and refinements both in continuous and discrete space, PSO has matured with immense scope of real-world applications ranging from neural-network training (first application), to medicine, to finance and economics, to communication and operations, to distribution networks, to graphic and visualization, to military and security, and the list can go on. The reason for such a diverse list of the application lies not only in the simplicity and ease of implementation but also the availability of the algorithm and its various hybrids in the public domain (see Table 3), whereby helping PSO reaching a wider audience even a non-technical background person can use PSO as a building block to mix with any tools they are familiar with and apply PSO through many open-source toolboxes.

Initially, PSO was only able to solve single-objective unconstrained problems, but it was evolved to solve constrained multi-objective problems and problems with dynamically changing landscape, parallel implementation further increased PSO acceptance. Since its first occurrence, many variants of PSO appeared in the literature addressing different aspects of PSO often refining and voiding weakness and combining elements of other methods proposing modifications, hybridizations, velocity update rules, population topologies, etc., and these variants keep growing rapidly. Despite the ongoing activity, swarm stagnation and dynamic environments are still identified as significant challenges for future development. PSO applications have seen nearly exponential growth in the last decade with many applications still appearing it seems to show no sign of slowing down in the year 2020.

Table 5 Selected applications areas of PSO

Application area	References
Neural-network training	[12, 56]
System design	[76, 77]
Multi-objective optimization	[26, 26]
Pattern recognition	[27, 78]
Signal processing	[60, 79]
Decision making	[80, 81]
Classification	[13, 82, 83]
Robotics	[84, 85]
Biological system modeling	[54, 86]
Games	[87, 88]
Control	[89–91]
Communication & operations	[42, 92, 93]
Civil engineering	[94–96]
Electrical	[65, 90]
Mechanical	[57, 97, 98]
Chemical	[99, 100]
Medicine	[101–103]
Finance and economics	[104, 105]
Combinatorial optimization	[106, 107]
Distribution networks	[108, 109]
Graphics and visualization	[110, 111]
Fuzzy and neuro-fuzzy	[14, 56, 64]
Image and video analysis	[112, 113]
Scheduling	[114, 115]
Prediction and forecasting	[116, 117]
Fault diagnosis	[118, 119]
Military and security	[120, 121]
Signal processing	[101, 122]
Power system/generation	[123–125]
LNG plant	[126, 127]

References

1. Kelley, T.: Optimization, an Important Stage of Engineering Design. Publications (2010). https://digitalcommons.usu.edu/ncete_publications/32/
2. Wets, R.J.-B.: On the Relation between Stochastic and Deterministic Optimization (1975). https://doi.org/10.1007/978-3-642-46317-4_26
3. Cavazzuti, M.: Optimization Methods. Springer Berlin Heidelberg, Berlin, Heidelberg (2013). https://doi.org/10.1007/978-3-642-31187-1
4. Andradóttir, S.: A global search method for discrete stochastic optimization. SIAM J. Optim. (1996). https://doi.org/10.1137/0806027
5. Iqbal, A., et al.: Metaheurestic algorithm based hybrid model for identification of building sale prices. In: Springer Nature Book: Metaheuristic and Evolutionary Computation: Algorithms and Applications. Studies in Computational Intelligence (2020). https://doi.org/10.1007/978-981-15-7571-6_32
6. Faiz Minai, A., et al.: Metaheuristics paradigms for renewable energy systems: advances in optimization algorithms. In: Springer Nature Book: Metaheuristic and Evolutionary Computation: Algorithms and Applications. Studies in Computational Intelligence (2020). https://doi.org/10.1007/978-981-15-7571-6_2
7. Yadav, A.K., et al.:Optimization of tilt angle for intercepting maximum solar radiation for power generation. In: Springer Nature Book: Optimization of Power System Problems (Methods, Algorithms and MATLAB Codes), pp. 203–232 (2020). https://doi.org/10.1007/978-3-030-34050-6_9
8. Bäck, T., Fogel, D.B., Michalewicz, Z.: Handbook of Evolutionary Computation. IOP Publishing Ltd (1997). https://stacks.iop.org/0750308958
9. Whitley, D.: A genetic algorithm tutorial. Stat. Comput.**4**(2) (1994). https://doi.org/10.1007/BF00175354
10. Price, K.V.: Differential Evolution. Intell. Syst. Ref. Libr. (2013). https://doi.org/10.1007/978-3-642-30504-7_8
11. Dorigo, M., Socha, K.: Handbook of Approximation Algorithms and Metaheuristics. Chapman and Hall/CRC (2007). https://www.taylorfrancis.com/books/9781420010749
12. Kennedy, J., Eberhart, R.: Particle swarm optimization. In: Proceedings of ICNN'95—International Conference on Neural Networks, vol. 4, pp. 1942–1948 (1995). https://doi.org/10.1109/ICNN.1995.488968
13. Zhu, C., Zhang, J., Liu, Y., Ma, D., Li, M., Xiang, B.: Comparison of GA-BP and PSO-BP neural network models with initial BP model for rainfall-induced landslides risk assessment in regional scale: a case study in Sichuan, China. Nat. Hazards **100**(1), 173–204 (2020). https://doi.org/10.1007/s11069-019-03806-x
14. Azad, A., et al.: Novel approaches for air temperature prediction: a comparison of four hybrid evolutionary fuzzy models. Meteorol. Appl. (2019). https://doi.org/10.1002/met.1817
15. Kramer, O.: Genetic Algorithm Essentials (2017). https://doi.org/10.1007/978-3-319-52156-5
16. Eberhart, Shi, Y.: Particle swarm optimization: developments, applications and resources. In: Proceedings of the 2001 Congress on Evolutionary Computation (IEEE Cat. No.01TH8546), vol. 1, pp. 81–86 (2001. https://doi.org/10.1109/CEC.2001.934374
17. AlRashidi, M.R., El-Hawary, M.E.: A survey of particle swarm optimization applications in electric power systems. IEEE Trans. Evol. Comput. **13**(4), 913–918 (2008). https://doi.org/10.1109/TEVC.2006.880326
18. Hassan, R.: Particle swarm optimization: method and applications. Present. https://ocw.mit.edu (2004). https://dspace.mit.edu/bitstream/handle/1721.1/68163/16-888-spring-2004/contents/lecture-notes/l13_msdo_pso.pdf
19. Ou, O., Lin, W.: Comparison between PSO and GA for parameters optimization of PID controller. In: 2006 International Conference on Mechatronics and Automation, pp. 2471–2475 (2006). https://doi.org/10.1109/ICMA.2006.257739
20. Li, C.: Particle Swarm Optimization in Stationary and Dynamic Environments (2010). https://bee22.com/resources/Li%202010%20thesis.pdf

21. Pedersen, M.E.H.: Tuning & simplifying heuristical optimization. University of Southampton (2010). https://eprints.soton.ac.uk/id/eprint/342792
22. Bai, Q.: Analysis of particle swarm optimization algorithm. Comput. Inf. Sci. **3**(1), 180 (2010). https://doi.org/10.5539/cis.v3n1p180
23. Schoeman, I.L.: Niching in particle swarm optimization. University of Pretoria (2010). https://repository.up.ac.za/handle/2263/26548?show=full
24. Liang, J.: Novel particle swarm optimizers with hybrid, dynamic and adaptive neighborhood structures (2008). https://bee22.com/resources/Jing%202008.pdf
25. Helwig, S.: Particle swarms for constrained optimization (2010). https://opus4.kobv.de/opus4-fau/frontdoor/index/index/docId/1328
26. Dasheng, L.I.U.: Multi objective particle swarm optimization: algorithms and applications (2009). https://scholarbank.nus.edu.sg/handle/10635/16724
27. Omran, M.G.H.: Particle swarm optimization methods for pattern recognition and image processing. University of Pretoria (2006). https://repository.up.ac.za/bitstream/handle/2263/29826/Complete.pdf?sequence=11
28. Birattari, M.: The Problem of Tuning Metaheuristics. PhD, Fac. des Sci. Appliquées, Univ. Libr. Bruxelles (2006). https://www.iospress.nl/book/the-problem-of-tuning-metaheuristics/
29. Schmitt, B.I.: Convergence analysis for particle swarm optimization (2015). https://kamenp enkov.files.wordpress.com/2016/01/schmitt-2015.pdf
30. Talukder, S.: Mathematicle modelling and applications of particle swarm optimization (2011)
31. Vis, J.K.: Particle Swarm Optimizer for Finding Robust Optima. LIACS, Holl. (2009). https://liacs.leidenuniv.nl/assets/Bachelorscripties/2009-12JonathanVis.pdf
32. Parsopoulos, K.E., Vrahatis, M.N.: Particle swarm optimization and intelligence: advances and applications (2010). https://www.igi-global.com/book/particle-swarm-optimization-int elligence/37246
33. Mikki, S.M., Kishk, A.A.: Particle swarm optimization: a physics-based approach. Synth. Lect. Comput. Electromagn. **3**(1), 1–103 (2008). https://doi.org/10.2200/S00110ED1V01Y20 0804CEM020
34. Zomaya, A.Y.: Handbook of Nature-Inspired and Innovative Computing: Integrating Classical Models with Emerging Technologies. Springer Science & Business Media, 2006.https://www.springer.com/gp/book/9780387405322
35. Clerc, M.: Particle Swarm Optimization, vol. 93. Wiley (2010). https://doi.org/10.1002/978 0470612163.fmatter
36. Poli, R.: Analysis of the publications on the applications of particle swarm optimisation. J. Artif. Evol. Appl.**2008** (2008). https://doi.org/10.1155/2008/685175
37. Poli, R., Kennedy, J., Blackwell, T.: Particle swarm optimization. Swarm Intell.**1**(1), 33–57 (2007). https://doi.org/10.1007/s11721-007-0002-0
38. Banks, A., Vincent, J., Anyakoha, C.: A review of particle swarm optimization. Part I: background and development. Nat. Comput.**6**(4), 467–484 (2007). https://doi.org/10.1007/s11047-007-9049-5
39. Banks, A., Vincent, J., Anyakoha, C.: A review of particle swarm optimization. Part II: hybridisation, combinatorial, multicriteria and constrained optimization, and indicative applications. Nat. Comput.**7**(1), 109–124 (2008). https://doi.org/10.1007/s11047-007-9050-z
40. Shi, Y., Eberhart, R.C.: Parameter selection in particle swarm optimization BT—Evolutionary Programming VII (1998). https://doi.org/10.1007/BFb0040810
41. Rini, D.P., Shamsuddin, S.M., Yuhaniz, S.S.: Particle swarm optimization: technique, system and challenges. Int. J. Comput. Appl.**14**(1), 19–26 (2011). https://citeseerx.ist.psu.edu/vie wdoc/download?doi=10.1.1.206.5070&rep=rep1&type=pdf
42. Zhang, Y., Wang, S., Ji, G.: A comprehensive survey on particle swarm optimization algorithm and its applications. Math. Probl. Eng.**2015**, 1–38 (2015). https://doi.org/10.1155/2015/931256. https://www.hindawi.com/journals/mpe/2015/931256/
43. Chatterjee, A., Siarry, P.: Nonlinear inertia weight variation for dynamic adaptation in particle swarm optimization. Comput. Oper. Res. **33**(3), 859–871 (2006)

44. Eberhart, R.C., Shi, Y.: Particle swarm optimization: Developments, applications and resources. Proc. IEEE Conf. Evol. Comput. ICEC **1**, 81–86 (2001). https://doi.org/10.1109/cec.2001.934374

45. Clerc, M., Kennedy, J.: The particle swarm-explosion, stability, and convergence in a multidimensional complex space. IEEE Trans. Evol. Comput. **6**(1), 58–73 (2002)

46. de Oca, M.A.M.: Particle swarm optimization introduction. IRIDIA-CoDE, Univ. Libr. Bruxelles (2007)

47. Dorigo, M., de Oca, M.A.M., Engelbrecht, A.: Particle swarm optimization. Scholarpedia **3**(11), 1486 (2008)

48. Selleri, S., Mussetta, M., Pirinoli, P., Zich, R.E., Matekovits, L.: Some insight over new variations of the particle swarm optimization method. IEEE Antennas Wirel. Propag. Lett. **5**, 235–238 (2006). https://doi.org/10.1109/LAWP.2006.874071

49. Kennedy, J.: Bare bones particle swarms. In: Proceedings of the 2003 IEEE Swarm Intelligence Symposium. SIS'03 (Cat. No. 03EX706), pp. 80–87 (2003)

50. Kennedy, J., Eberhart, R.C.: A discrete binary version of the particle swarm algorithm. In: 1997 IEEE International Conference on Systems, Man, and Cybernetics. Computational Cybernetics and Simulation, vol. 5, pp. 4104–4108 (1997)

51. Liu, G., Chen, W., Chen, H., Xie, J.: A quantum particle swarm optimization algorithm with teamwork evolutionary strategy. Math. Probl. Eng. **2019**, 1805198 (2019). https://doi.org/10.1155/2019/1805198

52. hydroPSO—Mathematical software—swMATH. https://www.swmath.org/software/24340. Accessed 28 June 2020

53. Zambrano-Bigiarini, M., Rojas, R.: A model-independent Particle Swarm Optimisation software for model calibration. Environ. Model. Softw. **43**, 5–25 (2013). https://doi.org/10.1016/j.envsoft.2013.01.004

54. Koyuncu, H., Ceylan, R.: Scout particle swarm optimization. In: 6th European Conference of the International Federation for Medical and Biological Engineering, pp. 82–85 (2015)

55. Elshamy, W., Emara, H.M., Bahgat, A.: Clubs-based particle swarm optimization. In: 2007 IEEE Swarm Intelligence Symposium, pp. 289–296 (2007)

56. Abdelbar, A.M., Abdelshahid, S., Wunsch, D.C.: Fuzzy PSO: a generalization of particle swarm optimization. In: Proceedings. 2005 IEEE International Joint Conference on Neural Networks, 2005, vol. 2, pp. 1086–1091 (2009). https://doi.org/10.1109/IJCNN.2005.1556004

57. Lee, C.M., Ko, C.N.: Time series prediction using RBF neural networks with a nonlinear time-varying evolution PSO algorithm. Neurocomputing (2009). https://doi.org/10.1016/j.neucom.2009.07.005

58. Wang, H., Li, H., Liu, Y., Li, C., Zeng, S.: Opposition-based particle swarm algorithm with Cauchy mutation (2007). https://doi.org/10.1109/CEC.2007.4425095

59. Jiang, B., Wang, N., Wang, L.: Particle swarm optimization with age-group topology for multimodal functions and data clustering. Commun. Nonlinear Sci. Numer. Simul. **18**(11), 3134–3145 (2013)

60. Xie, X.-F., Zhang, W.-J., Yang, Z.-L.: Adaptive particle swarm optimization on individual level. In: 6th International Conference on Signal Processing, 2002, vol. 2, pp. 1215–1218 (2002)

61. Lu, Y.C., Jan, J.C., Hung, S.L., Hung, G.H.: Enhancing particle swarm optimization algorithm using two new strategies for optimizing design of truss structures. Eng. Optim. (2013). https://doi.org/10.1080/0305215X.2012.729054

62. Shi, X.H., Liang, Y.C., Lee, H.P., Lu, C., Wang, L.M.: An improved GA and a novel PSO-GA-based hybrid algorithm. Inf. Process. Lett. **93**(5), 255–261 (2005)

63. Anand, A., Suganthi, L.: Hybrid GA-PSO optimization of artificial neural network for forecasting electricity demand. Energies **11**(4), 728 (2018)

64. Elloumi, W., Baklouti, N., Abraham, A., Alimi, A.M.: The multi-objective hybridization of particle swarm optimization and fuzzy ant colony optimization. J. Intell. Fuzzy Syst. **27**(1), 515–525 (2014)

65. Niknam, T., Narimani, M.R., Jabbari, M.: Dynamic optimal power flow using hybrid particle swarm optimization and simulated annealing. Int. Trans. Electr. Energy Syst. **23**(7), 975–1001 (2013)
66. Simon, D.: Biogeography-based optimization. IEEE Trans. Evol. Comput. **12**(6), 702–713 (2008)
67. Cheng, S., Chen, M.-Y., Fleming, P.J.: Improved multi-objective particle swarm optimization with preference strategy for optimal DG integration into the distribution system. Neurocomputing **148**, 23–29 (2015)
68. Zhang, G., Cheng, Y., Yang, F., Pan, Q.: Particle filter based on PSO. In: 2008 International Conference on Intelligent Computation Technology and Automation (ICICTA), Oct 2008, pp. 121–124. https://doi.org/10.1109/ICICTA.2008.262
69. Ramezani, F., Lu, J., Hussain, F.K.: Task-based system load balancing in cloud computing using particle swarm optimization. Int. J. Parallel Program. (2014). https://doi.org/10.1007/s10766-013-0275-4
70. Jordehi, A.R.: Enhanced leader PSO (ELPSO): a new PSO variant for solving global optimisation problems. Appl. Soft Comput. **26**, 401–417 (2015)
71. Parsopoulos, K.E.: UPSO: a unified particle swarm optimization scheme. Lect. Ser. Comput. Comput. Sci. **1**, 868–873 (2004)
72. Mendes, R., Kennedy, J., Neves, J.: The fully informed particle swarm: simpler, maybe better. IEEE Trans. Evol. Comput. **8**(3), 204–210 (2004)
73. Liang, J.J., Qin, A.K., Suganthan, P.N., Baskar, S.: Comprehensive learning particle swarm optimizer for global optimization of multimodal functions. IEEE Trans. Evol. Comput. **10**(3), 281–295 (2006)
74. Wang, H., Wu, Z., Rahnamayan, S., Li, C., Zeng, S., Jiang, D.: Particle swarm optimisation with simple and efficient neighbourhood search strategies. Int. J. Innov. Comput. Appl. **3**(2), 97–104 (2011)
75. Van den Bergh, F., Engelbrecht, A.P.: A cooperative approach to particle swarm optimization. IEEE Trans. Evol. Comput. **8**(3), 225–239 (2004)
76. Khan, M.S., Lee, M.: Design optimization of single mixed refrigerant natural gas liquefaction process using the particle swarm paradigm with nonlinear constraints. Energy**49**(1) (2013). https://doi.org/10.1016/j.energy.2012.11.028
77. Park, J., Choi, K., Allstot, D.J.: Parasitic-aware RF circuit design and optimization. IEEE Trans Circuits Syst. I Regul. Pap. (2004). https://doi.org/10.1109/TCSI.2004.835691
78. Ranaee, V., Ebrahimzadeh, A., Ghaderi, R.: Application of the PSO–SVM model for recognition of control chart patterns. ISA Trans. **49**(4), 577–586 (2010)
79. Venayagamoorthy, G.K., Zha, W.: Comparison of nonuniform optimal quantizer designs for speech coding with adaptive critics and particle swarm. IEEE Trans. Ind. Appl. (2007). https://doi.org/10.1109/TIA.2006.885897
80. Nenortaite, J., Simutis, R.: Adapting particle swarm optimization to stock markets (2005). https://doi.org/10.1109/ISDA.2005.17
81. Cabrerizo, F.J., Herrera-Viedma, E., Pedrycz, W.: A method based on PSO and granular computing of linguistic information to solve group decision making problems defined in heterogeneous contexts. Eur. J. Oper. Res. (2013). https://doi.org/10.1016/j.ejor.2013.04.046
82. Bianchi, L., Dorigo, M., Gambardella, L.M., Gutjahr, W.J.: Metaheuristics in stochastic combinatorial optimization : a survey. Gall. Rass. Bimest. Di Cult. 08, 1–58 (2006). [Online]. Available: https://citeseerx.ist.psu.edu/viewdoc/download?doi=10.1.1.70.3639&rep=rep1&type=pdf
83. Ahangarani, M.L., Aragh, N.O., Mojeddifar, S., Chegeni, M.H.: A combination of probabilistic neural network (PNN) and particle swarm optimization (PSO) algorithms to map hydrothermal alteration zones using ASTER data. Earth Sci. Inf.**13**(3), 929–937 (2020). https://doi.org/10.1007/s12145-020-00479-0
84. Chatterjee, A., Pulasinghe, K., Watanabe, K., Izumi, K.: A particle-swarm-optimized fuzzy-neural network for voice-controlled robot systems. IEEE Trans. Ind. Electron. (2005). https://doi.org/10.1109/TIE.2005.858737

85. Jatmiko, W., Sekiyama, K., Fukuda, T.: A pso-based mobile robot for odor source localization in dynamic advection-diffusion with obstacles environment: theory, simulation and measurement. IEEE Comput. Intell. Mag. **2**(2), 37–51 (2007). https://doi.org/10.1109/MCI. 2007.353419

86. Chuang, L.-Y., Chang, H.-W., Tu, C.-J., Yang, C.-H.: Improved binary PSO for feature selection using gene expression data. Comput. Biol. Chem. **32**(1), 29–38 (2008). https://doi.org/ 10.1016/j.compbiolchem.2007.09.005

87. Duan, H., Wei, X., Dong, Z.: Multiple UCAVs cooperative air combat simulation platform based on PSO, ACO, and game theory. IEEE Aerosp. Electron. Syst. Mag. **28**(11), 12–19 (2013)

88. Messerschmidt, L., Engelbrecht, A.P.: Learning to play games using a PSO-based competitive learning approach. IEEE Trans. Evol. Comput. **8**(3), 280–288 (2004)

89. Kolomvatsos, K., Hadjieftymiades, S.: On the use of particle swarm optimization and kernel density estimator in concurrent negotiations. Inf. Sci. (Ny) **262**, 99–116 (2014)

90. Pandey, S.K., Mohanty, S.R., Kishor, N., Catalão, J.P.S.: Frequency regulation in hybrid power systems using particle swarm optimization and linear matrix inequalities based robust controller design. Int. J. Electr. Power Energy Syst. **63**, 887–900 (2014)

91. Nedic, N., Prsic, D., Dubonjic, L., Stojanovic, V., Djordjevic, V.: Optimal cascade hydraulic control for a parallel robot platform by PSO. Int. J. Adv. Manuf. Technol. **72**(5–8), 1085–1098 (2014)

92. Zubair, M., Moinuddin, M.: Joint optimization of microstrip patch antennas using particle swarm optimization for UWB systems. Int. J. Antennas Propag.**2013** (2013)

93. Kim, Y.G., Lee, M.J.: Scheduling multi-channel and multi-timeslot in time constrained wireless sensor networks via simulated annealing and particle swarm optimization. IEEE Commun. Mag. **52**(1), 122–129 (2014)

94. Bozorgi-Amiri, A., Jabalameli, M.S., Alinaghian, M., Heydari, M.: A modified particle swarm optimization for disaster relief logistics under uncertain environment. Int. J. Adv. Manuf. Technol. **60**(1–4), 357–371 (2012)

95. Sadeghi, J., Sadeghi, S., Niaki, S.T.A.: Optimizing a hybrid vendor-managed inventory and transportation problem with fuzzy demand: an improved particle swarm optimization algorithm. Inf. Sci. (Ny) **272**, 126–144 (2014)

96. Wang, Y., Li, L.: A PSO algorithm for constrained redundancy allocation in multi-state systems with bridge topology. Comput. Ind. Eng. **68**, 13–22 (2014)

97. Zhang, Y., Gallipoli, D., Augarde, C.: Parameter identification for elasto-plastic modelling of unsaturated soils from pressuremeter tests by parallel modified particle swarm optimization. Comput. Geotech. **48**, 293–303 (2013)

98. Lee, C.-H., Shih, K.-S., Hsu, C.-C., Cho, T.: Simulation-based particle swarm optimization and mechanical validation of screw position and number for the fixation stability of a femoral locking compression plate. Med. Eng. Phys. **36**(1), 57–64 (2014)

99. Khajeh, M., Kaykhaii, M., Sharafi, A.: Application of PSO-artificial neural network and response surface methodology for removal of methylene blue using silver nanoparticles from water samples. J. Ind. Eng. Chem. **19**(5), 1624–1630 (2013)

100. Skvortsov, A.N.: Estimation of rotation ambiguity in multivariate curve resolution with charged particle swarm optimization (cPSO-MCR). J. Chemom. **28**(10), 727–739 (2014)

101. Subasi, A.: Classification of EMG signals using PSO optimized SVM for diagnosis of neuromuscular disorders. Comput. Biol. Med. **43**(5), 576–586 (2013)

102. Zhang, Y.-D., Wang, S., Wu, L.: A novel method for magnetic resonance brain image classification based on adaptive chaotic PSO. Prog. Electromagn. Res. **109**, 325–343 (2010)

103. Sharif, M., Amin, J., Raza, M., Yasmin, M., Satapathy, S.C.: An integrated design of particle swarm optimization (PSO) with fusion of features for detection of brain tumor. Pattern Recognit. Lett.**129**, 150–157 (2020). https://www.sciencedirect.com/science/article/pii/S01 6786551930337X

104. Dindar, Z.A., Marwala, T.: Option pricing using a committee of neural networks and optimized networks. In: 2004 IEEE International Conference on Systems, Man and Cybernetics (IEEE Cat. No. 04CH37583), vol. 1, pp. 434–438 (2004)

105. Xu, F., Chen, W.: Stochastic portfolio selection based on velocity limited particle swarm optimization. In: 2006 6th World Congress on Intelligent Control and Automation, vol. 1, pp. 3599–3603 (2006)
106. Pang, W., Wang, K.P., Zhou, C.G., Dong, L. J.: Fuzzy discrete particle swarm optimization for solving traveling salesman problem (2004). https://doi.org/10.1109/cit.2004.1357292
107. Shen, X., Li, Y., Wang, W., Zheng, B.: A dynamic adaptive particle swarm optimization for knapsack problem. In: 2006 6th World Congress on Intelligent Control and Automation, vol. 1, pp. 3183–3187 (2006)
108. Sedghi, M., Aliakbar-Golkar, M., Haghifam, M.-R.: Distribution network expansion considering distributed generation and storage units using modified PSO algorithm. Int. J. Electr. Power Energy Syst. **52**, 221–230 (2013)
109. Syahputra, R., Robandi, I., Ashari, M.: Reconfiguration of distribution network with distributed energy resources integration using PSO algorithm. Telkomnika **13**(3), 759 (2015)
110. Jornod, G., Di Mario, E., Navarro, I., Martinoli, A.: SwarmViz: an open-source visualization tool for Particle Swarm Optimization. In: 2015 IEEE Congress on Evolutionary Computation (CEC), pp. 179–186 (2015)
111. Solomon, S., Thulasiraman, P., Thulasiram, R.: Collaborative multi-swarm PSO for task matching using graphics processing units. In: Proceedings of the 13th Annual Conference on Genetic and Evolutionary Computation, pp. 1563–1570 (2011)
112. Zhang, Y., Huang, D., Ji, M., Xie, F.: Image segmentation using PSO and PCM with Mahalanobis distance. Expert Syst. Appl. **38**(7), 9036–9040 (2011)
113. Younus, Z.S., et al.: Content-based image retrieval using PSO and k-means clustering algorithm. Arab. J. Geosci. **8**(8), 6211–6224 (2015)
114. Liu, B., Wang, L., Jin, Y.-H.: An effective PSO-based memetic algorithm for flow shop scheduling. IEEE Trans. Syst. Man, Cybern. Part B**37**(1), 18–27 (2007)
115. Akjiratikarl, C., Yenradee, P., Drake, P.R.: PSO-based algorithm for home care worker scheduling in the UK. Comput. Ind. Eng. **53**(4), 559–583 (2007)
116. Wang, W., Xu, D., Chau, K., Chen, S.: Improved annual rainfall-runoff forecasting using PSO–SVM model based on EEMD. J. Hydroinformatics **15**(4), 1377–1390 (2013)
117. Bashir, Z.A., El-Hawary, M.E.: Applying wavelets to short-term load forecasting using PSO-based neural networks. IEEE Trans. Power Syst. **24**(1), 20–27 (2009)
118. Deng, W., Yao, R., Zhao, H., Yang, X., Li, G.: A novel intelligent diagnosis method using optimal LS-SVM with improved PSO algorithm. Soft Comput.**23**(7), 2445–2462 (2019). https://link.springer.com/article/10.1007%2Fs00500-017-2940-9
119. Yuan, X., Liu, Z., Miao, Z., Zhao, Z., Zhou, F., Song, Y.: Fault diagnosis of analog circuits based on IH-PSO optimized support vector machine. IEEE Access**7**, 137945–137958 (2019). https://ieeexplore.ieee.org/abstract/document/8846201
120. Cho, Y., Smith, J.S., Smith, A.E.: Optimizing tactical military MANETs with a specialized PSO. In: IEEE Congress on Evolutionary Computation, pp. 1–6 (2010)
121. Lin, C.J., Prasetyo, Y.T.: A metaheuristic-based approach to optimizing color design for military camouflage using particle swarm optimization. Color Res. Appl. **44**(5), 740–748 (2019)
122. Raj, S., Ray, K.C.: ECG signal analysis using DCT-based DOST and PSO optimized SVM. IEEE Trans. Instrum. Meas. **66**(3), 470–478 (2017)
123. Shayeghi, H., Safari, A., Shayanfar, H.A.: PSS and TCSC damping controller coordinated design using PSO in multi-machine power system. Energy Convers. Manag. **51**(12), 2930–2937 (2010)
124. Pan, I., Das, S.: Fractional order fuzzy control of hybrid power system with renewable generation using chaotic PSO. ISA Trans. **62**, 19–29 (2016)
125. Obukhov, S., Ibrahim, A., Diab, A.A.Z., Al-Sumaiti, A.S., Aboelsaud, R.: Optimal performance of dynamic particle swarm optimization based maximum power trackers for stand-alone PV system under partial shading conditions. IEEE Access**8**, 20770–20785 (2020). https://ieeexplore.ieee.org/document/8957566

126. Khan, M.S., Lee, M.: Design optimization of single mixed refrigerant natural gas liquefaction process using the particle swarm paradigm with nonlinear constraints. Energy **49**(1), 146–155 (2013). https://doi.org/10.1016/j.energy.2012.11.028
127. Qyyum, M.A., Qadeer, K., Lee, S., Lee, M.: Innovative propane-nitrogen two-phase expander refrigeration cycle for energy-efficient and low-global warming potential LNG production. Appl. Therm. Eng. (2018). https://doi.org/10.1016/j.applthermaleng.2018.04.105

AIML Applications for Monitoring System in Health and Management

Classification and Monitoring of Injuries Around Knee Using Radiograph-Based Deep Learning Algorithm

C. V. Praharsha and Pullabhatla Srikanth

Abstract In this chapter, a novel deep learning-based methodology for the classification of various types of fractures around the knee has been proposed. To train the deep learning algorithm, several radiographs of various types of fractures viz. both bone, tibial plateau, tibial shaft, fibula head, fibula shaft, patellae, and femur distal end have been fed. Before feeding these images to the deep learning algorithm, all the images were reoriented, rotated, and resized to a size of 600×300 pixels. These images are then populated to create 100 nos. of a dataset for each type of fracture. For the classification of various types of fractures, customized deep learning algorithm approach has been adopted. The proposed deep learning algorithm has been optimized after repeated validation and then has been used to classify the type of fractures. An effort has been put to train the network with different parameters and compare the individual performance. Finally, at an epoch of 10 and dropout value of 0.5, it was found that the network can classify all type of fractures with an accuracy of 100% without any overfitting issues. This chapter is novel in approach, and all types of fractures around the knee are identified with highest accuracy using the proposed deep learning algorithm. The work can further be extended to classify fractures of other areas of the human body.

Keywords Radiographs · Knee fractures · Deep learning · Classification · Monitoring

C. V. Praharsha (✉)
Musculoskeletal Clinical Physiotherapist, Defence Research and Development Organization, Secunderabad, India
e-mail: cpraharsha79@gmail.com

P. Srikanth
Scientist D, DRDO, Defence Research and Development Organization, Secunderabad, India
e-mail: srikanth.srikki@gmail.com

© The Author(s), under exclusive license to Springer Nature Singapore Pte Ltd. 2021   127
H. Malik et al. (eds.), *AI and Machine Learning Paradigms for Health Monitoring System*, Studies in Big Data 86,
https://doi.org/10.1007/978-981-33-4412-9_7

1 Introduction

In the last five years, physiotherapeutic practices had developed a lot due to the change in technology and digitalization. Also, huge research has been done in physical therapy to improve the efficiency in understanding the etiology of injury, assessing the subject, and providing appropriate treatment. The changes and improvements in these areas have reached very far into the physiotherapy society, and there is a rising awareness among the common people too. Recently, the evidence-based approach has gained popularity in the clinical practices which led to better management of various disorders. In the standard evidence-based approach of musculoskeletal physiotherapy, there is an interdependency between various medical fields like orthopedics, cardio-pulmonology, radiology, and other such departments. However, common to all these medical fields, a radiologist plays an essential role in clinical decision making to support the clinical assessment.

The radiographs along with its report provided for any type of disorders are vital in deciding the further prognosis. Specifically, in the field of musculoskeletal physiotherapy, a good radiological input is required regularly for a better follow up. However, such a requirement always increases the load on the radiologists which further delays the reporting by the radiologists. Often there are cases where only the radiographs with or without reports mislead the clinicians leading to erroneous diagnosis. Hence, there is always a requirement of some means through which the radiographs can be reassessed at the clinical end. It can be achieved by deploying a radiologist in the clinical setups at the cost of the operational budget. Thus, to optimize such cost burdens and achieve high quality reports, a computer-aided decision system is required. These systems are known as computer-assisted radiographic reporting system (CARRS) which assists the radiologists/clinicians by prompting the probable diagnosis as per its database. The CARRS approach has made the clinical interpretation to assist the physical therapists for assessments leading to decreased assessment time and increased physiotherapeutic management of the subjects.

Much research has been done in the area of computer-aided decision system or CARRS to aid the clinicians. Currently, the application of machine learning and deep learning is found to be more effective due to the robustness of the algorithm and near to human brain functioning. In this area, Ashinsky et al. have proposed a machine learning classification algorithm for identifying the symptoms of early osteoarthritis [1]. To train the machine Learning algorithm, they have magnetic resonance images of human articular cartilage of 68 subjects. By performing machine learning-based classification, accuracy of 75% was reported. However, the study was restricted to osteoarthritis but not explored for various types of fractures. Applications of artificial intelligence and machine learning in musculoskeletal physiotherapy were reported by Christopher Tack [2]. A brief discussion has been provided about supervised learning in medical imaging where a machine learning model was trained for identification of fractures in X-Ray. A review about various applications was also reported where it was shown that a 16-layer convolution neural network (CNN) had achieved an accuracy of 83% for identification of fracture. However, the classification is done to identify only the presence of fracture but not the type.

Similarly, application of deep neural networks was proposed by Rober Lindsay et al. to improve fracture detection by clinicians. In the paper, the authors have proposed a computer-aided decision-making system based on deep learning which can detect and classify the type of fracture through wrist radiographs. An accuracy of 93.9% has been reported with machine-aided classification and concluded that by using deep learning methods, the expertise of specialists could be transferred to the generalists [3]. Deep Patel et al. have proposed automatic detection of knee joints in radiographic images where they have reported an accuracy of 99.4% with their proposed methodology of You-Only-Look-Once (YOLO)-based deep learning algorithm [4]. However, the classification of knee fractures was not discussed. Balance evaluation of effective physical therapy using sensors and deep learning was proposed by Wei et al. [5] where they have used Wii balance boards and Kinect sensors. The highest accuracy of 97.7% was reported for balance level and 95.4% for fall risk.

A brief about deep learning workflow was described by Emmanuel Montagnon et al. [6]. The focus of the article was on classification of lesions in brain identified through magnetic resonance imaging (MRI) scans. The application of different types of CNNs viz. fully connected, CNNs, and U-Nets were discussed and concluded that deep learning shows excellent promise in radiological assessments. Kitamura et al. in 2020 had proposed a deep learning evaluation of pelvic radiographs for fracture detection along with the position [7]. In 2019 for the first time, efficacy of deep learning for thigh bone fracture detection has been reported by Bin Guan et al. They studied the effect of a new technique, dilated convolutional feature pyramid network (DCFPN), and obtained 82.1% accuracy [8]. The application of deep learning has been discussed by Mawatari et al. at an extent in [9] wherein they have used magnetic resonance images (MRIs) and computer tomographies (CTs) for detection of types of hip fractures. Also, David Naylor has described that there are high prospects of deep learning algorithms in the field of healthcare system [10]. Yang et al. did a systematic review in 2020. In this study, they have considered fourteen papers for review to study the accuracy of deep learning in fractures of various joints. They concluded that deep learning has high accuracy in feature identification but is not completely reliable for localizing fractures [11]. Similar review was done by Kalmet et al. wherein they have reviewed and concluded that deep learning application for detection of fractures is highly effective and presented few directions for future development [12]. However, in both the literature review papers, it was observed that till date a comprehensive system for knee fractures has not been reported. Given the above literature of significant articles, a novel radiograph-based deep learning algorithm has been proposed for classification of fractures around the knee. Few examples are given in [15, 16].

1.1 Novelty of the Work

As mentioned in the literature, many authors had proposed deep learning algorithm for applications in various types of radiographs. However, few areas have still been left unexplored which makes the proposed methodology novel and efficient. The novelties/innovations are as mentioned below:-

1. All fractures around the knee were classified in single proposed methodology.
2. Deep learning has been used for the first time for identification of fractures around the knee.
3. An accuracy of 100% has been reported for all types of fractures considered.
4. A customized CNN has been proposed for classification which is found to be highly efficient and accurate.

All these novelties are addressed in this chapter with proper results, and the major types of fractures around the knee have been considered for classification. For classification, a customized CNN based deep learning algorithm has been proposed, which, when trained, can classify any type of fracture around the knee with the highest accuracy. The chapter is organized in seven φions including introduction. Section 2 describes the importance of identifying fractures around the knee. The basics of deep learning and the design of proposed CNN is provided in Sect. 3. The image preprocessing and creation of datasets is provided in Sect. 4 with the description of the overall process of classification in Sect. 5. The results and discussions are provided in Sect. 6 with the conclusions in Sect. 7. The referred articles are presented at the end of the chapter.

2 Description of Fractures Around the Knee

The knee is an important weight-bearing joint which includes tibiofemoral joint and patellofemoral joint. While the tibiofemoral joint provides weight-bearing function, the patellofemoral joint provides transmission of force through quadriceps muscle. Since the injury to any of these joints disrupts the gait, and its related activities of daily living (ADLs), early diagnosis and further treatment plays a pivotal role in preventing future complications. The common fractures around the knee include femoral distal end fractures, patellar fractures, tibial shaft fractures, tibial plateau fractures, both bone fractures, fibular shaft fractures, and fibular head fractures. Out of these fractures, tibial fractures are the most commonly occurring fractures, whereas both bone fractures have the worst prognosis. However, the management of any type of fracture by a physiotherapist relies on the radiographs where the clinical assessments are not enough. In many instances, when the number of subjects is more, and the clinical interpretation needs to be done from the radiographs along with the clinical assessments, a radiographical reporting assistance will provide a faster clinical decision. As given in Table 1, the complications of the fractures vary

Table 1 Comprehensive details about the fractures around knee

S. No.	Name of the fracture	Mechanism of injury	Radiographical identification pattern	Complications	Treatment
1	Both bone fracture	High and low falls, motor vehicle collisions, slippery floor injuries, sport injuries (contact and non-contact)	Discontinuity in shaft of tibia and fibula	Weight-bearing inability, malunion, and nonunion	POP, surgery (displaced), rehab
2	Femur distal end fracture		Discontinuity in medial or lateral condyles of femur		
3	Patellar fracture		Discontinuity in patella	Improper transfer of force due to altered quadriceps femoris function	Knee arthroplasty, rehab
4	Tibial plateau fracture		Discontinuity on anterior or posterior aspect of lateral or medial plateau of tibia	Instability-ligamentous attachment damages	POP, surgery (displaced), Rehab
5	Tibial shaft fracture		Discontinuity in tibial shaft	Weight-bearing inability, malunion, and nonunion	
6	Fibular head fracture	Same as S No. 1–5 and osteoporosis	Discontinuity in fibular head	Common peroneal nerve injury, esthetic issues	
7	Fibular shaft fracture		Discontinuity in fibular shaft	Esthetic issues	Surgery—displaced, No procedure—Undisplaced

from esthetic issues to instability of the joint. Also, procedures viz. knee arthroplasty, Kirschner wires (K-wire fixation), and open reduction internal fixation (ORIF) shall be recommended at the earliest. Since a radiology department is not available in every clinical setup, a computer-aided radiographical reporting system (CARRS) can be supportive in such situations. The literature regarding such a system has already been discussed in the previous section. It was found that the present-day technological advancement is in the application of deep learning algorithm for classification of fractures. Since, the classification of fractures around the knee is very crucial, the same has been considered for developing a radiographs-based deep learning-based algorithm (DLA) to assist the physiotherapists and other clinicians.

3   Background and Design of Deep Learning Algorithm

3.1   Background of Deep Learning

There are many pretrained deep learning algorithms available in open source for training and utilizing it for classification or identification of various types of problem statements. To name a few, ResNet, AlexNet, VGGNet, and GoogleNet are found more frequently in most of the applications in the field of engineering. The accuracy levels, the number of computational variables, and floating-point operations per second are mentioned in Table 2 [13]. The best accuracy is 95.5% which is achieved by ResNet-152 pretrained network. However, the number of flops and computational parameters are high. The least computational time belongs to GoogleNet with a least no. of two flops but at the cost of accuracy. Hence, it can be concluded that these three parameters are very much interlinked, and any deep learning algorithm must go through the balance of these performance defining parameters. These nets can be used for individual application purpose with the help of transfer learning.

However, owing to the machine costs, computation overburden may make the algorithm not suitable for lighter applications. Also, due to the freedom in designing a customized deep learning algorithm, the authors of this chapter had proposed customized convolution neural network-based deep learning algorithm for classification of types of fractures around the knee of a human body. A typical architecture of a deep learning algorithm is shown in Fig. 1. It is visible that an input image goes through many levels of convolution, ReLU, max-pooling and reaches to a stage of flattening where the multidimensional matrix is converted into a single vector. This data then goes through the fully connected layer. These values then forwarded to the softmax layer, which gives the probability of identification of a class or type. The final classification layer gives the output as a categorical array, thus classifying the types of input fed to the network.

The individual mathematical representation of each layer is defined in Fig. 2 in the next page. It can be understood through such representation of how an image is converted to digital information and then processed through various mathematical operations to obtain the desired classification output. The performance of any deep learning algorithm (DLA) depends on the factors mentioned below: -

Table 2 Comparison of various parameters of the few best deep learning algorithms

S. No.	Name of the deep learning network	Computational parameters in millions	FLOPS in billions	Accuracy
1	AlexNet	62	1.5	84.7
2	GoogleNet	6.4	2	93.3
3	ResNet-152	60.3	11	95.5
4	VGGNet	138	19.6	92.3

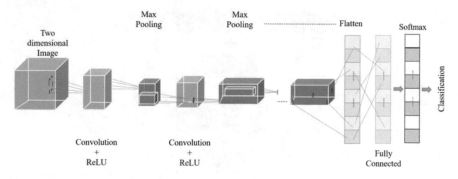

Fig. 1 Architecture of a typical CNN based deep learning algorithm

1. Size of the input image
2. Quality of the input image
3. Number of layers
4. Size of the convolution filter
5. Number of filters
6. Stride and padding
7. Training options.

Hence, to design a competent and efficient DLA, the above factors need to be considered. In this chapter, a customized DLA has been proposed, which is used for the classification of various types of fractures around the knee using the radiographic images as the input.

3.2 Design of the Proposed CNN

The proposed CNN based DLA is designed using MATLAB® 2019a software [14], and the model is shown in Fig. 3. The details and design architecture of the proposed CNN based DLA are mentioned in this section.

The proposed CNN contains two sets of convolution + ReLU + Max pooling + batch normalization layers. Followed by these layers, two sets of convolution + ReLU have been used with a drop out a layer at the end of convolution stage. After that, two sets of fully connected and ReLU are used. A softmax layer is introduced at the pre-final stage, and a classification layer has been added at the end for classification of various types of fractures around the knee. The size of the filter is defined as 5 × 5 with a stride of 1. Three (03) channels have been used for convolution with a dropout value of 0.5. The total number of learnbles of the proposed algorithm is given in Table 3. The size of the image is kept at a resolution of 600 × 300 pixels as the radiographs related to fractures which will be clearer in a rectangular dimension rather than a squared dimension because the bone structure is tall, and growth is vertical. However, all the images considered in the present chapter are not rectangular and clear. Also,

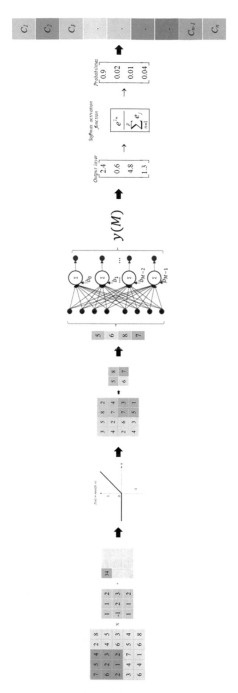

Fig. 2 Mathematical equivalents of the architecture of a typical CNN based deep learning algorithm shown in Fig. 1. (Rotate page for exact view)

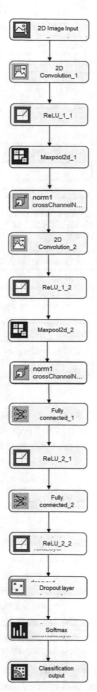

Fig. 3 Architecture of the proposed CNN designed in MATLAB

Table 3 Activations, learnables, and total learnables at each stage of the network

Name	Activations	Learnables	Total learnables
Data	$600 \times 600 \times 3$	–	0
Convolution 1	$600 \times 600 \times 3$	Weights $5 \times 5 \times 3 \times 3$; Bias $1 \times 1 \times 3$	228
ReLU 1	$600 \times 600 \times 3$	–	0
Normalization 1	$600 \times 600 \times 3$	–	0
Max pooling 1	$600 \times 600 \times 3$	–	0
Convolution 2	$600 \times 600 \times 3$	Weights $5 \times 5 \times 3 \times 3$; Bias $1 \times 1 \times 3$	228
ReLU 2	$600 \times 600 \times 3$	–	0
Normalization 2	$600 \times 600 \times 3$	–	0
Max pooling 2	$600 \times 600 \times 3$	–	0
Convolution 3	$600 \times 600 \times 3$	Weights $5 \times 5 \times 3 \times 3$; Bias $1 \times 1 \times 3$	228
ReLU 3	$600 \times 600 \times 3$	–	0
Fully connected 7	$600 \times 600 \times 3$	Weights 7×540000; Bias 7×1	3,780,007
ReLU 7	$600 \times 600 \times 3$	–	0
Drop 7	$600 \times 600 \times 3$	–	
SoftMax	$1 \times 1 \times 7$	–	0
Classification output	–	–	0
Total layers — 16		Total learnables ▬	3,780,691
			3.78×10^6

many of the radiograph images are preprinted with left-right indications, along with observations. Hence, these radiographs are preprocessed before feeding to the deep learning algorithm, which is discussed in the next section.

4   Image Preprocessing and Datasets

The DLA is trained with several radiographs related to various types of fractures around the knee, found in open source and ready to use have been downloaded. It is ensured that only those open source images are downloaded which are available without the details of the patients to respect privacy. A stepwise flow of the image preprocessing procedure is shown in Fig. 4. As presented in the figure, images, as shown in Step-1, are obtained from the Internet database, which does not have any details of the patients and open for download. However, it can be observed that the image orientation is not proper and few remarks like the brand of the radiograph machine, A side indication, R or L leg indication, etc., are present on the radiograph. Such images are firstly reoriented and rotated parallel with the vertical axis at an angle of $90°$ at Step-2, and then, removal of additional remarks using the image editing tools are done at Step-3. After this, the image is resized to a resolution of

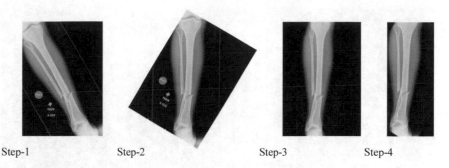

Step-1   Step-2   Step-3   Step-4

Fig. 4 Stepwise graphical description of the image preprocessing before feeding the images to the deep learning algorithm

Table 4 Details of the images preprocessed for training, validation and testing

Name	Class Name	No. of images processed for training	No. of images processed for validation	No. of images processed for testing
Both bone fracture	BBF	70	30	30
Femur distal end fracture	FDEF	70	30	30
Fibular head fracture	FHF	70	30	30
Fibular shaft fracture	FSF	70	30	30
Patellar fracture	PF	70	30	30
Tibial plateau fracture	THF	70	30	30
Tibial shaft fracture	TPF	70	30	30

600×300, as shown in Step-4, to focus the image only on the exposed white part of the radiograph. This procedure is repeated for all the images to create a database. However, there are few images which are free of such orientation and watermarks and are directly resized to a resolution of 600×300 pixels. Finally, the database size has been set to 100 images per type of fracture. The types of fractures and their respective class names are presented in Table 4.

5 Overall Process of DLA Based Classification

The overall process of classifying the type of fracture around the knee is shown in Fig. 5. The first stage is described in Sect. 2, which is the preprocessing stage. The images obtained at this stage are populated with different radiographs of a fracture

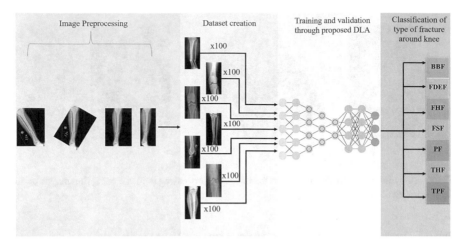

Fig. 5 Overall graphical description of the image preprocessing before feeding the images to the deep learning algorithm

which is done in stage 2. Later, these populated data are fed to the proposed deep learning algorithm for training and validation. The DLA extracts unique features for each type of fracture highlighted in red ellipses in Fig. 6. Once the DLA is trained, it is tested with 30 number of data for classification.

6   Results and Discussions

The proposed CNN based DLA is trained for different parameters and training options. Here, the importance of dropout layer is highlighted as this layer plays a crucial part in improving the accuracy. A dropout layer, when added to a DLA, passes only a part of the neuron samples received from the previous stage to the next stage. Due to this, all the neurons that are received from ReLU (in the proposed CNN case) layer will not contribute the weights and activations during the training process. By such action, the issues of overfitting can be avoided leading to a believable accuracy and lesser training loss. Hence, two CNNs are with, and without dropout, layers are considered for training, validation, and testing.

The training options for both the CNNs are given in Table 5. Further, in these two types of CNN, the number of epochs is varied to find out the best suitable training options for the proposed CNN. The number of epochs defines the training time as a greater number of epochs lead to higher training time but may lead to good accuracy. Since the performance of CNN is best defined with the balance between accuracy and training time, such cases are considered in this chapter. The training progress with every iteration is shown in Fig. 7, and the loss during the training is shown in Fig. 8 for all the four cases considered in Table 5.

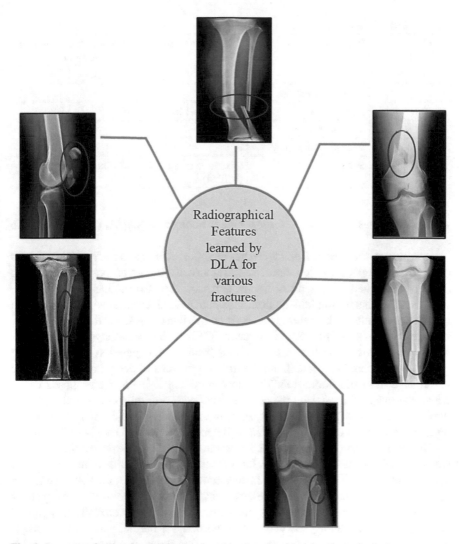

Fig. 6 Important features learned by the deep learning algorithm for (from clockwise top center) **a** Both bone fracture **b** Femur distal end fracture **c** Tibial Shaft fracture **d** Fibular head fracture **e** Tibial plateau fracture **f** Fibular shaft fracture **g** Patellar fracture

It is visible that a minimum of 85% validation accuracy has been achieved by using the proposed CNN in classifying the type of fracture around the knee, which is given in Table 6. The respective accuracy and loss during the training progress are shown in Fig. 7 and 8, respectively. By observing Fig. 7 and 8 together, it can be concluded that the CNN without dropout layer has produced 100% accuracy with epoch = 8. This is a clear case of overfitting as with very a smaller number of epochs and no dropout a 100% is achieved. It can further be established by observing Case-2

Table 5 Different cases considered for training

S. No.	Parameter	CNN without dropout layer		CNN with dropout layer and value of 0.5	
		Case 1	Case 2	Case 3	Case 4
1	Minimum batch size	120			
2	Max epochs	8	10	8	10
3	Initial learn rate	1e−3			
4	Validation frequency	3			
5	Solver	Stochastic gradient descent with momentum (SGDM)			

where 85.7% has been achieved for a higher number of epochs, i.e., 10, which is atypical.

However, in the case of CNN with dropout, a validation accuracy of 93.33% was obtained for an epoch 8 which shows the difference of adding a dropout layer. Further, the epoch has been increased to 10, where an accuracy of 100% has been achieved.

This shows that the implementation of dropout has reduced the overfitting problem in both Case-3 and 4. The training loss is smooth in these cases, and the loss is highest in Case-2 with a value of 0.556%. Since the CNN with dropout layer and an epoch of 10 had produced the best results with a balanced computation time, the same has been considered for visualizing the training features of every layer where there is a change in matrix dimension. The most important layers in the proposed CNN, where the image changes, are the convolution layers and fully connected layer. By observing the activations at the first, second, and third convolution layer, it can be understood whether a CNN has extracted the required features for classification.

The set of activations obtained for all the three convolution layers of the proposed CNN based DLA are shown in Fig. 9. It is visible that the input images are convoluted and fed forward to the next layer for further convolution. Briefly, the activated image after the first convolution layer is the representation of the structure of the leg along with fracture without background. In this stage, the DLA tried to omit the background and only read the highlighted white bony portion. At the next convolution stage, all the image with edges can be seen, thus filtering the background and extracting the bone structure. At the third stage, the extracted image is further learnt by the proposed DLA, and the finest details are passed to the fully connected layers for further classification.

The feature visualization has given a valid proof that the input images are well trained in each stage, and the proposed CNN is fully trained with the image database created. Hence, this trained CNN has been tested for the final classification of the type of fracture around the knee. For testing, 30 number of samples for each type of fractures have been used. The efficiency of a CNN depends on the number of events rightly identified out of the total number of events given as input. Such results as obtained are as shown in Fig. 10, which is a confusion matrix between the input and

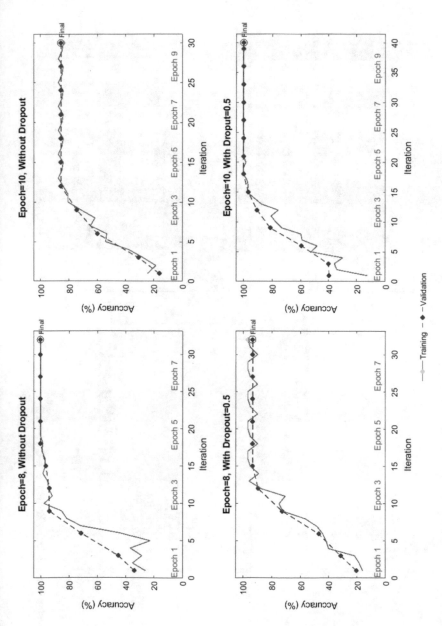

Fig. 7 Variation in accuracy for every iteration of **a** Case-1 **b** Case-2 **c** Case-3 **d** Case-4 as described in Table 5

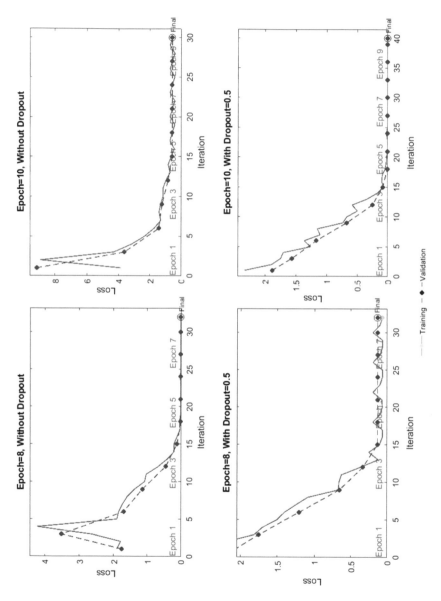

Fig. 8 Variation in loss for every iteration of **a** Case-1 **b** Case-2 **c** Case-3 **d** Case-4 as described in Table 5

Table 6 Performance comparison

S. No.	Parameter	CNN without dropout layer		CNN with dropout layer and value of 0.5	
		Case 1	Case 2	Case 3	Case 4
1	Training accuracy (in %)	100	84.71	96.67	100
2	Validation accuracy (in %)	100	85.71	93.33	100
3	Training loss (in %)	0.0001	0.556	0.0649	0.00007
4	Validation loss (in %)	0.0002	0.556	0.1297	0.00003
5	Training time (in s)	284	272	334	395

output categorical variables. The confusion plots for both the cases, i.e., with dropout layer at an epoch of 8 and 10 are shown.

As visible from the figure, the trained network had confused for both bone fracture (BBF) with tibial plateau and fibular shaft fracture for the case where epoch = 8. However, in the case of epoch = 10, i.e., Case-4 of Table 5, all types of fractures around the knee are successfully classified without any confusion. Such results are reported for the first time in the literature.

7 Conclusions

A novel convolution neural network (CNN)-based deep learning algorithm (DLA) for the classification of fractures around the knee has been proposed in this chapter. To train the DLA, radiographs of various types of fractures around the knee which are available in open source and not containing any private details have been downloaded. It was found that many of the images are having labels watermarked on the radiographs, and the resolution of these images is found to be different. For all such images, preprocessing has been done by clearing the watermarks, unnecessary details, and performing image modification like reorientation, rotation, and resizing, before feeding them to the DLA. The corrected images are resized to a resolution of 600×300 and then populated for training, validation, and testing. Two different DLAs have been proposed which are with and without the dropout layer. In both the CNNs, the number of epochs was varied with a value of 8 and 10.

It was observed that the CNN without dropout layer had produced a validation accuracy of 85.7% with an epoch of 10 but had produced an accuracy of 100% for an epoch of 8 which is suspected as a case of overfitting. However, in the case of CNN with dropout of 0.5 and epoch of 8, a validation accuracy of 93.3% has been reported, which is high for the case considered. Further, when the epochs have been increased to 10, a 100% validation accuracy has been achieved, which is outstanding and not reported till date in the literature. After the training of the DLA, 30 images of each type of fracture have been fed, and it was observed that DLA with dropout and epoch = 8 had identified 196 images correctly out of the 210 images with an accuracy of

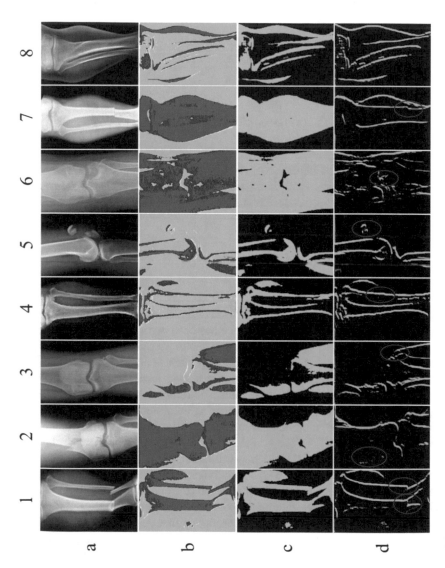

Fig. 9 Activations of the proposed CNN based DLA for the input image of **a** (1) Both bone fracture (2) Femur distal end fracture (3) Tibial shaft fracture (4) Fibular head fracture (5) Tibial plateau fracture (6) Fibular shaft fracture (7) Patellar fracture (8) Normal leg without fractures at various layers **b** Conv_1 **c** Conv_2 **d** Conv_3

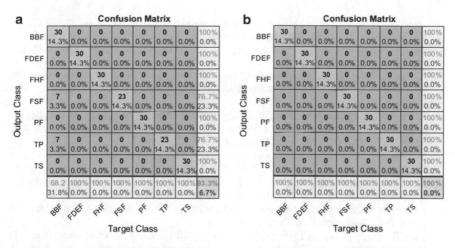

Fig. 10 Confusion matrices for the tested samples of 30 nos of each type of fracture based on the classification of the proposed CNN with **a** epoch = 8 **b** epoch = 10, i.e., case-4 of Table 5

93.3%. The DLA had confused the both bone fracture with tibia plateau and fibular shaft fracture. However, the DLA with dropout of 0.5, epoch 10, had classified all 210 images correctly with the type of fracture with an accuracy of 100%. It is concluded that due to the effective preprocessing of the images and design of DLA, an efficient model can be trained to achieve higher accuracies and shorter training time. The proposed method is novel in approach, able to identify all types of fractures around, and achieved the highest accuracy with a customized CNN. The work can be scaled for identification of fractures of different parts of the adult human body.

References

1. Ashinsky, B.G., Bouhrara, M., Coletta, C.E., Lehallier, B., Urish, K.L., Lin, P., Goldberg, I.G., Spencer, R.G.: Predicting early symptomatic osteoarthritis in the human knee using machine learning classification of magnetic resonance images from the osteoarthritis initiative. J. Orthop. Res. **35**, 2243–2250 (2017). https://doi.org/10.1002/jor.23519
2. Tack, C.: Artificial intelligence and machine learningl applications in musculoskeletal physiotherapy. Musculoskeletal Science & Practice **39**, 164–169 (2019). https://doi.org/10.1016/j.msksp.2018.11.012
3. Lindsey, R., Daluiski, A., Chopra, S., Lachapelle, A., Mozer, M.C., Sicular, S., Hanel, D.P., Gardner, M.F., Gupta, A., Hotchkiss, R.N., Potter, H.G.: Deep neural network improves fracture detection by clinicians. Proc. Natl. Acad. Sci. U.S.A. **115**, 11591–11596 (2018). https://doi.org/10.1073/pnas.1806905115
4. Patel, D.: Automatic Detection of Knee Joints in Radiographic Images (Doctoral dissertation). University of Florida, Gainesville. (2018). https://ufdcimages.uflib.ufl.edu/AA/00/06/32/24/00001/Patel_Deep.pdf
5. Wei, W., McElroy, C., Dey, S.: Using sensors and deep learning to enable on-demand balance evaluation for effective physical therapy. IEEE Access **8**, 99889–99899 (2020). https://doi.org/10.1109/ACCESS.2020.2997341

6. Montagnon, E., Cerny, M., Cadrin-Chênevert, A., Hamilton, V., Derennes, T., Ilinca, A., Vandenbroucke-Menu, F., Turcotte, S., Ka-doury, S., Tang, A.: Deep learning workflow in radiology: a primer. Insights Into Imaging, **11** (2020) https://doi.org/10.1186/s13244-019-0832-5
7. Kitamura, G.: Deep learning evaluation of pelvic radiographs for position, hardware presence, and fracture detection. Eur. J. Radiol. **130**, 109139 (2020). https://doi.org/10.1016/j.ejrad.2020.109139
8. Guan, B., Yao, J., Zhang, G., Wang, X.: Thigh fracture detection using deep learning method based on new dilated convolutional feature pyramid network. Pattern Recognit. Lett. **125**, 521–526 (2019). https://doi.org/10.1016/j.patrec.2019.06.015
9. Mawatari, T., Hayashida, Y., Katsuragawa, S., Yoshimatsu, Y., Hamamura, T., Anai, K., Ueno, M., Yamaga, S., Ueda, I., Terasawa, T., Fujisaki, A., Chihara, C., Miyagi, T., Aoki, T., Korogi, Y.: The effect of deep convolutional neural networks on radiologists' performance in the detection of hip fractures on digital pelvic radiographs. Eur. J. Radiol. **130**, 109188 (2020)
10. Naylor, C.: On the prospects for a (deep) learning health care system. JAMA **320**, 1099–1100 (2018). https://doi.org/10.1001/jama.2018.11103
11. Yang, S., Yin, B., Cao, W., Feng, C., Fan, G., He, S.: Diagnostic accuracy of deep learning in orthopaedic fractures: a systematic review and meta-analysis. Clin. Radiol. (2020). https://doi.org/10.1007/s11517-018-1915-z
12. Kalmet, P.H.S., Sanduleanu, S., Primakov, S., Guangyao, W., Jochems, A., Refaee, T., Ibrahim, A., Hulst, L.V., Hulst, P.L., Poeze, M.: Deep learning in fracture detection: a narrative review. Acta Orthop. **91**(2), 215–220 (2020). https://doi.org/10.1080/17453674.2019.1711323
13. https://towardsdatascience.com/the-w3h-of-alexnet-vggnet-resnet-and-inception-7baaaecccc96#:~:text=AlexNet%20and%20ResNet%2D152%2C%20both,training%20time%20and%20energy%20required
14. MATLAB/SIMULINK 7.6
15. Minai, F., et al.: Metaheuristics paradigms for renewable energy systems: advances in optimization algorithms. In: Springer Nature Book: Metaheuristic and Evolutionary Computation: Algorithms and Applications, Under Book Series Studies in Computational Intelligence (2020). https://doi.org/10.1007/978-981-15-7571-6_2
16. Iqbal, A., et al.: Metaheurestic algorithm based hybrid model for identification of building sale prices. In: Springer Nature Book: Metaheuristic and Evolutionary Computation: Algorithms and Applications, under book series "Studies in Computational Intelligence (2020). https://doi.org/10.1007/978-981-15-7571-6_32

Artificial Intelligence: Its Role in Diagnosis and Monitoring Against COVID-19

Vinay Kumar Reddy Chimmula, Lei Zhang, and Abhinay Kumar

Abstract Around December 2019, several pneumonia cases started to emerge from Wuhan, and later, it was known as COVID-19. Soon it spread all over china within few weeks, and by March 2020, it is labeled as global pandemic. Both SARS and COVID-19 outbreaks are from coronavirus and have no proper treatments or vaccines. The major difference between these outbreaks is that we have better Artificial Intelligence (AI) systems than we had 17 years ago during SARS. As of this writing, COVID-19 has infected around 5,401,222 people around the world with 343,800 fatalities. Since December 2019, the number of infections is increasing exponentially, and several attempts have been made to battle against the virus. The data collected from various resources are used to train the model and deployed on exclusive real-time tasks to help health care works and policy makers. However, we cannot restore human brain with an AI system. Within a short period of time, AI has been applied to a wide range of applications to fight against COVID-19, and in this chapter, we aim to review the recent successes. Lastly, after introducing different applications, we underline the common problems and limitations of the AI systems in COVID-19. In this short communication, we discussed the presence of AI to combat against the novel COVID-19 and its limitations.

Keywords Artificial intelligence · COVID-19 · Deep learning · Forecasting

V. K. R. Chimmula (✉) · L. Zhang
Electronics Systems Engineering, University of Regina, Regina, SK S4S 0A7, Canada
e-mail: vinayreddy911@gmail.com

L. Zhang
e-mail: lei.zhang@uregina.ca

A. Kumar
Electronics Engineering, Sreenidhi Institute of Science & Technology—SNIST, Hyderabad, India
e-mail: abhinayreddy2409@gmail.com

© The Author(s), under exclusive license to Springer Nature Singapore Pte Ltd. 2021   147
H. Malik et al. (eds.), *AI and Machine Learning Paradigms for Health Monitoring System*, Studies in Big Data 86,
https://doi.org/10.1007/978-981-33-4412-9_8

1 Introduction

In order to build effective AI systems, high-quality and reliable datasets are required. People around the world can access high-speed Internet through smartphones, and it is now one of the primary sources of COVID-19 information. Systems that are trained on such high-quality data reduce the load on healthcare professionals by speeding up the identification and tracking COVID-19.

Forecasting models considers several parameters or features to predict the transmission dynamics, and these models can assist governments while allocating medical supplies. Several models have been proposed and published since the outbreak ranging from statistical rule-based approaches to deep neural networks.

In the following section, we present the various AI platforms for COVID-19 and outline the standard machine learning (ML) and deep learning (DL) models that are being used to identify, segment, forecast, and monitor the outbreak. Lastly, we discussed the difficulties and limitations facing by the existing systems. Through this review, we anticipate to offer the enlightenment for biological and epidemiological researchers. In this chapter, we have reviewed the latest research methods until May 24, 2020.

Around December 2019, several pneumonia cases started to emerge from Wuhan, and later it was known as COVID-19. Soon, it spread all over china within few weeks, and by March 2020, it is labeled as global pandemic. Both SARS and COVID-19 outbreaks are from coronavirus and have no proper treatments or vaccines. The major difference between these outbreaks is that we have better AI systems than we had 17 years ago during SARS. As of this writing, COVID-19 has infected around 5,401,222 people around the world with 343,800 fatalities. Since December 2019, the number of infections is increasing exponentially, and several attempts have been made to battle against the virus. The data collected from various resources is used to train the model and deployed on exclusive real-time tasks to help healthcare works and policy makers. However, we cannot restore human brain with an AI system. Within a short period of time, AI has been applied to a wide range of applications to fight against COVID-19, and in this chapter, we aim to review the recent successes. Lastly, after introducing different applications, we underline the common problems and limitations of the AI systems in COVID-19. In this short communication, we discussed the presence of AI to combat against the novel COVID-19 and its limitations. Moreover, some AI has few drawbacks as mentioned in [1–4] (Fig. 1).

2 Artificial Intelligence in COVID-19

2.1 Medical Imaging

At present, nucleic acid test is widely used diagnostic method, and due to exponential increase of cases, there is shortage of testing kits. In order to overcome the shortage

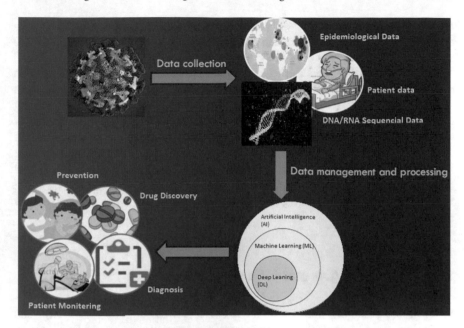

Fig. 1 Visual representation of different steps associated before deploying AI

of reagents, it is required to execute a possible alternative to classify infected people. Clinical examinations showed that majority of the COVID-19 infected people are suffering with lung infection. Most effective ways to determine lung infections is either by CT scan or X-ray.

As the total number of infections are increasing exponentially, physical severity evaluation is getting laborious and leading toward delayed diagnosis. When a fast diagnosis is required, CT scans of lungs are one of the quickest ways to detect the traces of coronavirus. If CT scans are manually inspected by medical practitioners, it would take a lot of time for inspecting each scan manually. While patients are waiting for scan results, they could infect the disease to other patients and medical staff around them. In contrast, computer vision (CV)-based systems can take less than 10 s to read an image. By integrating DL methods with real-time CT scans, we can automate the COVID-19 evaluations. Through this method, we can witness least contact exposure with patients and also ensures the safety of radiology technicians.

In the process of CT scan-based diagnosis, first a pre-scan arrangement is made before obtaining scan and finally its inspection for diagnosis. Most of the recent CT systems are provided with high-quality cameras to enable contactless diagnosis. In order to train the network to classify the COVID-19 from healthy person, a convolutional neural network (CNN) is trained on pre-labeled dataset. This method of training is called supervised learning setup. Now, the trained networks are fed with CT images to make real-time classification. However, with the limited training data, it is difficult to train the network. To overcome this issue, researchers in [5] used transfer learning techniques by fine tuning the pre-trained network. A Bayesian network trained using transfer learning achieved 92% classification accuracy. In [6], three CNN models are trained on multiple datasets, and among three networks, ResNet50 architecture achieved highest accuracy of 98%. Similarly, in [7], a ResNet architecture was used classify COVID-19 patients from a sample of 1078 X-ray images where 70 of them are infected and 1008 are healthy subjects. In addition to classification, researchers in [7] detected anomalies in the data to improve the classification accuracy. Wang and Wong in [8] proposed a novel architecture called COVID-Net tailored to classify COVID-19 from healthy and other bacterial pneumonia and achieved 83.5% accuracy. Even though the accuracy of Wang et al. is low, it is worth noting that, they classified COVID-19 pneumonia from bacterial pneumonia which is hard and difficult. An RF model in [9] predicted the severity with 87.5% accuracy and stated that attributes collected from right lungs are more important while making severity assessments.

2.2 Textual Analysis and Virtual Assistants

In the globalization era, misinformation is considered as similar threat of virus and can intervene health strategies and can cause dangerous consequences. For instance, conspiracy theories on COVID-19 are caused by 5G towers, and this misinformation led toward burning of 5G towers in UK [10]. In [11], data collected using Twitter showed the direct correlation between number of tweets and spread of virus at a particular country. Sear et al. used ML models to quantify the online discussions of antivaccination groups and spread of misinformation [12]. A latent dialect allocation (LDA) is used in [12] to identify the conversations around vaccines and provided the solid foundation to trace out the online misinformation without human intervention.

As the current pandemic progressing day by day, several countries have started dedicated hotline numbers to pre-screen COVID-19 infections. However, these networks are flooded with several people and resulting hours of waiting and in some cases, people are unable to reach these hotlines. In [13], authors proposed a digital health assistant to classify 20,000 plus diseases with more than 90% confidence. Trained using natural language processing (NLP) techniques, "Symptoma" can classify COVID-19 with 96.3% accuracy based on multiple questionnaires.

2.3 Drug Discovery

Several researchers are now attempting to find a new mixture targeting COVID-19. In [14], different models were developed to compile protein structures, ligands, and nature of protein molecules as model inputs. Each input feature is further processed through advanced deep learning (DL) algorithms like generative autoencoders [15]. Furthermore, in [14] researchers explored the reward-based AI system called reinforcement learning (RL). Such reward-based learning takes lot of computational resources but gives fruitful outcomes [16]. In [17], a crucial antiviral enzyme called 3C protease was analyzed using Q-learning network to predict crucial sequence of the compound that can attack SARS-CoV-2 virus. Using Q-network, they were able to find 47 new compounds that have potential to use as drugs against current virus. One of the main advantages of using AI in drug research is that with in short period of time, DL networks can find multiple sequences or compounds targeting viral protein sequences.

Similarly, in [18] a generative language model, where it treats protein sequences as characters. The objective function this model is to predict the next variable of protein sequence. The model was trained on 1.6 million atoms from ChEMBL database [19], and by using transfer learning, the network is trained on protease data. Combinations developed by primary networks will be filtered by several subnetworks to result a few possible combinations for testing. After final filtering, Bung et al. came up with 31 potential compounds out of which aurantiamide was proposed for clinical trials.

2.4 Modeling COVID-19 Outbreak

Outbreak modeling and simulations can assist to minimize the impact of COVID-19 in many ways [20]. For instance, precise forecasting model can help in planning and distributing of medical resources like masks and personal-protective equipment (PPE), and could assist while making policy changes. Several forecasting models have been proposed since the outbreak to predict the future cases. Forecasting models are classified into three categories, i.e., epidemiological models, statistical approaches, and deep learning methods. In traditional epidemiological models [21–24], forecasting is made by making several assumptions, and these models do not include the temporal components while forecasting. In statistical model-based predictions, temporal components are included yet, several parameter assumptions are made to estimate the parameters [25, 26]. Deep learning models such as long short-term memory networks (LSTMS) [27, 28] predicted future cases with better accuracies. LSTMs are inherently good at capturing time-series patterns and can be modeled without any assumptions. Each forecasting model has its own advantages, so it is recommended to implement different models to answer diverse questions. By looking into different predictions, underlying uncertainties can be estimated to aid policy makers decisions.

2.5 Data and Privacy

In the process of tracing infected patients, several existing methods should be read-dressed. For example, navigation history of infected person is important to trace out the infections; however, such data should not be shared with public. Sharing the traveling history with public is fundamental breach of privacy in many countries.

So, instead of sharing the exact location, a granular data should be shared. In addition to the above concerns, several concerns could be raised by public about lack of during the outbreak situation, and such issues should be addressed by making privacy guidelines.

Sharing data of COVID-19 infected people within research community, clinical experts and government policy makers help to curb the growth of highly contagious COVID-19. By integrating various datasets into a single system can help health departments to automate overall procedures. At this moment, entire world is going through a massive outbreak, and it is a legitimate cause to gather and distribute the data. Once after this pandemic end, a robust legal regulation should be implemented to promote personal privacy of people and also to prevent data misuse. Every country can develop its own laws based on their interests; however, an information should balance between tests, tracking, and self-isolating people while addressing privacy disputes.

3 Conclusion

It is clear that AI has huge impact on healthcare especially in fighting against COVID-19. As we are witnessing a rapid growth of infections every day, the data sources of current outbreak are also increasing. With more and more data, systems can learn to represent the data efficiently to make predictions. In the current situation, AI has been integrated as a part of system to combat against the current COVID-19 outbreak. However, a cautious stand should be taken between data privacy and public health regulations while collecting user data. Meanwhile, in the current pandemic situation, it is unlikely to address them because the data collected from infected persons can save lives and can restrict the economic destructions.

References

1. Iqbal, A., et al.: Big-data analytics based energy analysis and monitoring for multi-story hospital buildings: case study. In: Springer Nature Book: Soft Computing in Condition Monitoring and Diagnostics of Electrical and Mechanical Systems, pp. 325–343 (2019). https://doi.org/10.1007/978-981-15-1532-3_14
2. Faiz Minai, A., et al.: Metaheuristics paradigms for renewable energy systems: advances in optimization algorithms. In: Springer Nature Book: Metaheuristic and Evolutionary Computation: Algorithms and Applications. Studies in Computational Intelligence (2020). https://doi.org/10.1007/978-981-15-7571-6_2
3. Iqbal, A., et al.: Metaheurestic algorithm based hybrid model for identification of building sale prices. In: Springer Nature Book: Metaheuristic and Evolutionary Computation: Algorithms and Applications. Studies in Computational Intelligence (2020). https://doi.org/10.1007/978-981-15-7571-6_32
4. Chimmula, V.K.R., et al.: Novel application of relief algorithm in cascade ANN model for prognosis of photovoltaic maximum power under sunny outdoor condition of Sikkim India: a

case study. In: Springer Nature Book: Soft Computing in Condition Monitoring and Diagnostics of Electrical and Mechanical Systems, pp. 387–405 (2019). https://doi.org/10.1007/978-981-15-1532-3_17

5. Ghoshal, B., Tucker, A.:Estimating uncertainty and interpretability in deep learning for coronavirus (COVID-19) detection (2020).arXiv preprint arXiv:2003.10769
6. Narin, A., Kaya, C., Pamuk, Z.:Automatic detection of coronavirus disease (covid-19) using x-ray images and deep convolutional neural networks (2020).arXiv preprint arXiv:2003.10849
7. Zhang, J., Xie, Y., Li, Y., Shen, C., Xia, Y.:Covid-19 screening on chest X-ray images using deep learning based anomaly detection (2020).arXiv preprint arXiv:2003.12338
8. Wang, L., Wong, A.:COVID-Net: a tailored deep convolutional neural network design for detection of COVID-19 cases from chest radiography images (2020).arXiv preprint arXiv: 2003.09871
9. Tang, Z., Zhao, W., Xie, X., Zhong, Z., Shi, F., Liu, J., Shen, D.:Severity assessment of coronavirus disease 2019 (COVID-19) using quantitative features from chest CT images (2020).arXiv preprint arXiv:2003.11988
10. Ahmed, W., Vidal-Alaball, J., Downing, J., Seguí, F.L.:Dangerous messages or satire? Analysing the conspiracy theory linking 5G to covid-19 through social network analysis.J. Med. Internet Res. (2020)
11. Singh, L., Bansal, S., Bode, L., Budak, C., Chi, G., Kawintiranon, K., Padden, C., Vanarsdall, R., Vraga, E., Wang, Y.:A first look at COVID-19 information and misinformation sharing on Twitter (2020).arXiv preprint arXiv:2003.13907
12. Sear, R.F., Velásquez, N., Leahy, R., Johnson Restrepo, N., El Oud, S., Gabriel, N., Lupu, Y., Johnson, N.F.:Quantifying COVID-19 content in the online health opinion war using machine learning (2020).IEEE Access
13. Martin, A., Nateqi, J., Gruarin, S., Munsch, N., Abdarahmane, I., Knapp, B.:An artificial intelligence-based first-line defence against COVID-19: digitally screening citizens for risks via a chatbot (2020).bioRxiv
14. Zhavoronkov, A., Aladinskiy, V., Zhebrak, A., Zagribelnyy, B., Terentiev, V., Bezrukov, D.S., Polykovskiy, D., et al.Potential COVID-2019 3C-like protease inhibitors designed using generative deep learning approaches.Insilico Medicine Hong Kong Ltd. A 307: E1 (2020)
15. Blaschke, T., Olivecrona, M., Engkvist, O., Bajorath, J., Chen, H.: Application of generative autoencoder in de novo molecular design. Mol. Inform. 37(1–2), 1700123 (2018)
16. Benhenda, M. (2017).ChemGAN challenge for drug discovery: can AI reproduce natural chemical diversity? (2017).arXiv preprint arXiv:1708.08227
17. Tang, B., He, F., Liu, D., Fang, M., Wu, Z., Xu, D.:AI-aided design of novel targeted covalent inhibitors against SARS-CoV-2 (2020).bioRxiv
18. Bung, N., Krishnan, S.R., Bulusu, G., Roy, A.:De novo design of new chemical entities (NCEs) for SARS-CoV-2 using artificial intelligence(2020)
19. Gaulton, A., Bellis, L.J., Patricia Bento, A., Chambers, J., Davies, M., Hersey, A., Light, Y., et al.:ChEMBL: a large-scale bioactivity database for drug discovery.Nucleic Acids Res. 40(D1), D1100–D1107 (2012)
20. Currie, C.S.M., Fowler, J.W., Kotiadis, K., Monks, T., Onggo, B.S., Robertson, D.A., Tako, A.A.:How simulation modelling can help reduce the impact of COVID-19.J. Simul. 1–15 (2020)
21. Liu, Y., Gayle, A.A., Wilder-Smith, A., Rocklöv, J.:The reproductive number of COVID-19 is higher compared to SARS coronavirus.J. Travel Med. (2020)
22. Peng, L., Yang, W., Zhang, D., Zhuge, C., Hong, L.:Epidemic analysis of COVID-19 in China by dynamical modeling (2020).arXiv preprint arXiv:2002.06563
23. Zhang, S., Diao, M.Y., Yu, W., Pei, L., Lin, Z., Chen, D.:Estimation of the reproductive number of novel coronavirus (COVID-19) and the probable outbreak size on the Diamond Princess cruise ship: a data-driven analysis.Int. J. Infect. Dis. 93, 201–204 (2020)
24. Choi, S., Ki, M.:Estimating the reproductive number and the outbreak size of COVID-19 in Korea.Epidemiol. Health 42 (2020)

25. Ceylan, Z.:Estimation of COVID-19 prevalence in Italy, Spain, and France.Sci. Total Environ. 138817 (2020)
26. Ribeiro, M.H.D.M., da Silva, R.G., Mariani, V.C., dos Santos Coelho, L.:Short-term forecasting COVID-19 cumulative confirmed cases: perspectives for Brazil.Chaos Solitons Fractals 109853 (2020)
27. Chimmula, V.K.R., Zhang, L.:Time series forecasting of COVID-19 transmission in Canada using LSTM networks.Chaos Solitons Fractals 109864 (2020)
28. Tomar, A., Gupta, N.:Prediction for the spread of COVID-19 in India and effectiveness of preventive measures.Sci. Total Environ. 138762 (2020)

Predicting Future, Past, and Misinterpreted COVID-19 Cases Using Bidirectional LSTM Model for Proper Health Monitoring: Advances in Data Analytics

Abhinay Kumar

Abstract The first coronavirus case was reported in Hubei province of China, and within three months, it affected almost all the countries in the world. under such circumstances, World Health Organization (WHO) declared 2019 novel coronavirus as a global pandemic. Even though its fatality is low, the transmission rate makes it more dangerous. Similar to previous disease outbreaks in the human history, COVID-19 also exhibits certain transmission patterns. Mathematical models can be used to analyze these patterns and forecast the upcoming COVID-19 cases. Such forecasting methods could help governments to take further actions to stop those cases from occurring. Most of the previous studies used past infections to forecast future infections. However, they completely neglected the unreported cases while making predictions. By knowing the initially reported cases, we can understand the dynamics of the epidemic more precisely. In order to capture the transmission dynamics, we proposed a novel deep learning model called a B-LSTM (Bidirectional Long Short-Term Memory) model. In order to recalculate the past or missing infections, we applied a masking technique to our B-LSTM model. Results obtained from our model shows that end point of this pandemic in India will be around next year. However, by November the rate of infections will decrease linearly. In addition to that, we compared the forecasting accuracies of B-LSTM with statistical-based ARIMA and LSTM models.

Keywords Artificial neural networks · Deep learning · Infectious disease modeling · Time-series analysis

1 Introduction

Novel coronavirus (2019-nCoV) belongs to same family of SARS (severe acute respiratory syndrome) virus that was outbroke in south china during the period of 2002–2003 [1]. The first COVID-19 infection was reported in Hubei province of

A. Kumar (✉)
Sreenidhi Institute of Science & Technology—SNIST, Hyderabad, India
e-mail: abhinayreddy2409@gmail.com

© The Author(s), under exclusive license to Springer Nature Singapore Pte Ltd. 2021   155
H. Malik et al. (eds.), *AI and Machine Learning Paradigms for Health Monitoring System*, Studies in Big Data 86,
https://doi.org/10.1007/978-981-33-4412-9_9

China. This virus is believed to be originated from a wet market in Wuhan city. Even before scientists realized that it will spread through bodily fluids of infected persons comes in contact with the healthy person, the virus started spreading rapidly all over the world. Up until March, there were several uncertainties regarding its symptoms and incubation period. Differentiating novel coronavirus is difficult because of its symptoms are similar to that of the common flu while some patients had difficulty in breathing. The main victims of this virus are elderly people, people with less immunity power, and subjects with prior medical conditions. Despite of preventive measures like social distancing, closing public transportation, and traveling between cities, the number of infections is growing every day. However, these factors can be used as parameters while making predictions.

During initial stages of outbreak, there was no proper data available, so forecasting number of cases at the initial stages was either difficult or not possible. The quality of predictions directly depends on the data availability. While some people argued that data provided by governments are not reliable because countries tried to cover the actual infections. Absence of transparency is one of the main reasons why we were unable to stop the nCoV-19 during the early stages of its origin. Due to pressure from public health associations and media, government started to report original number of infections. In this chapter, we have analyzed the transparency of these datasets using mathematical models.

In epidemiology, mathematical models have been very helpful to model the dynamics of infectious diseases. When compared with previous pandemics, the existing mathematical model with high performance computing can forecast epidemic timing and severity, so that we can allocate resources and make decisions to improve intervention strategies. There are few models like phenomenological growth model and sub-epidemic growth model [2], where these models can be used to formulate the actual parameters of previous pandemics like SARS (2002–2003), Spanish flu (1918–1920), influenza, and Ebola. In [3], a mathematical model with logistic, Bertalanffy, and Gompertz models were used to forecast the number of infections in Wuhan. An LSTM model is used in [4] to forecast COVID-19 transmission in Canada. However, it does not used temporal components of infections. In this chapter, we proposed a novel B-LSTM architecture to predict future infections as well as previous missing or unreported cases. The results of B-LSTM model are compared with previous state-of-the-art statistical and deep learning models (Fig. 1).

2 Forecasting Models

2.1 Differential Equation Model

These models are based on differential equations and show the dynamic properties of infectious disease depending upon the properties of increasing population, occurrence of disease in the particular area, and laws of transmission in that area.

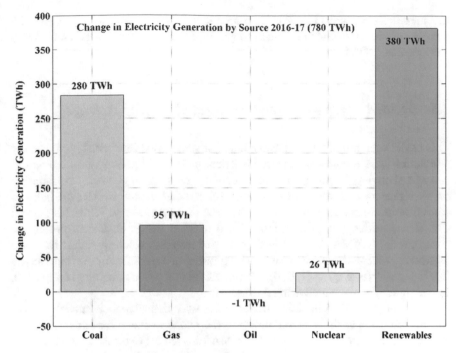

Fig. 1 Change in electricity generation in the 2016–17 [5]

Differential equation prediction model is most commonly used when age structure is considered [3]. Population of the region must be a constant in this model. The most common models that are based on these differential equations are SI (susceptible infectious), SIS (susceptible infectious susceptible), SIR (susceptible infectious recovery), and SEIR (susceptible exposed infectious recovered susceptible). The main drawback in this model is that it considers population as constant while predicting. In practice, population changes in given area because people move in and out of that area.

2.2 Statistical Time-Series Prediction Models

This model is a series of data points with separation of specific time period. In such models, data may or may not be collected with regular interval of time. These models are generally used in predicting the stock price, weather, and economics. But this model can also be used in field of epidemiology in order to predict the future spread of disease that can be used to warn public, and to alert government as well health workers to take necessary preventive measures. This model can make predictions only if the data is stationary. A data is said to be stationary if it is mean and variance are constant, and it must not exhibit any trends and seasonal properties. There are various prediction models like AR (auto-regressive), MA (moving average), ARIMA (auto-regressive integrated moving average), LSTM (long short-term memory), and bidirectional LSTM.

2.3   ARIMA (Auto Regression Integrated Moving Average)

This model was initially used in economics for stock price forecasting and whether monitoring. It is a combination two statistical models, i.e., AR (Auto Regression) and MA (Moving Average) models. AR model uses the dependency relationship between present and lagged observations. Integrated function in ARIMA helps in converting non-stationary time-series (TS) data into stationary. While MA model uses the dependency between observed and residual values obtained from lagged observations, ARIMA (p, d, q) is the standard notation where p stands for auto-regressive process, d stands for integrative process, and q stands for moving average [6]. Using AR $(p, d, q) = (1, 0, 0)$, we can model AR process, and by taking $(0, 0, 1)$, MA model can obtained using ARIMA.

Even though ARIMA model outperformed most statistical models, models that are constructed using artificial neural networks help us in realizing the expensive flaws in ARIMA. Forecasting accuracy of ARIMA was almost decreased by 30% when compared with deep learning-based LSTM networks. This could make the huge difference while forecasting rate of COVID-19 transmission. Accuracy of LSTM model can go even higher if the number of epochs is increased after each training cycle [5]. Due to the above reasons, LSTM models are widely employed for TS forecasting when compared to ARIMA.

2.4   RNN (Recurrent Neural Networks)

These models are designed to process sequential data by sharing the parameters between different layers of the network, and this enables to include past information to make predictions. Sequential memory is the key part in RNN because, it helps to store the information from previous time steps and pass to next time steps sequentially [7]. RNN has a loop which helps to flow information to move in reverse direction, and this loop is considered as hidden layer; hence, the information carried by it is also hidden. This network performs same operation on every input, and the result of the present input depends on past results. One of the main disadvantages of this RNN is vanishing or exploding gradients. When RNN computes information for present time step, the information farther from the current step diminishes. Another reason for short-term memory and vanishing gradients is due to back propagation (used to optimize and train neural networks) [8]. If tanh is used as activation function, then these networks cannot process very long sequences.

Current state equation:

$$h_t = f(h_{t-1}, x_t) \tag{1}$$

h_t is current state
h_{t-1} is previous state
x_t is input state

Formula for activation:

$$h_t = \tanh(w_{hh}h_{t-1}, w_{xh}x_t) \tag{2}$$

w_{hh} is weight of recurrent neuron
w_{xh} is weight of input neuron

Formula for output:

$$y_t = w_{hy}h_t \tag{3}$$

y_t is output
w_{hy} is weight at output layer

2.5 *LSTM (Long Short-Term Memory)*

The reason for introducing LSTM is to remove the long-term dependency problem, and this is solved by introducing a memory block. In this model, each LSTM unit is combination system module [5]. Differential storage systems of digital systems and memory blocks of LSTM have similar architecture. Vanishing gradient problem is resolved in LSTM. This model has chain-like structure, but the module which is repeating have completely different structure. LSTMs can add or remove the information from the cell state with the help of gates. There are total three gates in LSTM.

Removing the information from the cell state is done by the forget gate. Sigmoid function looks at h_t and x_t and gives a result as a number between 0 and 1, 1 represents "keep this information completely," and 0 represents "get rid of this information completely."

$$f_t = \text{sigmoid}(w_f.[h_{t-1}, x_t], b_f) \tag{4}$$

f_t Function of forget gate
w_x Coefficient of neuron at gate (x)
h_{t-1} Result from previous time step
b_x Bias of neuron at gate (x).

In the next step, we are going to add the new information to cell state. This step has two sub-steps, first input gate decides which value is to be updated, and then, tanh layer creates a new candidate value.

$$i_t = \text{sigmoid}\left(w_i.[h_{t-1}, x_t], b_i\right) \tag{5}$$

i_t Function of input gate

$$\tilde{c}_t = \tanh\left(w_c.[h_{t-1}, x_t], b_c\right)$$

$\tilde{c}_t$ Candidate value.

Finally, the output of the cell state is given by the output gate. We run the sigmoid function first, then, we run the tanh function, and finally, we multiply both tanh and sigmoid functions to get the output.

$$o_t = \text{sigmoid}\left(w_o.[h_{t-1}, x_t], b_o\right)$$

o_t Function of output gate

$$h_t = o_t * \tanh(c_t)$$

h_t Output required by us

$$c_t = f_t * c_{t-1} + i_t * \tilde{c}_t \tag{6}$$

c_t Candidate function
c_{t-1} Candidate function from previous time step.

2.6   Bidirectional LSTM (Long Short-Term Memory) and RNN

The most important reason for choosing this network is because it has no limitation on data flexibility that is input data can be accessed from both forward and backward direction. This architecture can overcome all the limitations that existed in unidirectional RNN and LSTM. This bidirectional network can also increase the computational cost by introducing dropout between the LSTM layers. Previous research on COVID-19 forecasting mainly focused on predicting upcoming COVID-19 infections and completely ignored previous or missing cases that occurred during the initial stages of pandemic. If the missing cases are as null values, LSTM model will fail to extract the sequential patters from input data. However, fitting the model with null values results the biased estimates and results overfitting LSTM network. After obtaining the initial number of missing cases, we can obtain more accurate forecasting results. Initial missing cases are obtained by using masked B-LSTM.

Bidirectional networks consist of two unidirectional networks where one of the networks takes input in the forward direction of data and other takes data from backward direction. Theoretically, these networks use all of the input data while computing future and past values [9]. Instead of conventional method where single network is split, so that half of neurons responsible for positive time direction and the other half are responsible for negative time direction [10], here we have modified the network by taking two separate networks with more number of neurons in negative time direction (reverse direction), so that predictions for the initial data are more accurate.

A special function (summation) is used to combine the final outputs of both states, so that we can get the future predictions [11]. By applying similar functions on input side, we can obtain the initial data that is date when the first COVID-19 case was reported accurately. The outputs of both forward and backward layers are calculated with the help of standard LSTM equations. To solve the missing value problem, we are going to consider $\varnothing$ as the missing value. For each x_t, the missing value which is equal to $\varnothing$ during the training process. This tth step is skipped by proceeding to the $t + 1$th step, and later, all these missing values are predicted after the algorithm is completely trained to make future and past predictions (Fig. 2).

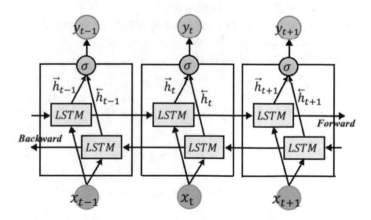

Fig. 2 Architecture of BDLSTM used for training the network

3 Architecture and Training

In this chapter, we have used two hidden layers and 97 single cell memory blocks in forward LSTM while for backward LSTM, 97 single cell memory blocks with skip connections. A target delay between 0 and 10 is applied for both forward and backward directions. Hidden layers are connected to fully connected neurons, and a logistic sigmoid is used as activation function for input with the range of [−2, 2], and Squashing function is used in the activation of output with the range of [0, 1]. Both forward and backward networks are trained with the target delay from 0 to 10. These networks can be trained with the same algorithms as that of the unidirectional algorithms because there is no connection between the forward and backward networks [10]. Any form of back propagation through time (BPTT) is not used because that would have complicated the forward and backward pass. Forward state inputs of time-series at the starting point and backward state inputs are calculated through the learning process. There are three steps in training procedure of bidirectional networks. A forward pass, during which, the network parameters of LSTM are calculated. Secondly, during backward pass, coefficients of backward LSTM are determined. Finally, the weights of both LSTM layers are updated.

Hidden state is calculated by the following equation:

$$h_t = \sigma_h(w_{rh}x_t + w_{hh}x_{t-1} + b_h) \tag{7}$$

where

σ_h is activation function of hidden state

w_{xh}, w_{hh} are weights matrices of input layer-to-hidden layer and hidden layer-to-hidden layer, respectively, and

b_h is the bias vector of hidden layer.

$$f_t = \sigma_g\left(w_f x_t + u_f h_{t-1} + b_f\right) \tag{8}$$

$$i_t = \sigma_g(w_i x_t + u_i h_{t-1} + b_i) \tag{9}$$

$$o_t = \sigma_g(w_o x_t + u_o h_{t-1} + b_o) \tag{10}$$

$$\widetilde{c}_t = \tanh(w_c x_t + u_c h_{t-1} + b_c) \tag{11}$$

$$c_t = f_t * c_{t-1} + i_t * \widetilde{c}_t \tag{12}$$

$$h_t = o_t * \tanh(c_t) \tag{13}$$

Here

σ_g	is gate activation function, and
f_t, i_t, o_t	are the forget, input, and output gates, respectively
w_x	is the weight matrix, mapping the hidden layer input to all the three gates and also to the input gate, and
b_x, c_t, h_t	are bias vector, cell output state, and layer outputs, respectively.

Forward layer output $\vec{h}$ is calculated by taking the inputs in forward direction and applying all the above equations that is through standard LSTM. In the same way, $\overleftarrow{h}$ is calculated by taking the input in the reverse direction.

The output layer vector y_t which is generated by B-LSTM is given by the equation

$$y_t = \sigma(\vec{h}, \overleftarrow{h}).$$

where σ can be any of the following function summation, multiplication conjugation, and average. After trying all the functions mentioned above, we finalized summation because it yielded low error when compared with other functions.

3.1 Data

The COVID-19 data used in this study is obtained from John Hopkins University and ICMR (Indian Council of Medical Research). The data is collected every day since February, 2020, in the time-series format. The data that we collected include number of deaths, confirmed cases, and recoveries. While training the network, temporal components of the dataset are not neglected. ADF (augmented Dickey–Fuller) [12] test has been performed on input data to check whether the data is stationary or non-stationary, and it is interpreted by using the P-value. If the value of P is in between 5 and 1%, then it does not have unit root, and such series is said to be in stationary. If the P-value is greater than 5% or 0.005 with a unit root, then it is considered as non-stationary series. The data that we used in this prediction model are stationary. We have divided the input data into three parts, i.e., training (60%), cross-validation (20%), and testing dataset (20%) (Figs. 3 and 4).

Main components of WECS are rotor (which consists of WT blades and hub), gearbox, main shaft, generator, bearing of gearbox and generator, power electronic convertors, and so on. The wind energy is arrested and converted into mechanical energy by the rotor blades, and then, the electrical generator is being driven by this mechanical energy in close aid with gearbox and main shaft connecting all the rotating bodies.

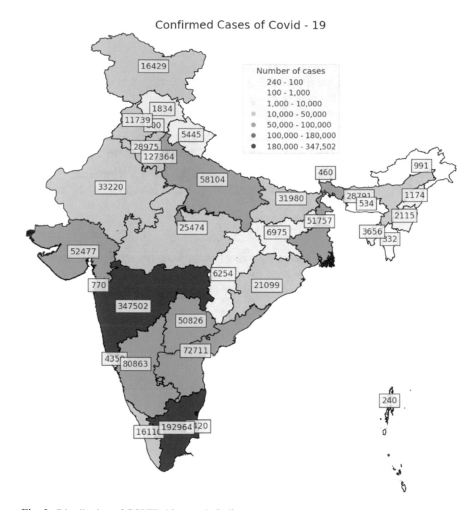

Fig. 3 Distribution of COVID-19 cases in India

4   Results and Discussion

All the previous studies on predicting the COVID-19 are primarily focused on future cases. This is the first research work to use deep learning architecture to forecast future and past missing infections of COVID-19. We also introduced the several new features which were not discussed in most of the previous studies. By finding past and missing cases, we reduced bias and increase the accuracy of predictions. We calculated missing values by analyzing trends with certain time gap between them and compared it with the present-day values. The predicted values that are obtained using our dataset are compared with the actual values, the trends are observed, and some values are flagged and considered mismatched values as missing values. We

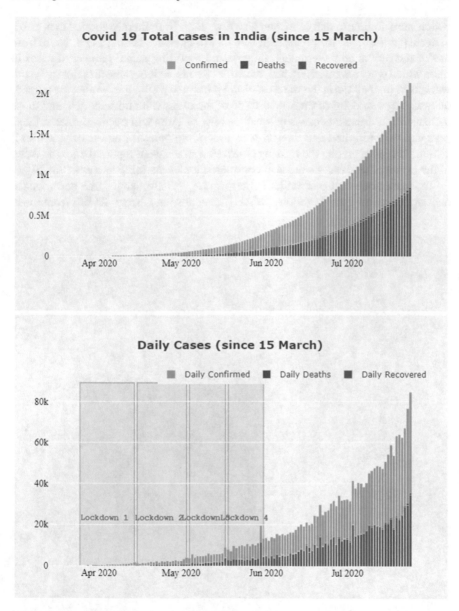

Fig. 4 Graphical representation of COVID-19 in India during different phases of lockdown

obtained graph of flagged values and located the mismatched cases of previous graph in new graph and obtained a perfect dataset for our predictions. We found our initially reported number of cases by feeding our data to LSTM in the reverse direction. The reason for predicting the past cases is, during initial stages of spread, some cases were not reported in India, due to lack of awareness and also because of the symptoms which were similar to that of flu and also few states in India misreported their cases to avoid panic among the public. But later due to intensive testing and pressure from media and public on government, they started reporting actual number of cases in India which were not matching with the initial trends, so it became difficult for health workers to treat all the at the same time, and it became difficult to predict the number of cases at given point of time. And some of the cases were not reported, and those patients left untreated because of which spread of virus will occur, and later, those case will be multiplied and directly gets added into present number of cases, so it also important to predict the missing cases. Few cases were reported after the death of the person, these cases were also considered under the missing cases (Fig. 5).

To check how well our model is performing, we are using three performance measures, and they are as follows, MAE (mean absolute error), RMSE (root mean

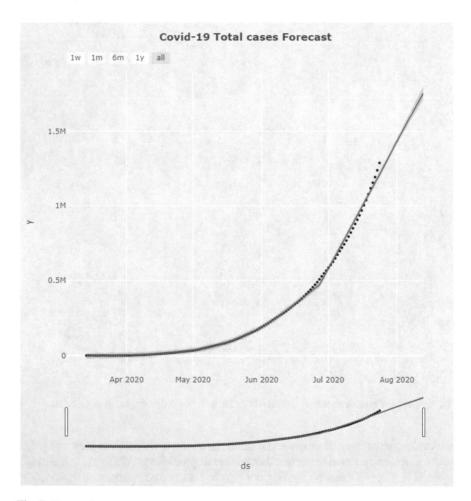

Fig. 5 Forecasting results of BDLSTM model

square error), and coefficient of determination which is represented by R^2

$$\text{MAE} = 1/n \sum_{t=0}^{n-1} |y_t - \tilde{y_t}| \tag{14}$$

$$\text{RMSE} = \sqrt{1/n \sum_{t=0}^{n-1} (y_t - \tilde{y_t})^2} \tag{15}$$

$$R^2 = 1 - \frac{1/n \sum_{t=0}^{n-1} (y_t - \tilde{y_t})^2}{1/n \sum_{t=0}^{n-1} (y_t - \overline{y_t})^2} \tag{16}$$

Here y_t is actual value, $\tilde{y_t}$ is predicted value, and $\overline{y_t}$ is the average value of predicted values. We used short-term scales to predict the next day's cases and long-term scales to predict next 30 days cases. Training and test values of our model using above performance measures are as follows:

Short-term prediction: MAE-0.00695, RMSE-0.00854, R^2-0.996.
Long-term prediction: MAE-0.05103, RMSE-0.05987, R^2-0.94.

5 Conclusion

With the help of these accurate predictions, we can alert healthcare workers and governments, so that it will be easy for them to allocate resources and to take further preventive measures. If we predicted future cases today, those cases are certain to occur and nothing can be done about those cases, unless public start taking seriously preventive measures implemented by government. As the number of cases is increasing exponentially, government needs to introduce the strict rules, so that people can stay indoors and practice social distancing. We already saw the increase in trends in exponential order from the starting of May first week, and prior to May, these trends are predicted to increase linearly. By performing simulations and data fitting with currently available data and present policies implemented by government, we have estimated that number of cases in India may reach the peak number of infections during the third week of September. In order to curb the infections, governments must introduce more strict policies, and also must increase the number of tests performed per day. No other model can give such detailed predictions of COVID-19.

References

1. Kwok, K.O., Tang, A., Wei, V.W.I., Park, W.H., Yeoh, E.K., Riley, S.:Epidemic models of contact tracing: systematic review of transmission studies of severe acute respiratory syndrome and middle east respiratory syndrome. Comput. Struct. Biotechnol. J. **17**, 186–194 (2019)
2. Roosa, K., Lee, Y., Luo, R., Kirpich, A., Rothenberg, R., Hyman, J.M., Yan, P., Chowell, G.: Short-term forecasts of the COVID-19 epidemic in Guangdong and Zhejiang, China: February 13–23, 2020. J. Clin. Med. **9**(2), 596 (2020)
3. Jia, L., Li, K., Jiang, Y., Guo, X.:Prediction and analysis of coronavirus disease 2019 (2020). arXiv preprint arXiv:2003.05447
4. Chimmula, V.K.R., Zhang, L.:Time series forecasting of COVID-19 transmission in Canada using LSTM networks.Chaos Solitons Fractals 109864 (2020)
5. Siami-Namini, S., Namin, A.S.:Forecasting economics and financial time series: ARIMA vs. LSTM.. arXiv preprint arXiv:1803.06386 (2018)
6. Brownlee, J.: Introduction to Time Series Forecasting with Python: How to Prepare Data and Develop Models to Predict the Future. Machine Learning Mastery (2017)
7. Sherstinsky, A.: Fundamentals of recurrent neural network (RNN) and long short-term memory (LSTM) network. Phys D **404**, 132306 (2020)
8. Chan, L.-W., Fallside, F.:An adaptive training algorithm for back propagation networks.Comput. Speech Lang. **2**, (3–4), 205–218 (1987)
9. Salehinejad, H., Sankar, S., Barfett, J., Colak, E., Valaee, S.:Recent advances in recurrent neural networks (2017).arXiv preprint arXiv:1801.01078
10. Schuster, M., Paliwal, K.K.: Bidirectional recurrent neural networks. IEEE Trans. Signal Process. **45**(11), 2673–2681 (1997)
11. Cui, Z., Ke, R., Pu, Z., Wang, Y..Deep bidirectional and unidirectional LSTM recurrent neural network for network-wide traffic speed prediction (2018).arXiv preprint arXiv:1801.02143
12. Cheung, Y.W., Lai, K.S.: Lag order and critical values of the augmented Dickey–Fuller test. J. Bus. Econ. Stat. **13**(3), 277–280 (1995)

Data-Driven Analysis to Identify the Role of Relational Benefit in Developing Customer Loyalty and Management: A Case Study

Asif Sanaullah

Abstract The purpose of this study was to examine the relationship of relationship benefit (confidence benefit) in developing customer loyalty. Survey methodology was used to gather data from restaurant. A sample of 200 customers and responses was collected randomly. Correlation analysis by using SPSS 20 was applied to analyze the data collected. The finding of the study revealed that confidence benefit had direct positive influence on customer loyalty. Obtained results reveals, that confidence benefit can be instrumental in developing long-lasting relationship with the service provider.

Keywords Relationship benefit (RB) · Customer loyalty (CL) · Confidence benefit (CB)

1 Introduction

The approach of relationship benefit in marketing literature has been used extensively by the researcher [1]. To measure the outcome of customer behavior, relationship benefit has been used. In service industry, loyalty of customer is positively associated with relational benefit. Furthermore, these benefit led organizations to double their revenue through customer loyalty [2].

In this hyper-competitive era in service industry, companies tend to retain loyal customer because of economic viability. According to Richeld and Sasser [3], loyal customer will pay additional amount to stay in relationship with organization because of the benefits. Additionally Henning-Thurau [1] suggested that these benefits are considered as antecedents of satisfaction and repurchase intentions in service industry.

A. Sanaullah (✉)
Department of Business Management, UNiSZA, Kuala Terengganu, Malaysia
e-mail: asifbaltee@gmail.com

Department of Business Management, Karakoram International University, Gilgit-Baltistan, Pakistan

© The Author(s), under exclusive license to Springer Nature Singapore Pte Ltd. 2021   169
H. Malik et al. (eds.), *AI and Machine Learning Paradigms for Health Monitoring System*, Studies in Big Data 86,
https://doi.org/10.1007/978-981-33-4412-9_10

Elements like loyalty, positive word of mouth, price insensitivity, complaints behavior, and bad word of mouth are the outcome of relationship between organization and customer. These outcomes are directly linked with the success and failure of any organization [4]. Researches carried out on relationship benefit mainly focused on the reason of success and failure of relationship between organization and customer [5, 6].

Consumer perception regarding relational benefit varies with respect to the type of product and service. In services like restaurant, customers are more toward getting relational benefits than other services [7]. In fact, Henning-Thurau [1] confirmed this positive association between confidence benefit and repurchase intentions. Customer bears opportunity cost of forgoing other service provider in anticipation of getting relational benefits from the preferred service provider, and this helps in fostering committed relationship with service provider [8].

Loyalty is one of the most important and wanted behavior of a customer for organization. Companies indulge themselves in a relationship with customers to get maximum benefit in terms of monetary benefit [8]. In service industry, companies are offering different benefits to customers in order to get competitive advantage [9]. Empirical research proves that benefits are strongly associated with loyalty behavior of customers [1].

Number of researchers attempted to identify the relationship among relational benefit and loyalty outcomes like positive word of mouth and repurchase intentions [5, 6]. However, there is a lack of study in the context of restaurant industry in Pakistan. All the previous results in this context are with some limitation and specifications, so to fill the gap this research attempts to find out the impact of confidence benefit on repurchase intention in restaurant industry.

This chapter is organized into four sections, which have some sections. Section 1 describes the introduction part of the study which motivates the researchers to do so. Section 2 represents the brief state of the art of the related work, which includes the confidence benefits, customer loyalty, and theoretical framework. Research methodology used in this study has been represented in Sect. 3. Finally, conclusion and recommendation have been presented in Sect. 4.

2 Literature Review

2.1 Confidence Benefits

Confidence benefit is favorable state of mind toward any object which could be any organization, person, or anything that led to develop trust and confidence at touch points [5]. In creating a loyal and committed customer, confidence benefit plays a very important role. Confidence benefit helps in reducing psychological cost associated with service industry [1].

2.2 Customer Loyalty

Customer loyalty has been termed as "a deeply held commitment to rebuy or repatronize a product or service consistently in the future, despite situational influences and marketing efforts having the potential to cause switching behavior" [10]. Oliver [10] describes four stages of customer loyalty beginning with belief or cognitive sense. The second stage is affective sense in which consumer satisfaction level after repeat purchase use to be increasing. Third stage is referred as cognitive stage which depicts behavioral commitment toward service provider. The last and the fourth stage of customer loyalty is action. In this stage, irrespective of different competitors' offers or price increase by the firm customer remains stick to its service provider.

Customer loyalty can also be defined as a positive attitude toward any organization or brand. In marketing, customer loyalty usually judged on two levels behavioral and attitudinal. Behavioral aspect covers customer actions like repurchase and positive word of mouth. Loyalty of customers tends to communicate offering of service provider in a more but influential way.

2.3 Theoretical Framework

The benefits will help customer in a service setting to minimize the distress and improve comfort with the organization as well as to diminish risk and enhance knowledge of service expectation, confidence benefit helps customer in increasing relationship efficiency through decreasing transactional cost [1, 11].

Confidence of having minimum risk is the ultimate essence of relationship [12]. Consumer may also get benefit by getting closer to employees and developing good relations with employees [13]. With the passage of time in a relationship, customer can get financial and customized benefits through the relationship [5].

The factor which drives customers to repurchase a service remained in shadow for long. It has been proved in research [14], that to strengthen customer behavior to repurchase firm should provide relationship benefit. Specifically, Dagger et al. [14] suggested that service manager must ensure that customer should feel minimal risk and maximum comfort while using service.

Lee et al. [15] showed that relation benefit affects customer loyalty positively. According to them, relationship benefit is significantly related to customer loyalty. To get consequences like loyalty, repurchase intention and positive word of mouth for a firm can be possible through providing relational benefit to their customer. Impact of relationship benefits observed to have the highest effect in getting positive consequences. Customer and Service Provider Relationships.

The length of relationship does effect on the output of relation benefits provided by the service provider. Impact of relational benefit on customer is greater on a long-term customer than that of a novice customer. On consequences like loyalty impact of confidence benefit is greatest on novice customer's mind [16].

Customer relationship management supposed to be different with respect to cultural context based on different dimensions of culture. The amount of similarity in results across to two different cultures, i.e., east and west regarding relationship benefit found to be identical and replicable [8].

Understanding the role of relationship benefit on service quality, i.e., technical and functional quality is another dimension. Impact of benefits varies on the perception of service quality, and relational benefits are positively associated with perception of both functional and technical quality aspect of service. Confidence benefit is more objective oriented in diminishing risk [5].

Relationship benefit has been consistently associated positively with consequences like showing loyal behavior, positive word of mouth, and commitment by customer [1, 5]. Prior studies found that confidence benefit is associated with positive effects like loyalty and satisfaction in face-to-face encounter services [1, 5]. Yen and Gwinner [17] confirm these findings that relationship benefits in online transaction but with weaker effect than that of face-to-face encounters. The absence of physical infrastructure (Internet transactions) and its impact on relationship building has been discussed by Colgate et al. [12]; its impact varies with respect to the perception of customer. Some consider physical contact with service provider as important source for being in long-lasting relationship and some argued that convenience in Internet transaction drive them to be in relationship with the service provider. Nevertheless most of the Internet banking satisfied user extract relational benefit from the physical existence of bank. Initially, Gwinner [2], relational dimension were tested in a qualitative research for Internet-based relationship benefit for a bank. However, later on they found new relational dimension in Internet context.

As the literature suggested, the impact of relationship benefit has mainly revolved around the service settings [1, 8, 12]. Customization characteristics of service help us to understand the impact of such functional and emotional benefits in getting positive outcomes for a service firm.

However, researches on business like commercial distribution of goods regarding relationship benefit depict almost same the result. Impact of confidence benefit in a business setting like commercial distribution on getting consequences like satisfaction is greatest than that of others. Relationship benefits are important and source of satisfaction in physical distribution business as it is important in other intangible business [18].

Research setting by Dimitriafis [19] included new dimension of trust-related benefits of competence, benevolence along with special treatment, social and convenience as the driver construct in getting satisfaction and positive outcome behaviors like word of mouth, intention to continue, and cross-buying in retail banking service. In this setting, convenience benefit has been included as a distinct item, although convenience has been used as benefit measure but not as distinct measure [5, 6]. Convenience benefit has been referred as convenient repeat interaction of customer and service provider. Like in previous research findings [1], among the all previous benefits classified by Gwinner [5], confidence benefit came up as the strongest driver of positive outcomes for a company.

In consistent with previous research, Dimitriafis [19] confirmed that confidence benefit influences satisfaction and loyalty. Interestingly, the new trust-related dimension of benefits competence (includes predictability) and convenience confirms its association and impact on satisfaction in banking setup. Finally, result revealed that among the operationalized concept of trust-based relationship benefit, competence benefit offered by bank enhanced customer satisfaction. Furthermore, the study aligning with previous studies of [1, 6, 7] found that satisfaction act as mediator in relationship between relationship benefit and positive outcomes. Contradictory to the findings of Henning-Thurau et al. [1] the finding showed no direct relationship between relationship benefit and positive outcomes like positive word of mouth, strong relationship for banking industries.

According to Henning-Thurau [1] confidence benefit is instrumental in developing loyal customer in service industries. Relationship benefit increases relationship competence by minimizing the cost associated in using services. The above discussion suggested that through confidence benefit service can earn behavioral as well as loyalty from their customer. In this case, we formally develop hypothesis that,

H1 (a): confidence benefit has positive and significant impact on customer loyalty.

3   Research Methodology

This research work is designed to examine the role of relationship benefit in developing loyalty in customer of restaurants. The nature of study is hypothesis testing. Due to natural environment and had less control, this study is carried out in non-contrived environment. Because of the environment researcher interference was minimal. Data has been collected through using instrument and at once.

Service organizations of high contact customized personal service category include the restaurants. Restaurants used in this research are Bar.B.Q tonight, Chaye Khana, Loshey Restaurant, Jahangir Balti, Cave Inn, Kabuli Restaurant, Nadia Restaurant, Savour, Lahore Restaurant, and Data Kabana.

Participants were selected based on non-probability/convenience sampling from the restaurants. The reason for using customer from restaurants as sample is to measure the level of customer loyalty through confidence benefits that the data was collected randomly from more than 350 customers of above-mentioned groups, while after scrutiny only two hundred customer's response has been analyzed.

Confidence benefit scale was used as measuring instrument, used by Gwinner et al. [1]. To measure customer loyalty, instrument by Zeithaml et al. [20] has been used. Seven-point Likert scale is used to measure the constructs. According to Fullerton [27], all the scales fulfill Nunnally and Bernstein [21] requirement by having Cronbach alpha greater than 0.80.

Data was analyzed through descriptive statistics and correlation by using SPSS. The role of confidence benefit in developing loyalty behavior in restaurant industry was the basic aim of the study. The analyses are conducted on the response of

200 customers collected from different restaurants, although some advance data processing techniques are presented in [22–26] (Fig. 1).

Table 1 depicts the demographic statistic of study. Demographic variable consists of gender and marital. Table 1 shows statistic of frequency and percentage of demographic variables.

The above descriptive statistic table reveals the value and standard deviation. Using mean value response, positions can be identified. Mean value of confidence benefit and customer loyalty are, respectively, 4.7121 and 4.641 and standard deviation are 1.33886 and 1.43043 based on 200 responses (Table 2).

Fig. 1 Approach used in this study

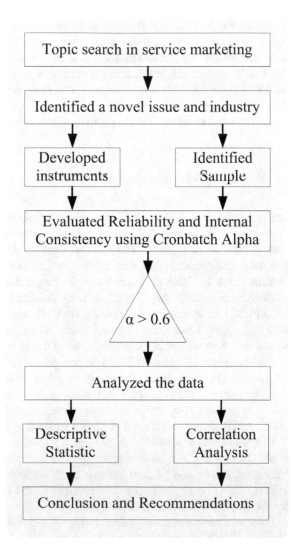

Table 1 Demographic variable

Demographic variables	Groups	Frequency	Percentage (%)
Gender	Male	98	49
	Female	102	51
	Total	200	100
Marital status	Single	78	39
	Married	122	61
	Total	200	100

Table 2 Descriptive statistics

Measures	Confidence benefit	Customer loyalty
Mean	4.7121	4.6414
Std. deviation	1.33886	1.43043
Minimum	1.25	1.00
Maximum	6.75	7.00

Cronbatch alpha (α) is the most acceptable, widely, and frequently used key to measure the reliability of items of the variables [28]. Instruments having $\alpha \geq .7$ are considered as fit to use for measuring a construct. It indicates the consistency in responses with the items proposed.

The range of construct used in this study suggested by the analysis is useable. Table 3 depicts that instrument used in this study to measure constructs is reliable. The internal consistency and reliability of items in this study are 0.824 and 0.712. That shows that instruments are fit to use in measuring confidence benefit and customer loyalty.

The result of correlation indicates that confidence benefits and purchase intention are positive associated and this association is also statistically significance. Correlation among variables is displayed. This correlation analysis is applied to evaluate the strength and path among independent and dependent variable. Table 4 revealed that confidence benefit is strongly associated and an antecedent of customer loyalty, as the details mentioned in the table depicts that confidence benefit has a strong impact on customer loyalty ($r = 0.919**, p < 0.01$). The result showed significant positive relationship among the constructs. This reveals that loyalty of customer is outcome

Table 3 Reliability analysis

Variables	No. of items	Alpha coefficient
Confidence benefit	04	0.82
Customer loyalty	12	0.71
Total	16	–

Table 4 Correlation analysis

Correlations test			
Measures		Confidence benefit	Customer loyalty
Confidence_benefit	Pearson's correlation	1	0.919[**]
	Sig. (2-tailed)		0.000
	N	99	99
Purchase intention	Pearson's correlation	0.919[**]	1
	Sig. (2-tailed)	0.000	
	N	99	99

** Correlation is significant at the 0.01 level (2-tailed)

of relational benefit customer received during transaction. Positive and strong correlation of 0.919** is found between confidence benefit with customer loyalty. That led us to accept the assumption established.

4 Conclusion and Recommendation

Purpose of the study was to analyze the relationship of relational benefit in terms of confidence on loyalty behavior of customer. The study was conducted by taking the customers of restaurants. The sample was taken randomly. Study revealed that confidence benefit has significant positive impact in building loyalty among the customer. In the contemporary era when customer became savvier, it is very important for organizations to build loyalty among their customers. This study revealed the fact that irrespective of nature of business in service industry, customer gets attracted toward service providers who offer them more benefit. In pertinent to previous research, it has also been proved that customers who are enjoying relational benefit from the service provider are more affectively committed to the service providers. So, we can conclude that customers who were satisfied with the relational benefits offered by the service provider are more committed and obliged to stay for long period of time with the company. When a customer enjoys relational benefit from the service provider, company gave more attention, dedication, and time to the customers and in return service provider attempts to have committed and loyal customers for their own benefit. This study is based on relationship benefit (confidence benefit), and customer loyalty model is designed with the aim to generalize the result in different service settings but there are hurdles in this study. The research will be carried out in a particular demographic setting, so the finding will remain stick to this very cultural context and generalizability will remain an issue. The number of service organization in our cultural context is numerous and to select all of them in our study is near to impossible so it is beyond the scope of this study.

References

1. Henning-Thurau, T., Gwinner, K.P., Gremler, D.D.: Understanding relationship marketing outcomes: an integration of relational benefits and relationship quality. J. Serv. Res. **4**(3), 230–247 (2002)
2. Hennig-Thurau, T., Klee, A.: The impact of customer satisfaction and relationship quality on customer retention: a critical reassessment and model development. Psychol. Mark. **14**, 737–764 (1997)
3. Reichheld, F.F, Sasser, W.E.: Zero defections: quality comes to services. Harvard Bus. Rev. 68(September-October), 105-111 (1990)
4. Szczepanska, K., Gawron, P.P.: Changes in approach to customer loyalty. J. Contemp. Econ. **5**(1), 60–69 (2011)
5. Gwinner, K.P., Gremler, D.D., Bitner, M.J.: Relational benefits in services industries: the customer's perspective. J. Acad. Mark. Sci. **26**(2), 101–114 (1998)
6. Reynolds, K.E., Beatty, S.: Customer benefits and company consequences of customer-salesperson relationships in retailing. J. Retail. **75**(1), 11–32 (1999) (users', European Journal of Marketing, 44(9/10): 1528–1552)
7. Kinard, B., Capella, M.: Relationship marketing: the influence of consumer involvement on perceived service benefits. J. Serv. Mark. **20**(6), 359–368 (2006)
8. Patterson, P.G., Smith, T.: Relationship benefits in service industries: a replication in a southeast asian context. J. Serv. Mark. **15**(6), 425–433 (2001)
9. Verhoef, P., Franses, P., Hoekstra, J.: The effect of relational constructs on customer referrals and number of services purchased from a multiservice provider: does age of relationship matter. J. Acad. Mark. Sci. **30**(3), 202–216 (2002)
10. Oliver, R.L.: Satisfaction: A Behavioral Perspective on the Consumer. McGraw-Hill, New York, NY (1997)
11. Bitner, M.J.: Building service relationships: it's all about promises. J. Acad. Mark. Sci. **23**(4), 246–251 (1995)
12. Colgate, M., Buchanan-Oliver, M., Elmsly, R.: Relationship benefits in an internet environment. Managing Serv. Qual. **15**(5), 426–436 (2005)
13. Berry L.L.: Relationship marketing of services—growing interest, emerging perspectives benefits, satisfaction, trust, commitment and loyalty for novice and experienced service. J. Acad. Mark. Sci. 236–245 (1995)
14. Dagger, T.S., David, M.E., Sandy, N.: Do relationship benefits and maintenance drive commitment and loyalty. J. Serv. Mark. **25**(4), 273–281 (2011)
15. Lee, H.Y., Ahn, S.J., Yang, I.S.: Case study of menu satisfaction index in business & industry food service. J. Korean Soc. Food Sci. Nutr. **37**(11), 1443–1451 (2008)
16. Dagger, T.C., O'Brien, T.K.: Does experience matter? Differences in relationship (2010)
17. Yen, H.J., Gwinner, K.: Internet retail customer loyalty: the mediating role of relational benefits. Int. J. Serv. Ind. Manag. **14**, 483–500 (2003)
18. Martín Consuegra, D., Molina, A., Esteban, Á.: An integrated model of price, satisfaction and loyalty: an empirical analysis in the service sector. J. Prod. Brand Manage. **16**(7), 459–468 (2007)
19. Dimitriadis, S.: Testing perceived relational benefits as satisfaction and behavioral outcomes drivers. Int. J. Bank Mark **28**(4), 297–313 (2010)
20. Zeithaml, V.A., Berry, L.L., Parasuraman, A.: The behavioral consequences of service quality. J. Mark. **60**, 31–46 (1996)
21. Nunnally, J.C., Bernstein, I.H.: The assessment of reliability. Psychom. Theor. **3**, 248–292 (1994)
22. Iqbal, A., et al.: Metaheurestic algorithm based hybrid model for identification of building sale prices. In:Metaheuristic and Evolutionary Computation: Algorithms and Applications. Studies in Computational Intelligence. Springer (2020). https://doi.org/10.1007/978-981-15-7571-6_32

23. Minai, A.F., et al.: Metaheuristics paradigms for renewable energy systems: advances in optimization algorithms. In: Metaheuristic and Evolutionary Computation: Algorithms and Applications. Studies in Computational Intelligence. Springer (2020). https://doi.org/10.1007/978-981-15-7571-6_2

24. Iqbal, A., et al.: Big-data analytics based energy analysis and monitoring for multi-story hospital buildings: case study. In: Soft Computing in Condition Monitoring and Diagnostics of Electrical and Mechanical Systems, pp. 325–343 (2019). https://doi.org/10.1007/978-981-15-1532-3_14

25. Fatema, N., et al.: Data-driven occupancy detection hybrid model using particle swarm optimization based artificial neural network. In: Metaheuristic and Evolutionary Computation: Algorithms and Applications. Studies in Computational Intelligence. Springer (2020). https://doi.org/10.1007/978-981-15-7571-6_13

26. Iqbal, A., et al.: Data driven intelligent model for sales prices prediction and monitoring of a building. In: Soft Computing in Condition Monitoring and Diagnostics of Electrical and Mechanical Systems, pp. 407–421. Springer (2019). https://doi.org/10.1007/978-981-15-1532-3_18

27. Fullerton, G.: Creating advocates: the roles of satisfaction, trust and commitment? J. Retail. Consum. Serv. **18**(1), 92–100 (2011)

28. Cronbach, L. J.: Coefficient alpha and the internal structure of tests. Psychometrika **16**, 297–334 (1951)

Interpretation of EEG Signals During Wrist Movement Using Multi-resolution Wavelet Features for BCI Application

Mohd Wahab, Abdulla Shahid, Nidal Rafiuddin, Omar Farooq, and Yusuf Uzzaman Khan

Abstract The proposed signal processing approach investigates the effectiveness of wavelet transforms in classifying different motion attributes using non-invasive MEG recording for brain–computer interface applications. The dataset used accompanied MEG recording of two healthy people executing their wrist in four directions. Wavelet analysis using discrete wavelet transform and wavelet packet transform was carried out to extract features. Features were ranked, and best performing was selected for classification. Mahalanobis distance metric was used for classification of two different classes at a time. The average performance obtained with this method is 72.28%.

Keywords Signal processing · Wavelet transform · Brain–computer interface · Magneto–encephalogram · Mahalanobis distance

1 Introduction

A brain–computer interface (BCI) accompanies a software-based system and hardware that aims user inherent brain activity to control external device independent from the peripheral nerves and muscles. These systems rely on real-time recognition of different mental states from brain activity. The aim of BCI is accomplished in five successive stages namely signal acquisition and processing, extraction of features, their selection, and finally classification. Various works have been reported for application of non-invasive modality in BCI. Imagination of movement of different parts

M. Wahab
Arizona State University, Tempe, AZ, USA
e-mail: mdwahab1509@gmail.com

A. Shahid
Mazaya Group, Dammam, Saudi Arabia
e-mail: abdullahshahid19721@gmail.com

N. Rafiuddin (✉) · O. Farooq · Y. Uzzaman Khan
Aligarh Muslim University, Aligarh, India
e-mail: nidal.rafi@gmail.com

© The Author(s), under exclusive license to Springer Nature Singapore Pte Ltd. 2021   179
H. Malik et al. (eds.), *AI and Machine Learning Paradigms for Health Monitoring System*, Studies in Big Data 86,
https://doi.org/10.1007/978-981-33-4412-9_11

of the body and self-regulation of evoked potentials, e.g., slow cortical potentials. Decoding of wrist movement using MEG using the same dataset was reported by [1]. They used a combination of SVM and LDA classifier and obtained an accuracy of 59.5 and 34.3% for subject-1 and subject-2. Various results have also been quoted directly on the same dataset at BCI competition-IV.

2 Signal Acquisition

A BCI system fetches the electrical signals in brain using either invasive or non-invasive modality [2]. The invasive technique involves recording these electrical signals by surgically implanting an array of microelectrodes into the cortex to obtain single unit activity, multiple unit activities, and local field potential (LFP) [3]. Non-invasive modality that records the activity by placing on the surface of scalp to capture electrical activity involves functional magnetic resonance imaging (fMRI), electroen-cephalography (EEG), magneto-encephalogram (MEG), near-infrared spectroscopy (NIRS). Electrodes here are placed on the scalp of the subject in accordance with International 10–20 system [4, 5].

2.1 BCI Competition

This paper uses data from the BCI competition-IV dataset-3, which pertains with a recording of MEG signals during different hand movement directions. The dataset-3 of BCI competition-IV pertains with directionally modulated MEG signal of two subjects performing wrist movement in four different directions namely right, left, forward, and backward. Ten MEG channels were placed above motor cortex. The MEG data recorded a total of 160 trials on each subjects S1 and S2 separately, accompanying 40 trials corresponding to classes of right, left, backward, and forward wrist movement. The test data for subjects S1 and S2 comprises 74 and 73 test trials, respectively. The subjects were right-handed healthy people. The data was recorded at a sample rate of 625 Hz and resampled at 400 Hz as presented in Table 1. The proposed work for classification utilizes two directions of movement at a time for classification hence making it a 2-class problem instead of 4. The 4-class data is

Table 1 Dataset-3 BCI competition-IV

	Recording sample rate (Hz)	Resampling rate (Hz)	Training set (Trials in s)				Test set (trials in s)
			Right	Left	Forward	Backward	
Subject 1	625	400	40	40	40	40	74
Subject 2			40	40	40	40	73

Fig. 1 Sensors placed
following 10–20 electrode
placement technique

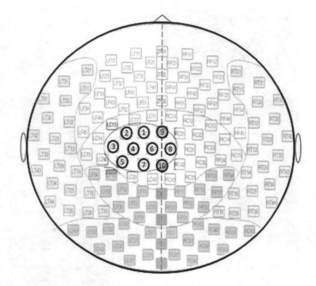

segregated into a pair of 2-class, each comprising of class set namely right–left and forward–backward.

The subject sat relaxed on a special chair integrated with MEG system. To prevent unnecessary movement, the elbows and head were stabilized by a pillow. The recording was done by placing 10 electrodes in accordance with the international 10–20 electrode system [6] (see Fig. 1).

The assignment was to shift a joystick in any of the four given directions perpendicular to each other. All the targets were arranged horizontally in a form of a rhombus with the corners as left, right, backward, and forward. The movement was done by the right wrist with 4.5 cm displacement from the rest position. The subject chooses the target with his own will. The subject was instructed to achieve the target within 0.75 s after initiating the movement and then had to remain still for 1 s at the target to improve temporal consistency and to reduce interference. The trials were slit to hold the data from 0.4 s prior to and 0.6 s post movement onset. Data was further resampled at 400 Hz. The proposed work used MEG brain maps to understand the zone of the brain where the superior and inferior activities take place and to understand the brain physiology during the wrist movement. The plot of 10 channels MEG signal waveforms (see Fig. 2) of subject-1 is related to all the four classes, and the duration of the plot is 5 s along with the brain maps depicting activity of the brain during the period. In order to correctly train the algorithm, the signal corresponding to the movements was mined out from the raw signal which otherwise encompasses both rest and movement related data, therefore movement data spanning 0.6 s was sorted out from each class.

Figure 3 portrays the averaged 10 trials MEG plot of channel-1 obtained from subject-1.

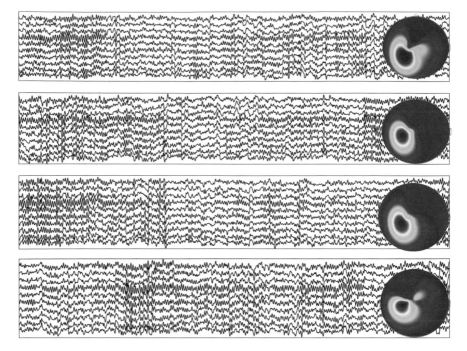

Fig. 2 MEG waveform sections with 10 channels and respective brain maps of subject-1 corresponding to movements: **a** right, **b** forward, **c** left, and **d** backward

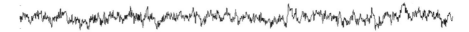

Fig. 3 MEG plot of averaged 10 trials of subject-1, channel-1 after removal of the portion corresponding to resting state

3   Wavelet Transform

A digital signal processing technique used extensively for extracting information that is not readily available in raw signal is the wavelet transform. It is a mathematical transformation used for data that is highly random in nature. The wavelet transform is explicitly acceptable when signals are non-stationary. MEG is a non-stationary signal; hence, wavelet technique includes discrete wavelet transform (DWT) and wavelet packet decomposition (WPD) to extract the features of the signal. The advantage of using wavelet technique is it allows a multi-resolution analysis to traverse the hidden information from the raw signal. Furthermore, wavelet transform allows decimation in time and frequency simultaneously. The definition of continuous wavelet transform on a signal can be found as in [7].

$$\text{CWT}(\tau,a) = \int\limits_{-\infty}^{\infty} x(t)\frac{1}{\sqrt{|a|}}\Psi\left(\frac{t-\tau}{a}\right)dt \tag{1}$$

where a and τ are the scaling and shifting parameter, respectively, ψ is the basic wavelet or mother wavelet given by:

$$\Psi(t) = \frac{1}{\sqrt{|a|}}\Psi\left(\frac{t-\tau}{a}\right) \tag{2}$$

Because of high computational cost associated with wavelet transforms at every scale, a different technique is used to ease the computational complications. This is done by discretizing scaling factor and shifting factor as $a = 2^j$ and $\tau = 2^{j*k}$, where j and $k \in z$ (integer). By discretizing the scaling and shifting factor, the wavelet analysis thus becomes much more systematic which defines discrete wavelet transform (DWT) as:

$$\text{DWT}_{j,k}(\tau.) = \frac{1}{\sqrt{|2^j|}}\int\limits_{-\infty}^{\infty} x(t)\Psi\left(\frac{t-2^{j*k}}{2^j}\right)dt \tag{3}$$

In this method, signal is decomposed to the fifth level using Daubechies 'db4' wavelet (see Fig. 4a) shows DWT transform of the signal shown in Fig. 3 up to the fifth level of decomposition. Here, 'Ca' represents approximate coefficient and 'Cd' represents detailed coefficient while the number associated with it represents the level of decomposition. Moreover, the proposed method also extracts features by applying WPT approach in addition to DWT, where decomposition is done on both lower and higher frequencies forming a balanced binary tree. This process leads to a higher degree of possibilities for signal analysis than the DWT [8–11]. Figure 4b shows the first thirty wavelet packets acquired from the signal shown in Fig. 3.

4 Feature Extraction

After acquiring a set of wavelet coefficients by applying DWT and WPT technique to the MEG signals, features are extracted from the wavelet coefficients as well as raw signals. These features are temporal and time-spectral domain-based. Most features employed in this work were obtained from the literature, and a brief discussion of statistical measures to extract features is carried out below. In all, 296 features were obtained by computing measures on the raw signal as well as discrete wavelets coefficients and wavelet packet coefficients.

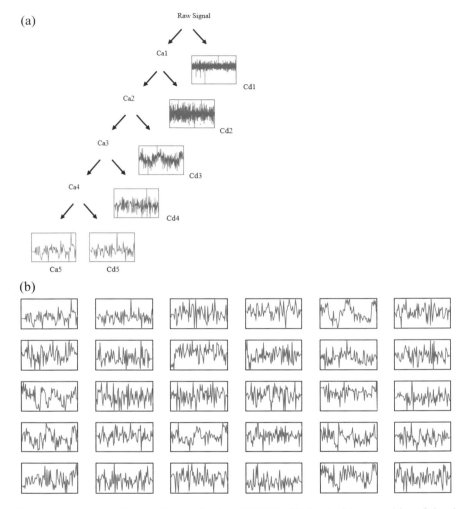

Fig. 4 a Retained coefficients after application of DWT to fifth level of decomposition of signal in Fig. 3. **b** Plot of first 30 wavelet packets of the MEG signal up to the fifth level of decomposition

4.1   Inter-quartile Range

IQR measures the range of score in the middle eliminating the top 25% and bottom 25% of the distribution, thus is a strong and impressive measure of inconsistency [12]. The general formula to calculate IQR is:

$$IQR = Q_3 - Q_1 \qquad (4)$$

where the first and third quartile are evaluated, respectively, as $Q_1 = \frac{n+1}{4}$ term and $Q_3 = \frac{3(n+1)}{4}$ term.

4.2 Energy

The energy was given as the sum of squares of amplitude. If x_i is the value signal, m is samples and k is levels, and energy is computed as:

$$e(k) = \sum_{i=1}^{m} x_i^2 \tag{5}$$

4.3 Normalized Coefficient of Variation (NCV)

NCV was calculated by initially changing the coefficient of variation by analyzing ratio of the epoch variance to absolute values mean given as:

$$NCV = \sigma^2 / \mu_a \tag{6}$$

where σ is standard deviation and μ_a is absolute value mean. WPT coefficient at the same frequency can averaged as:

$$NCV(k) = \frac{1}{q} \sum_{k=1}^{q} (\sigma^2 / \mu_a)(k) \tag{7}$$

where k represents the decomposed level.

4.4 Normalized Coefficient of Variation-2 (NCV2)

NCV2 was evaluated by computing proportion of the epoch variance to the square of mean calculated on absolute values as:

$$NCV2 = \sigma^2 / \mu_a^2 \tag{8}$$

The WPT coefficient of the same frequency can be averaged as:

$$\text{NCV2}(k) = \frac{1}{q} \sum_{k=1}^{q} (\sigma^2 / \mu_{a^2})(k) \tag{9}$$

4.5 Normalized Covariance (COVFF)

COVFF was evaluated by the proportion of epoch variance to the square of mean as:

$$\text{COVFF} = \frac{\sigma}{\mu^2} \tag{10}$$

4.6 Covariance (Cov)

COV was evaluated by the proportion of epoch variance to square of absolute values mean of x as:

$$\text{COV} = \frac{\sigma}{\mu_a^2} \tag{11}$$

5 Feature Selection

Feature ranking technique aims to choose the best-performing feature that can differentiate dissimilar classes of data more effectively [13]. In this work, features were ranked and top 10 best-performing features out of the total 296 features were selected for classification. The proposed system ranks the features using independent evaluation criterion for binary classification. Out of the total extracted features, 10 best-performing features were selected based on their ranks shown in Table 2; WP stands for wavelet packet and DW stands for discrete wavelet. Since the present work relates to a two-class problem, the feature ranking results in Table 2 is shown for both the classes separately. The order of appearance of features in the table signifies its discriminative performance.

Table 2 Features ranking results with 10 best-performing features

Rank	Subject-1		Subject-2	
	Right–left	Forward–backward	Right–left	Forward–backward
	Feature/frequency range (Hz)	Feature/frequency range (Hz)	Feature/frequency range (Hz)	Feature/frequency range (Hz)
1	WP_IQR/25–31.25	WP_NCV2/193.75–200	WP_NCV2/106.25–112.5	WP_NCV/150–156.25
2	WP_NCV2/187.5–193.75	WP_IQR/143.75–150	DW_NCV/12.5–25	DW_IQR/25–50
3	WP_IOR/81.25–87.5	WP_NCV/75–81.25	DW_MAV/12.5–25	COVFF/RAW SIGNAL
4	WP_ENERGY/87.5–93.75	WP_NCV2/100–106.25	WP_COV/137.5–143.75	DW_VAR/25–50
5	WP_NCV2/87.5–93.75	DW_NCV/25–50	WP_NCV2/125–131.25	WP_IQR/162.5–168.75
6	WP_COV/156.25–162.5	WP_IOR/125–131.25	DW_VAR/12.5–25	WP_ENERGY/112.5–118.75
7	WP_NCV2/25–31.25	WP_NCV/112.5–118.75	COV/RAW SIGNAL	DW_MAV/25–50
8	WP_ENERGY/175–181.25	WP_COV/81.25–87.5	WP_NCV/0–6.25	WP_NCV/125–131.25
9	WP_NCV/175–181.25	WP_NCV/25–31.25	WP_NCV2/37.5–43.75	WP_NCV/168.75–175
10	WP_ENERGY/56.25–62.5	WP_NCV/125–131.25	WP_NCV/131.25–137.5	WP_NCV2/6.25–12.5

6 Classification

The main focus of classification in BCI system is to identify the human intention on the principle of feature vector characterization. Feature vector being furnished by feature extraction method is used to classify the brain activity [14]. Classification algorithm or regression method can be used to attain the desired goal. A number of methods for classification have been proposed for the recognition of the state like the linear discriminant analysis (LDA), quadratic discriminant analysis (QDA), etc. The stated method can produce a completely inaccurate result in the presence of dominating artifacts [15]. In the present work, a classifier based on Mahalanobis distance [16] is employed which gives better results than LDA and QDA classifiers.

A Mahalanobis distance-based classifier technique reports the variance of each variable and covariance between variable. Geometrically, it transforms the data into uncorrelated standardized data and determines the Euclidean distance from the data obtained. It is scale-invariant, unitless, and considers the correlation between given data. We used Mahalanobis distance-based method to divide the class of the feature vector accompanying two sets of two different classes. If x is a feature vector containing 10 best features of a class of the training set, Mahalanobis distance is given as [17]

$$d - (x - m_I)^t M_I^{-1} (x - m_I) \tag{12}$$

where M_I is the covariance matrix, while t stands for transposition matrix. m_I stands for the mean of a particular class, and let say m_r and m_l are the means of right and left movement taken into consideration. We classify the given vector x by computing the Mahalanobis length d between x and means (m_r and m_l) and allocate x to a particular group to which d is minimal.

7 Results

The dataset consists of two subjects carrying out wrist motion in four dissimilar directions. Training and test set were processed through wavelet transform technique, and coefficient of each subband is computed through WPT and DWT. In order to examine the potential to discriminate, feature vectors are subjected to Mahalanobis distance-based classifier. The accuracy rate of classifier used is evaluated as [18, 19].

$$\text{Accuracy Rate} = \frac{\text{Correctly classified test trial}}{\text{number of all test trial}} \times 100 \tag{13}$$

Additionally, to scrutinize the efficacy of the classifier, the confusion matrix is used. Confusion matrix helps in contrasting between the actual and predicted classifications of the data. Accuracy was computed as

Table 3 Confusion matrix

Predicted					
		Backward	Forward	Left	Right
Actual	Backward	TP_B	$E_{(B,F)}$	$E_{(B,L)}$	$E_{(B,R)}$
	Forward	$E_{(F,B)}$	TP_F	$E_{(F,L)}$	$E_{(F,R)}$
	Left	$E_{(L,B)}$	$E_{(L,F)}$	TP_L	$E_{(L,R)}$
	Right	$F_{(R,B)}$	$E_{(R,F)}$	$E_{(R,L)}$	TP_R

Table 4 Results from different literature

S. No.	Research	No. of classes taken	Average accuracy (%)
1	Sepideh Hajipour et al.	4 class in 1 set	46.9
3	Nasim Montazeri et al.	4 class in 1 set	23.9
4	Jinjia Wang et al.	4 class in 1 set	20.4
5	Our work	2 class in 2 sets	72.28

$$\text{Accuracy Rate} = \frac{TP + TN}{TP + TN + FP + FN} \times 100 \tag{14}$$

where TN and TP are the entirety of true negative and true positive events, respectively, while FN and FP are the total numbers of false negative and false positive. Table 3 provides confusion matrix representation of the actual wrist movements mapped to predicted movements for left, right, forward, and backward.

In the present work, the accuracy obtained for subject-1 taking only right–left wrist movement is 79.31% while for forward–backward wrist movement is 77.78% averaging to 78.54%. For subject-2, the results obtained for right–left wrist movement is 67.74% while in case of forward–backward wrist movement the accuracy is 64.29% leading to an average accuracy of 66.02%. The overall average accuracy for both the subjects is 72.28%. The outcome of this method is juxtaposed with [20, 21] as shown in Table 4 below. The previous studies took 4 classes altogether for classification results.

8 Discussion and Conclusion

Different activity results in a different pattern of brain signal. The required information of brain signals is concealed in a state full of artifacts. Desired signal may be contaminated in space and time by several signals invoked due to simultaneous performance of the different tasks by brain. For this reason, we do not use conventional approach such as bandpass filter. We implemented a pattern recognition technique which classified the features into different classes. The statistical features are calculated from the signal thus finding discriminative information needed to distinguish classes. Using Mahalanobis distance-based classifier on the feature vector obtained after ranking different features on raw data, WPT and DWT resulted in overall average classification accuracy for both the subjects of 72.28%. Moreover, this work may be extended by employing some more key features, removing artifacts arising due to simultaneous performance of the different activity, and using classifiers like SVM or another nonlinear classifier.

References

1. Hajipour Sardouie, S., Sham-sollahi, M.B.: Selection of efficient features for discrimination of hand movements from MEG using a BCI competition IV data set. Front Neurosci. **6**, 42 (2012)
2. Georgieva, P., Silva, F., Figueiredo, N.: IEETA brain computer interface technologies. Int. J. Comput. Intell. Stud. **2**(3/4), 314–332 (2013)
3. Kipke, D.R., Shain, W., Buzsaki, G., Fetz, E., Henderson, J.M., Hetke, J.F., Schalk, G.: Advanced neurotechnologies for chronic neural interfaces: new horizons and clinical opportunities. J. Neurosci. **28**(46), 11830–21183 (2008)
4. Jasper, H.H.: The ten-twenty electrode system of the international Federation. Electroencephalogr. Clin. Neurophysiol. **10**, 371–375 (1958)
5. Shahid, A., et al.: Decrypting wrist movement from MEG signal using SVM classifier. J. Intell Fuzzy Syst. **35**(5), 5123–5130 (2018). https://doi.org/10.3233/JIFS-169796
6. Wanchai: 10/20 System Positioning Manual. Hong Kong Trans Cranial Technologies Ltd. (2012)
7. Rafi, N., Khan, Y.U., Farooq, O.: Epileptic seizure detection: reformation of the traditional method on scalp recorded electroencephalogram. In: International Conference on Emerging Trends in Electrical Engineering, (ICETREE 2014), Kollam, Kerala (2014)
8. Khan, Y.U., Gotman, J.: Wavelet based automatic seizure detection in intracerebral electroencephalogram. Clin. Neurophysiol. **114**(1), 898–908 (2003)
9. Rafiuddin, N., Khan, Y.U., Farooq, O.: Feature extraction and classification of EEG for automatic seizure detection. In: International Confrence on Multimedia, Signal Processing and Communication Technologies (IMPACT-2011), Aligarh
10. Rafiuddin, N., Tabrez, M., Khan, Y.U., Farooq, O.: Wavelet packet-based classification of brain states during English and mother tongue script writing. Int. J. Biomed. Eng. Technol. **22**(4), 325–337 (2016)
11. Ocak, H.: Automatic detection of epileptic seizures in EEG using descrete wavelet transform and approximate entropy. Expert Syst. Appl. **36**, 2027–2036 (2009)
12. Dekking, F.M., Kraaikamp, C., Lopuhaa, H.P., Meester, L.E.: A modern introduction to probability and statistics: understanding why and how, p. 236. Springer, London (2005)
13. Hidayat, R., Kristomo, D., Togarma, I.: Feature extraction of the Indonesian Phonemes using discreet wavelet and wavelet packet transform. In: 2016 8th International Conference on Information Technology and Electrical Engineering (ICITEE), Yogyakarta, Indonesia
14. Vazquez, R.R., Perez, H.V., Ranta, R., Dorr, V.L., Maquin, D., Maillard, L.: Blind source separation, wavelet denoising and discriminant analysis for EEG artefacts and noise cancelling. Biomed. Signal Process. Control **7**, 389–400 (2012)
15. Muller, K.R., Anderson, C.W., Birch, G.E.: Linear and nonlinear methods for brain–computer interfaces. IEEE Trans. Neural Syst. Rehabil. Eng **11**, 165–169 (2003)
16. Angari, H.M.A., Kanitz, G., Tarantino, S., Cipriani, C.: Distance and mutual information methods for EMG feature and channel subset selection for classification of hand movements. Biomed. Signal Process. Control **27**, 24–31 (2016)

17. Babilone, F., Bianchi, L., Semeraro, F., Millan, J.R., Mourino, J., Cattini, A., Salinari, S., Marciani, M.G., Cincotti, F.: Mahalanobis distance based classifiers are able to recogize EEG patterns by using few EEG electrodes. In: 23rd Annual Conference—IEEE/EMBS, 25–28 October 2001, Istanbul, Turkey
18. Ghaemi, A., Rashedi, E., Pourrahimi, A.M., Kamandar, M., Rahdari, F.: Automatic channel selection in EEG signals for classification of left or right hand movement in brain computer interfaces using improved binary gravitation search algorithm. Biomed. Signal Process. Control **33**, 109–118 (2017)
19. Shahid, A., Wahab, M., Rafiuddin, N., Farooq, O.: Classification of seizure through SVM based classifier. In: International Conference on Computer Communication and Informatics (ICCCI 2017), Coimbatore, India
20. Montazeri, N., Shamsollahi, M.B., Hajipour, S.: MEG based classification of wrist movement. In: Annual Inter-national Conference of the IEEE Engineering in Medicine and Biology Society. IEEE Engineering in Medicine and Biology Society. Annual Conference, vol. 2009
21. Jinjia, W., Lina, Z., Yuchao, Z.: Feature extraction method for MEG-based brain computer interface. Chin. J. Sci. Instrum. (7), 6 (2010)

Validation of Road Traffic Noise Prediction Model CoRTN for Indian Road and Traffic Conditions

Pervez Alam, Kafeel Ahmad, S. S. Afsar, and Nasim Akhtar

Abstract Noise prediction explains the method of calculating ranges of noise theoretically within an area of interest for an explicit type of situation. Many researchers have developed plenty of noise prediction models for their respective countries such as (CoRTN) (UK), EMPA (Stl 86) (Switzerland), and RLS-90 (Germany). CoRTN has been progressed by Hood, Harland, Delany, and Scholes in the Department of Environmental Engineering, United Kingdom (UK). The validation of any model provides its applicability and appropriateness in various road and traffic condition. Therefore, the main objective of this paper is to carry out validation of road traffic noise prediction model CoRTN for Indian road and traffic conditions. The standard deviation between monitored and predicted level of noise before and after applying correction factor has been found to be in the range of 0.62 to 4.99 and 0.06 to 3.47, respectively. The results clearly indicate that the CoRTN model cannot be directly used for forecasting the extent of noise in Indian traffic conditions. However, after applying some correction like correction for honking noise, noise of bicycle and noise due to vintage of vehicle predicted results improve considerably which point toward the applicability and fitness of the model in Indian traffic and road conditions.

Keywords Model validation · CoRTN · Indian conditions · Road traffic

1 Introduction

Noise models are the exercise to predict the noise level around any source, at any distance and at any time. Noise modeling explains the method of calculating the ranges of noise theoretically within an area of interest for a given set of conditions. The particular set of situations for which the noise is being predicted could be a fixed

P. Alam (✉) · K. Ahmad · S. S. Afsar
Department of Civil Engineering, Jamia Millia Islamia, New Delhi, India
e-mail: pervezjmi@gmail.com

N. Akhtar
CSIR, CRRI, Mathura Road, New Delhi, India

© The Author(s), under exclusive license to Springer Nature Singapore Pte Ltd. 2021   193
H. Malik et al. (eds.), *AI and Machine Learning Paradigms for Health Monitoring System*, Studies in Big Data 86,
https://doi.org/10.1007/978-981-33-4412-9_12

illustration for a physical surrounding of interest. Although, practically, the part of physical environment will not generally be fixed, it will be characterized by constantly variable situations. Recognizing a model for estimating noise for a selected type of condition could be done easily, but currently the attention is required to shape these conditions. The important conditions, to which a noise model relates, are as follows:

1. Traffic condition: heterogeneous and traffic flow.
2. The physical environment during which the noise spreads from source(s) to the location.
3. Estimation of the way by which sound travels from the input noise source(s) through the input physical environment.

This method is a distinctive process after the instructions given by ministries to restrict the environmental noise, where maps for noise have been recommended for urban agglomerations and transportation sources. Therefore, many relevant models have been created for the prediction of sound as of late focussing on this angle and introducing only the source out flow and observation details of producing the sound. Many researchers have developed and validated numerous noise prediction models for their respective countries, such as RLS-90 (Germany) in 1990, DIN 18,005 road (Germany), Temanord 525 (Scandinavia), (CoRTN) (UK), EMPA (Stl 86) in 1986 (Switzerland), RVS 3.02 (Austria), TNM (USA), ENEA (Italy), Federal Highway model (USA), FHWA Model (Australia), and STOP and GO Model, MITHRA (France) in 1982. These models are used for forecasting the level of noise in different conditions of traffic. These models have been outstanding and implemented by different organizations for the progress of maps drawn for noise. To resolve the sound engendering impacts, advanced numerical planning, including equation of continuity and wave conditions, is implemented, apart from the source interpretation. Therefore, for traffic noise modeling, it is very important to compare and examine these models to obtain the best methodology among them and to discover their reasonableness on the whole.

Steele [1] did a detailed analysis of the paramount noise traffic model in 2001 but some of them have been revised between 2007 and 2013 and the same has been modified by Garg and Maji [2] in 2014. In another study, a critical study of various noise traffic forecasting models was done by Rajakumara and Gowda [3]. They found that most of these models are either deterministic or arithmetical in nature. A research work carried out by Parida [4] presents an analytical modeling approach for predicting road traffic noise for Indian conditions. He presents a model based on the FHWA Model, CoRTN Model, and Regression Model. Devender [5] used three models for noise prediction, namely FHWA, CoRTN and STOP and GO Model to predict the level of noise in an urban area for interrupted traffic flow. He reported that both the models 'FHWA and CoRTN' could be satisfactorily applied for Indian road traffic conditions as the predicted results are satisfactory, with a deviation of 7–10 dB (A) for FHWA and 5–8 dB(A) for CoRTN. The above literature review shows that the validation of noise model for road traffic model has been carried out for developed countries but found to be missing in India road and traffic conditions, particularly for CoRTN model in urban environment. Therefore, the main objective of this paper is to carry out validation of CoRTN model in Indian road traffic conditions. Some recent example of this domain is given in [6].

2 Material and Methods

Delany, Harland, Scholes, and Hood have developed the noise prediction model CoRTN, for Department of Environmental Engineering, United Kingdom (UK) [7]. For the design of the road, it is generally used as assistance and also used for forecasting the degree of noise around the source of noise. The only tool which CoRTN takes into consideration for the determination of impact on environment due to road traffic in UK is constant speed of traffic and line source. Amore handy, Predicting Road Traffic Noise (PRTN) [8], which considered Delany et al. [9] explanation for the process has replaced the method of calculation of Road Traffic Noise (CoRTN) [10]. The level of noise (forecasted or determined) is measured hourly in terms of L_{10} having units as dB (A) and L_{10} (18-h) units as dB (A): 6:00 to 24:00 h. CoRTN can be implemented to determine the values of $L(A)_{10}$ hourly, if data of traffic will be hourly available which can be later transformed to Leq(A) hourly values. But, in case of non-motorway roads where flow of hourly traffic during the period of 24:00 to 06:00 h is less than 200 vehicles, the below mentioned equation should be followed:

Leq(A), hourly $= 0.57 * L_{10}(A),1$ h $+ 24.46$ dB

The Leq may be calculated using below mention formula (motorways)

L(day) $= 0.98 * L_{10},18$ h $+ 0.09$ dB
L(Eve.) $= 0.89 * L_{10},18$ h $+ 5.08$ dB
L(Nig.) $= 0.87 * L_{10},18$ h $+ 4.24$ dB
L(den) $= 0.90 * L_{10},18$ h $+ 9.69$ dB
The Leq may be calculated using below mention formula (Non motorways)
L(day) $= 0.95 * L_{10},18$ h $+ 1.44$ dB.
L(eve.) $= 0.97 * L_{10},18$ h $- 2.87$ dB
L(nig.) $= 0.90 * L_{10},18$ h $- 3.77$ dB
L(den) $= 0.92 * L_{10},18$ h $+ 4.20$ dB

2.1 Assumption for Model Validation

The below conditions have been presumed during the prediction of level of noise.

1. The carriage level has to be 0.5 m below the height of source.
2. The edge distance of source should be 3.5 m from the nearest side carriage way.
3. Noise has been calculated in front of the most exposed part, i.e., external window or door, at a distance of 1 m.
4. The meteorological conditions are ignored.

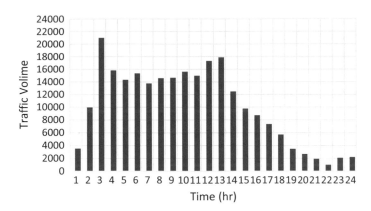

Fig. 1 Variation of hourly average traffic volume

5. Background noise is neglected.

2.2 Input Data Used for Validation

Features of traffic including the traffic volume, speed of vehicle, composition, and traffic noise have been recorded for verifying the CoRTN model. Composition of traffic is generally classified into heavy and light vehicles. For this study, heavy vehicles comprise of trucks and buses, whereas light vehicles consist of local taxis, vans, personal cars, and motorized two-wheelers, as shown in Fig. 1.

The L_{10} noise level is one of the input factors implemented to predict the level of noise. The monitoring of L_{10} average hourly level of noise has been carried out for Ashram which is further used for the purpose of validation of CoRTN model. As shown in Fig. 2, the maximum L_{10} level of noise has been registered at 9 a.m. (85.42 dB) and minimum has been observed at 4 a.m. (72.24 dB). This may be due to the maximum and minimum traffic volume found at 8–9 a.m. (daytime) and 3–4 a.m. (nighttime), respectively.

The volume of traffic for each category of vehicles has been counted on regular basis, see Fig. 3. The speed of each kind of vehicle (heavy and light) has been calculated and the average speed of vehicles has been estimated. Geometrical measurement of road section and layout of site have also been prepared in addition to the noise and traffic data.

3 Result and Discussion

The monitored and predicted level of noise for Ashram Chowk monitoring station has been shown in Table 1. The validation of model for noise prediction CoRTN has

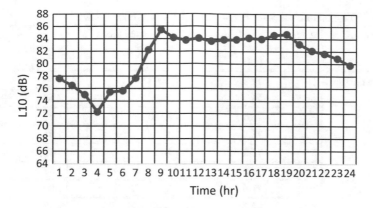

Fig. 2 Variation of hourly average L10 noise level

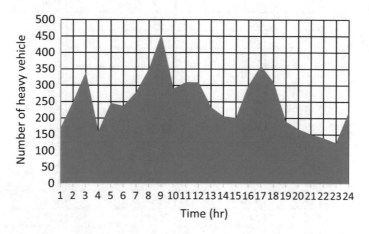

Fig. 3 Variation of number of heavy vehicles

been carried out by equating the observed noise level and predicted level of noise using CoRTN. As shown in Table 1, the variation between the monitored noise level and the level of noise predicted remains between 2.1 dB and 10.97 dB. The maximum variation has been observed at 7 a.m., i.e., 10.97. The variation of standard deviation between monitored and level of noise predicted remained in the range of 0.61 to 5.48, maximum at 5 PM. So, the results indicate that the CoRTN model cannot be directly implemented for predicting the level of noise in Indian traffic condition. However, after applying some correction like correction for honking noise, bicycle noise, and noise due to faulty engines, it may give better predicted results.

After addition of honking noise, noise of bicycle, and noise due to faulty engine in the predicted noise level, the maximum standard deviation of noise level monitored, and noise level predicted has been reduced to 3.47 at 5 PM instead of 4.99 at 8 PM, shown in Table 2. Furthermore, most of the time in a day the standard deviation

Table 1 Validation of noise prediction model CoRTN at Ashram Chowk

Location	Time (h)	Monitored noise level (dB)	Predicted noise level (CoRTN)	SD (monitored and predicted)
Ashram Chowk	1	77.8	71.03	3.38
	2	76.3	71.92	2.19
	3	76.5	72.80	1.85
	4	75.5	73.68	0.91
	5	75.8	74.57	0.62
	6	78.6	75.45	1.57
	7	79.9	71.90	4.00
	8	82.5	74.65	3.92
	9	85.5	77.04	4.23
	10	83.8	75.82	3.99
	11	82.1	75.57	3.26
	12	78.9	75.78	1.56
	13	78.8	75.24	1.78
	14	79.8	75.35	2.23
	15	78.7	75.35	1.67
	16	81.3	75.81	2.74
	17	86.8	75.83	5.48
	18	86.4	76.16	5.12
	19	85.3	75.98	4.66
	20	84.7	74.71	4.99
	21	82.6	73.86	4.37
	22	79.8	73.45	3.17
	23	79.1	72.83	3.14
	24	78.8	72.62	3.09

remains less than 2 which clearly shows that the correction of predicted noise is really helpful in achieving the accurate predicated noise level.

Figure 4 shows the difference of predicted level of noise, monitored noise level, and corrected level of noise for Indian traffic condition. The figure clearly depicts that the difference between monitored noise level and predicted noise level remains very high. Correction is required because the CoRTN model has been developed for uniform traffic flow without considering honking noise, bicycle noise, and noise due to faulty engines. Therefore, after applying correction for Indian condition like addition of honking noise, bicycle noise, and noise due to engine/poor vehicle, the graph coincides at many places.

Table 2 Validation of noise prediction model CoRTN after applying correction for Indian traffic conditions

Location	Time (h)	Monitored noise level (dB)	Predicted noise level (CoRTN)	Corrected noise level (Indian condition)	SD (monitored and corrected)
Ashram Chowk	1	77.8	71.03	74.75	1.53
	2	76.3	71.92	75.69	0.31
	3	76.5	72.80	76.63	0.06
	4	75.5	73.68	77.57	1.03
	5	75.8	74.57	78.51	1.35
	6	78.6	75.45	79.45	0.42
	7	79.9	71.90	75.67	2.11
	8	82.5	74.65	78.60	1.95
	9	85.5	77.04	81.14	2.18
	10	83.8	75.82	79.84	1.98
	11	82.1	75.57	79.57	1.26
	12	78.9	75.78	79.80	0.45
	13	78.8	75.24	79.22	0.21
	14	79.8	75.35	79.34	0.23
	15	78.7	75.35	79.34	0.32
	16	81.3	75.81	79.83	0.73
	17	86.8	75.83	79.85	3.47
	18	86.4	76.16	80.20	3.10
	19	85.3	75.98	80.01	2.64
	20	84.7	74.71	78.66	3.02
	21	82.6	73.86	77.75	2.42
	22	79.8	73.45	77.32	1.24
	23	79.1	72.83	76.66	1.22
	24	78.8	72.62	76.44	1.18

4   Conclusion

This study has been conducted to validate the CoRTN model for Indian conditions. For noise prediction, input data such as features of traffic including volume of traffic, its composition, and speed of vehicle have been recorded. Validation of CoRTN model for Indian road and traffic conditions has been carried out. The results clearly indicate that the model cannot be directly used for predicting the level of noise in Indian road and traffic conditions. However, after applying a correction to the CoRTN model (addition of honking noise, noise due to old engines, etc.), the predicted noise level improves considerably and remains very near to monitored noise level. Hence,

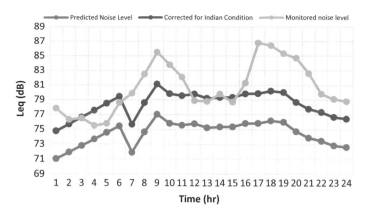

Fig. 4 Validation of noise prediction model CoRTN

it has been concluded that the CoRTN model can be used for the determination of traffic noise after applying some correction.

References

1. Steele, C.: A critical review of some traffic noise prediction models. Appl. Acoust. **62**, 271–287 (2001)
2. Garg, N., Maji, S.: A critical review of principal traffic noise models: strategies and implications. Environ. Impact Assess. Rev. **46**, 68–81 (2014)
3. Rajakumara, H.N., Gowda, R.M.M.: Road traffic noise prediction models—a review. Int. J. Sustain. Dev. Plan. **3**(3), 257–271 (2008)
4. Parida, M.: Modelling of metropolitan traffic noise in Delhi. ITPI J. **21**(1) (2003)
5. Devender, V.: Modelling of interrupted traffic flow noise. M. Tech, Thesis, University of Roorkee (2002)
6. Mahto, T., et al.: Traffic signal control to optimize run time for energy saving: a smart city paradigm. In: Metaheuristic and Evolutionary Computation: Algorithms and Applications. Studies in Computational Intelligence. Springer (2020). https://doi.org/10.1007/978-981-15-7571-6_21
7. Anon: Calculation of road traffic noise. United Kingdom Department of the Environment and Welsh Oce Joint Publication/HMSO, London (1975)
8. Delany, M.E., Harland, D.G., Hood, R.A., Scholes, W.E.: The prediction of noise levels L10 due to road traffic. J. Sound Vib. **48**(3), 305–325 (1976)
9. Anon.: FHWA. Traffic noise predictions model US. Department of Transportation, Federal Highway Administration National Technical Information Service, Washington (1978)
10. Anon.: Predicting road traffic noise. United Kingdom Department of the Environment/HMSO, London (2004)

AIML Applications for Monitoring System in Engineering and Automation

Deep Learning and Statistical-Based Daily Stock Price Forecasting and Monitoring

Vinay Kumar Reddy Chimmula, Lei Zhang, Hasmat Malik, and Amit Kumar Yadav

Abstract Designing a machine learning algorithm to predict stock prices is a subject of interest for economists and machine learning practitioners. Financial modeling is a challenging task, not only from an analytical perspective but also from a psychological perspective. After 2008 financial crisis, many financial companies and investors shifted their interest toward predicting future trends. Most of the existing methods for stock price forecasting are modeled using nonlinear methods and evaluated on specific datasets. These models are not able to generalize for diverse datasets. Financial time series data is highly dynamic in nature and makes it difficult to analyze through statistical methods. Recurrent neural network (RNN)-based long short-term memory (LSTM) networks were able to capture the patterns of the sequences data meanwhile statistical methods tried to generalize by memorizing data instead of recognizing patterns. In this book chapter, we examined the performance of LSTM model and statistical models over stock prices of different companies to generalize the model. The experimental results of this study show that, LSTM networks outperformed traditional statistical methods like ARIMA, MA, and AR models. Furthermore, we have noticed that, LSTM networks were able to perform consistently on different datasets while statistical methods showed varied performance. Through this project, we addressed the gaps in current models of stock price prediction in both economic and machine learning perspective.

V. K. R. Chimmula (✉) · L. Zhang
Electronics Systems Engineering, University of Regina, Regina, Saskatchewan S4S 0A7, Canada
e-mail: vinayreddy911@gmail.com

L. Zhang
e-mail: lei.zhang@uregina.ca

H. Malik
Electrical Engineering, Indian Institute of Technology (IIT) Delhi, New Delhi, India
e-mail: hasmat.malik@gmail.com

A. Kumar Yadav
Electrical Engineering, National Institute of Technology (NIT), Sikkim, Ravangla, India
e-mail: amit1986.529@rediffmail.com

© The Author(s), under exclusive license to Springer Nature Singapore Pte Ltd. 2021
H. Malik et al. (eds.), *AI and Machine Learning Paradigms for Health Monitoring System*, Studies in Big Data 86,
https://doi.org/10.1007/978-981-33-4412-9_13

Keywords Deep learning · Stock price forecasting · Statistical models · Machine learning · Financial forecasting

1 Introduction

Decoding information from the financial data and making meaningful decisions is a research hotspot in financial sector. Over the last decade, with an increase in computation power, collection of data from various sources (satellite imaging [1], smart devices [2], smart phone sensors [3], etc.) has also been increased which led to rise of machine learning. Today, machine learning is applied in almost in every field from medical [4] to space applications [5]. In this research, we have discussed, one such application, i.e., role of machine learning in finance sector with specific application and stock price forecasting.

Stock price forecasting is a big data problem, because millions of data points are generated during each session. Real-time data analysis without losing temporal components is not achieved completely. In this complex world, it is difficult to predict stock prices with high accuracies because of their dynamic and volatile nature. Even top financial companies, like Morgan Stanley, J.P Morgan, etc., failed many times in market analysis. Despite all the difficulties, prospective investors are continuously trying to predict the future markets, one of such examples is Warren Buffet, who succeeded in beating markets since last two decades. Stock price forecasting can be done in two ways. In the first method, investors will analyze the current market scenarios, political stability of the country, climatic conditions, and other human-itarian factors. While in the other method, investors will only consider statistical analysis of the historical data and the data patterns.

In [6], Malkiel addressed market monopoly in investment community during 1980s and proposed stock prices can be predicted efficiently using the trading data. Over the last decade, many models have been proposed to predict stock prices. Initially stock price forecasting started with basic regression methods like linear regression. When stock price information/data is classified as time series data, entire world shifted toward using nonlinear machine learning models like artificial neural networks and support vector machines. When machine learning started taking off in financial sector, Ayodele et al. [7] published a model called auto-regressive integrated moving average (ARIMA), a traditional statistical approach for finding short-term stock predictions and performed better than existing models at that time. Auto-regressive integrated moving average method came into existence in early 1970s to tackle time series data, and output of this model is linear combination of previous results and previous loss metric. Soon after its discovery, this model was used many times for short-term forecasting and many hybrid approaches along with ARIMA models are being used in stock price forecasting and other wide range of applications. Jigar et al. in [8] compared four models (support vector machines, ANN, random forest, and Naïve Bayes) on 10-year stock data and achieved maximum accuracy

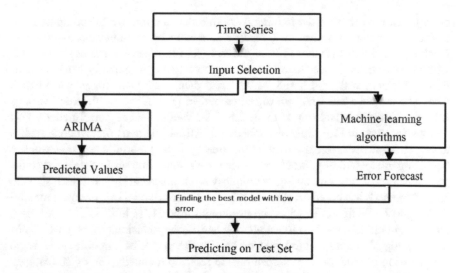

Fig. 1 Graphical abstract of the proposed methodology

using random forest technique and the accuracy of each model increased even further with the use of trend deterministic layers (Fig. 1).

Lately, use of deep learning for predicting sequential data has increased due to its fruitful results [9], decoding hidden patterns in complex datasets and is faster to train a model. Deep neural networks with multiple hidden layers are proved to be efficient to learn the patterns in the data and are able to extract complex features even from the large datasets. Recurrent neural networks (RNNs) are one of the deep learning architectures designed to handle sequential time series data and achieved good results [10]. One of the major drawbacks of RNN is if we go deeper into the network's gradients they will either explode or vanish. To overcome the vanishing gradient problem, an LSTM block with memory cells and additional gates are introduced into RNNs. As we are moving away from traditional neural networks with multilayers to recurrent networks, we still have to include the advantages of statistical models proposed in late 90 s like parameter sharing, which is one the major factors behind the success of RNNs. By sharing parameters between different layers, multilayer deep neural networks can process datasets of different sequences and generalize them. Without this, there would be different weights for each time step and make it difficult to extrapolate the test set data sequences that are not seen during training. Such sharing is extremely necessary when there are abrupt changes in the given time series data. Each layer will generate output in such a way that, similar weight update rules are applied to all the previous outputs.

Dev Shah et al. applied long short-term memory (LSTM) networks and deep neural networks (DNN) to make weekly stock price forecasting. LSTM networks outperformed DNNs in terms of accuracy. They may able to reduce the overfitting in both the models [11]. To minimize prediction errors, LSTM models should be tested with different parameters and a number of units are needed to be increased in order to learn more from the training data. In order to minimize the computational cost and maximize learning rate, batch size should be as minimum as possible. Hochreiter and Schmidhuber [12] proposed LSTM to replace some of the neurons with memory cells. Inside the memory cells, two gates prominently work on error flow in memory cells and based on the input data, third gate (forget gate) learns what to remember and what not to remember. In [13], Klaus et al. tested various LSTM architectures and out of many LSTMs, Vanilla LSTM performed well on various datasets. In [13], they also discussed optimal methods for hyperparameter tuning and how to save experimentation time by tuning learning parameter at the beginning model building. Stock prices vary with time (time series data), and so for generalization of data windowing technique was introduced in [14], while most of the current methods are based on short-term predictions. Nikola [15] proposed method for long-term prediction in which he used eight models for long-term forecasting. Out of eight models, random forest method has higher precision (75.1%) over SVM (63.9%), logistic regression (64.3%), and Naïve Bayes (54.5%). In order to increase the precision of random forests, features are selected manually, out of 28 features, after iterative process only 11 features were selected [15].

The related works discussed above clearly show that, each algorithm/model can solve the forecasting problem in its own methods and each model has its own limitations. From the above survey, we can observe that, there is an improvement in stock forecasting if LSTM networks are used in prediction models. However, in most cases, existing networks are tested and evaluated on particular datasets and these models often perform badly on other datasets. Yoojeong et al. used filtering with 715 input features in their models and got better predictions than before [16]. Finding important features and using those features as inputs will improve the model accuracy. Therefore, we developed stock price forecasting model using LSTM and compared it with traditional models. In addition to that, we tested the effectiveness on different datasets and evaluated the accuracy by changing the hyperparameters (number of hidden neurons, learning rate, epochs, etc.) after every training cycle to find the optimum hyperparameters.

Generalized neural network for forecasting stock prices is challenging work because of complexity and volatile nature of time series. So far, very few researchers have attempted to solve this problem by modeling hybrid networks and transfer learning approaches. Yet, they could not able to preserve the temporal components, which are crucial for financial time series models. In this chapter, we have addressed the problem and proposed a novel RNN-based LSTM architecture with skip connections to preserve temporal components. Moreover, for understanding of other forecasting approaches, reader may refer [17–21].

This chapter is organized as follows: In Sect. 2, we have discussed the background work and theoretical knowledge behind the stock price forecasting in terms of machine learning context and I have also discussed some previous works done in this domain. In Sect. 3, the description about the model used in this project is discussed and the parameter selection. In Sect. 4, our experimental results are discussed and the report ends with conclusion and future work in section.

2   Methodology

2.1   Time Series Analysis of Financial Data

Many companies rely on forecasting before making the policy changes. For instance, airlines will observe the passenger data and future forecasts of how many people will travel in their airlines so that they can order new planes. It is very important application for government to use birth and death rates as multivariate features to forecast population growth so that they can plan or take necessary measures like immigration or budget planning, etc.

TS data is further classified into two categories: univariate and multivariate TS data. In our model, we have only considered closing prices of the stock data with respect to time and modeled using the univariate TS techniques, where only one value (closing price) is observed at each time step. After classifying the nature of given TS, we now have to apply the data on different models for forecasting.

2.2   Statistical Methods for TS Analysis

Moving average (MA): This statistical approach gives the general direction of trends and patterns by exploring historical data. For a window size of K, moving average is calculated by adding most recent data points and divide them by K and iterated until it converges. The MA is commonly used to smoothen the prices by eliminating white noise from the given dataset. A typical moving average is written by the following equation:

$$M_i = (1/k) \sum_{i=0}^{k-1} (P_{t-i}) \tag{1}$$

where k is the window size

Autoregression (AR) model: AR model uses the past values to predict future patterns. An AR(P) is an autoregressive process where it uses previous p values to predict future values. These models are built upon the assumption that, past values do not change with respect to time. Most of the times it can lead to wrong predictions if the input data is strictly temporal. Yet these models are still used for predicting non-temporal data. For instance, before 2008 financial crises, most shareholders used AR models to forecast US stock prices before investing. Surprisingly, most of them were successful to capture the trends and made profits using this model. In this chapter, we have used AR model to compare our results with other statistical models and neural networks.

ARIMA model: Autoregressive integrated moving average method is often referred as ARIMA model. A non-seasonal data without white nose can be modeled using this model. This model is distinguished by three variables, i.e., p, d, q, where p is the order of autoregressive term, q is the order of moving average term, and q is the quantity used when time series needed to be converted into stationary form.

$$\hat{y}_t = k + \Omega_1 y_{t-1} + \cdots + \Omega_p y_{t-p} - \beta_1 e_{t-1} - \cdots - \beta_q e_{t-} \qquad (2)$$

where $\hat{y}_t$ is the prediction at time step t, β is the moving component, and Ω is the autoregressive component. Moving average parameters (β) in the above equation is initiated as negative variables to follow the standard convention of Box and Jerkins method presented in [22]. In order to improve the efficacy of the model, we removed the aggregate features of seasonality by using variance transformation technique. Stationary series obtained after transformation may still have some autocorrected noise and it is mitigated by adjusting AR and MA terms greater than unity.

2.3 Datasets

Stock price data is collected at specific time in various forms like open, close, high, low, and volume in the time span of a day. For this project, data has been collected from Goldman Sachs, Facebook, AMD, Apple, and IBM from 1999 to 2017 through Yahoo finance. Initial processing of data includes finding the missing values and normalization and finding the mean and median of the data with respect to time. The transformation function used in this project is given by the equation below:

$$\text{Log}\ (p_i) - \log\ (p_{i-1}) \qquad (3)$$

A dropout is used to reduce the computational load on the model by removing the unused neurons while training and the dropout parameter used in this network is 0.2 for first hidden layer and 0.25 for second hidden layer. Each dataset is divided into training, testing, and validation sets with 6:2:2 ratio. Missing values in the given datasets are filled using temporal interpolation [23].

2.4 LSTM Hyperparameter Selection

One of the most important tasks of any machine learning algorithms is hyperparameter selection. The number of layers, which is fundamental choice for building a neural network, must be decided before building the network. Before finalizing our network architecture, we have searched over several possibilities of errors and overfitting, with the help of validation set. Especially, we varied the LSTM architecture

Table 1 LSTM results

LSTM units	Epochs	Batch size	Optimizer	RMSE	Time (Sec)
50	10	16	adam	6.77	61
40	10	80	adamax	5.4	16
10	10	80	adamax	6.5	18
80	10	150	adamx	3.95	22
100	5	50	adam	3.71	18

from 1 to 4 layers and the number of epochs to be used for better results. After all this experimental analysis, we concluded to use a 2-layer LSTM network with tanh activation function. It is to be noted that, we haven't used batch gradient which most people used for hyperparameter tuning. Using batch gradient will eventually increase the computational load on the network and it will take long time to converge.

Since we are using mini-batch gradient decent optimization technique to update the weights, training data is passed multiple times for convergence. Nevertheless, it is still unknown how many epochs are required to get the optimal weights. We trained our networks several rounds with different epochs each time. At the end of each training cycle, RMSE values are noted.

After handful of experiments on various LSTM network architectures, the model that returns lowest RMSE was selected for forecasting. After each experiment, RMSE and the simulation time is noted. The results of experiment are shown in below Table 1. We observed that LSTM network with 100 units, 5 epochs, batch size of 50 with Adam optimizer gave the accurate predictions and took 18 s to converge.

2.5 Network Structure

After selecting necessary hyperparameters from the above section, my final neural network consists of LSTM and dense artificial neural networks. We have used simple 3-layer network with 2 LSTM blocks and the final block is connected to output to get the predicted values. The main reason for selecting LSTM is because of the temporal data and to overcome regression problems. Unlike other neural networks, LSTM has its own advantages like the flexibility to accept sequential data (data is processed in such a way that, previous data point is related to past data) and its three internal gates that allows and forgets data where it is unrelated to our network. This functionality allows us to use the previous data. For training our network I have used Adam optimizer and mean square error as loss metric.

Furthermore, to reduce the computational load on the network, a data preprocessing method was used by normalizing the input data. Training, testing, and validation datasets are normalized to bring the dataset to the same values without distorting

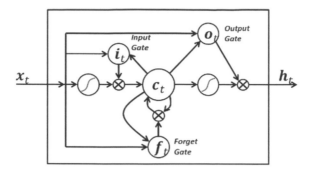

Fig. 2 Internal structure of LSTM cell

the distribution range of data. An exponential smoothing technique is used on training data to extract the seasonal patterns behind the data (Fig. 2).

Our dataset consists of various columns such as opening price, closing price high, and low; we have focused on opening and closed prices for our evaluation and compared its performance with the traditional statistical method. Prediction accuracy is defined by mean square error (MSE)

$$\text{MSE} = \text{mean}\left(\left(\sum_t \text{actual value} - \text{predicted value}\right)^2\right) \quad (4)$$

In this project, we have used MSE as our main quality metric function for testing the model performance and sometimes Mean absolute percentage error (MAPE) is also used.

3 Experimental Results

In this chapter, five different datasets are selected for experimental analysis. The motivation behind using multiple datasets is to test the stability, generalization, and the correlation between the datasets for understanding market dynamics using the proposed models. Statistical methods mainly focus on data points that are close to the predicting values. Meanwhile, LSTM networks consider all the previous data points by updating weights frequently.

We compared the results of four networks presented in this chapter in the context of temporal framework. In order to decrease the complexity and computational load, we considered univariate datasets. However, in our initial experimental setup, we compared the results of univariate and bivariate datasets. In our comparisons, both datasets almost resulted same RMSE error, but bivariate network took longer time

Table 2 Comparison between univariate and bivariate LSTM models

	Univariate	Bivariate
RMSE (LSTM)	1.6512	1.6409
Training time	76.35 s	104.08 s

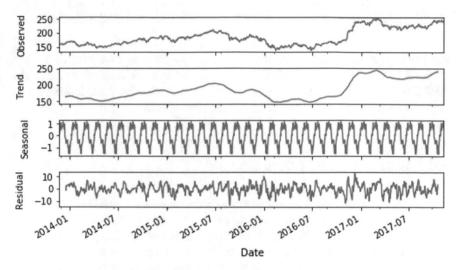

Fig. 3 Time series decomposition, where it divided into trend, seasonal, and residual components

for training. Table 2 shows the training time and RMSE of LSTM networks with univariate and bivariate datasets.

3.1 Time Series Decomposition

A time series is the combination of three main components, i.e., trend, seasonality, and noise. Decomposition of time series involves extracting trends, seasonality, and noise and helps us to discover the underlying patters. A multiplicative decomposition technique [24] is used for this purpose which transforms nonlinear data into linear. The output of decomposition algorithm used in this project is presented in the following Fig. 3.

3.2 Average or Mean Method

In this method, the stock prices are predicted based upon the average of the training data. $\hat{y} = \sum_{i=1}^{N} Xi$, where X_i = input data, $\hat{y}$ = predicted outputs, and N = total

Table 3 RMSE values of different models on similar datasets used for testing

	Goldman sachs	Apple	Facebook	AMD	IBM
MA model	8.268	5.668	7.145	6.037	6.845
AR model	7.11	6.844	7.796	5.389	7.264
ARIMA	5.369	4.923	5.099	5.197	6.294
LSTM	3.236	3.089	2.904	3.036	3.166

number of samples. Time index and closing prices are used as attributes for MA model. Moving averages are calculated using fixed window sizes of 20 days. The RMSE of 5 datasets is shown in below Table 3. The results show that this method is highly inaccurate and failed to deliver the expected results.

3.3   Autoregression Method

Autoregression is a method for interpreting time series data which takes input from the past time steps as source and forecasts the future time step values. It is one of the basic time series models which can deliver precise results and also proved to be one the best models to evaluate time series data. The autoregression function used in this project is imported from statistical library in the name of AR class. The RMSE for this model is surprisingly low (2.56) when compared to the above average model. The results of predictions are shown in the following figure.

3.4   ARIMA Model

In the below Table 3, we can see the performance of ARIMA model on five datasets. Based on the model predictions, we can say that, a constant variable K from Eq. 2 is added to the previous values at each time step to predict future variables. This model outperformed AR and MA model as the RMSE of ARIMA is relatively lower than other statistical proposed in this chapter. We examined our model with various parameters of p and q to find the optimal model. Autoregressive moving average method is the statistical method for time series analysis. This model performed well on the dataset we have used, with 2.5 RMSE we can clearly say that ARIMA can be used for short-term predictions.

3.5   LSTM Model

LSTM network is implemented using deep learning framework called Keras, which is built on top of TensorFlow. While processing the stock prices, LSTM networks unwrap the data along the time axis. Cell states from the previous time steps will be saved and used for calculating the current cell state. In order to ensure the reproduction of same results, we fixed the random seed to 8. The model starts training after calling "model.fit" command. Fit command takes training data, epochs, number of LSTM units, learning rate, optimization method, and loss function as the input variables.

3.6   Comparison of Different Models

From the heuristic results presented in the below table, we can say that LSTM network outperformed statistical in terms of forecasting accuracy. It can be argued that all the statistical models showed almost similar performance however produced mixed results when these models are evaluated on different datasets.

For generalizing the model to find the series data, I modified input data into a categorical price and that authorizes us to find the optimal solutions at all the instances. Meanwhile the output price or the closing price does not necessarily vary with the demand price or peak price of that day and this permits us to deal with similar data points. This also reduces the computational cost by 15% additionally we can converge in less time when compared with other methods. The seasonal trends in the data are observed in different levels (day, week, month) by using regularization and based on this our network will perform better in finding patterns in time series by using seasonal trends as a feedback.

The network we have modeled is designed in such a way that it can execute tick-level data which is collected from previous stock prices. Main motivation behind using tick-level data is it is less computationally expensive to train our model by providing a good feedback signal to the network. After conducting experiment on stock prices of different companies on different models, results of each models are given in the Table 3. Form the experimental results, it is clear that statistical models are bad at generalizing and showed varied performance on different datasets. One of the key findings of our research is statistical models are able to detect the patterns of time series where the data has strong trend and weak seasonality also, and they failed to detect dynamical fluctuations in datasets. Meanwhile, LSTM networks were able to produce same results on different datasets. Our results clearly show that previous lags are also played important role in modeling LSTM networks. It also helped us to detect the dynamical patterns (Fig. 4).

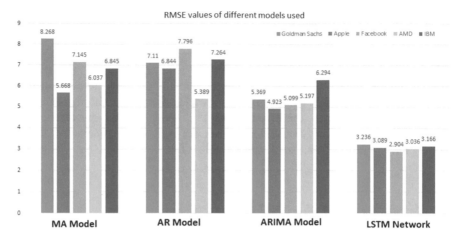

Fig. 4 Comparison of different models used in the study with respect to their RMSE values

4 Conclusion

Stock price forecasting is a challenging task. Nonlinear relationships, dynamic changes, and unpredictable are some of the factors made forecasting laborious. With the help of deep learning, we were able to solve the nonlinear patterns of stock price data and a successful model is developed for efficient predictions.

Regardless of the favored belief that deep RNN's performs better than statistical methods, our experimental results prove that belief as true. In this chapter, we have proposed and discussed various methods to forecast the stock prices. To find how accurate and reliable are these LSTM methods when compared with statistical methods like ARIMA, AR, MA methods. In our approach, we modeled different networks and compared accuracies of different models. Results indicated that LSTM-based recurrent neural networks was able to capture the non-stationary patterns from the given time series datasets. Experimental outcomes showed that we can predict stock prices with several methods and each method or network architecture is good at predicting specific patterns in data. For example, the model we have developed in this project can be used for long term prediction like weekly forecasting. In our case studies we have found that, stock prices are greatly affected by news and blogs. More specifically, the LSTM-based algorithm improved the prediction by 85% on average compared to ARIMA. Furthermore, this chapter reports no improvement when the number of epochs is changed.

References

1. Jean, N., Burke, M., Xie, M., Davis, W.M., Lobell, D.B., Ermon, S.: Combining satellite imagery and machine learning to predict poverty. Science **353**(6301), 790–794 (2016)
2. Weiss, G. M., Timko, J.L., Gallagher, C.M., Yoneda, K., Schreiber, A.J.: Smartwatch-based activity recognition: a machine learning approach.In : 2016 IEEE-EMBS International Conference on Biomedical and Health Informatics (BHI), pp. 426–429. IEEE (2016)
3. Jahangiri, A., Rakha, H.A.: Applying machine learning techniques to transportation mode recognition using mobile phone sensor data. IEEE Trans. Intell. Transp. Syst. **16**(5), 2406–2417 (2015)
4. Kourou, K., Exarchos, T.P., Exarchos, K.P., Karamouzis, M.V., Fotiadis, D.I.: Machine learning applications in cancer prognosis and prediction. Comput. Struct. Biotechnol. J. **13**, 8–17 (2015)
5. Ribli, D., Pataki, B.A., Csabai, I.: An improved cosmological parameter inference scheme motivated by deep learning. Nat. Astrono. **3**(1), 93–98 (2019)
6. Malkiel, B.G., Fama, E.F.: Efficient capital markets: A review of theory and empirical work. the Journal of Finance **25**(2), 383–417 (1970)
7. Ariyo, A.A., Adewumi, O.A., Ayo, C.K.: Stock price prediction using the ARIMA model. In: 2014 UKSim-AMSS 16th International Conference on Computer Modelling and Simulation, pp. 106–112. IEEE (2014)
8. Patel, J., Shah, S., Thakkar, P., Kotecha, K.: Predicting stock and stock price index movement using trend deterministic data preparation and machine learning techniques. Expert Syst. Appl. **42**(1), 259–268 (2015)
9. Qin, K., Li, C., Pavlu, V., Aslam, J.A.: Adapting rnn sequence prediction model to multi-label set prediction. arXiv preprint, arXiv:1904.05829 (2019)
10. Chimmula, V.K.R., Zhang, L.: Time series forecasting of COVID-19 transmission in Canada using LSTM networks. Chaos Solitons Fractals 109864 (2020)
11. Shah, D., Campbell, W., Zulkernine, F.H.: A Comparative study of LSTM and DNN for stock market forecasting. In: 2018 IEEE International Conference on Big Data (Big Data), pp. 4148–4155. IEEE (2018)
12. Hochreiter, S., Schmidhuber, J.: Long short-term memory. Neural Comput. **9**(8), 1735–1780 (1997)
13. Greff, K., Srivastava, R.K., Koutník, J., Steunebrink, B.R., Schmidhuber, J.: LSTM: a search space odyssey. IEEE Trans. Neural Netw. Learn. Sys. **28**(10), 2222–2232 (2016)
14. Bifet, A., Gavalda, R.: Learning from time-changing data with adaptive windowing. In: Proceedings of the 2007 SIAM international conference on data mining, pp. 443–448. Society for Industrial and Applied Mathematics (2007)
15. Milosevic, N.: Equity forecast: predicting long term stock price movement using machine learning. arXiv preprint arXiv:1603.00751 (2016)
16. Song, Y., Lee, J.W., Lee, J.: A study on novel filtering and relationship between input-features and target-vectors in a deep learning model for stock price prediction. Appl. Intell. **49**(3), 897–911 (2019)
17. Iqbal, A., et al.: Metaheurestic algorithm based hybrid model for identification of building sale prices. In: Metaheuristic and Evolutionary Computation: Algorithms and Applications. Studies in Computational Intelligence. Springer (2020). https://doi.org/10.1007/978-981-15-7571-6_32
18. Fatema, N., et al.: Data-driven occupancy detection hybrid model using particle swarm optimization based artificial neural network. In: Metaheuristic and Evolutionary Computation: Algorithms and Applications. Studies in Computational Intelligence. Springer (2020). https://doi.org/10.1007/978-981-15-7571-6_13
19. Minai, A.F., et al.: Metaheuristics paradigms for renewable energy systems: advances in optimization algorithms. In: Metaheuristic and Evolutionary Computation: Algorithms and Applications. Studies in Computational Intelligence. Springer (2020). https://doi.org/10.1007/978-981-15-7571-6_2

20. Iqbal, A., et al.: Data driven intelligent model for sales prices prediction and monitoring of a building. In: Soft Computing in Condition Monitoring and Diagnostics of Electrical and Mechanical Systems, pp. 407–421. Springer (2019). https://doi.org/10.1007/978-981-15-1532-3_18

21. Chimmula, V.K.R., et al.: Novel application of relief algorithm in cascade ANN model for prognosis of photovoltaic maximum power under sunny outdoor condition of Sikkim India: A case study. In: Soft Computing in Condition Monitoring and Diagnostics of Electrical and Mechanical Systems, pp. 387–405, Springer (2019). https://doi.org/10.1007/978-981-15-1532-3_17

22. Tang, Z., De Almeida, C., Fishwick, P.A.: Time series forecasting using neural networks vs. Box-Jenkins methodology. Simulation **57**(5), 303–310 (1991)

23. Shahar, Y.: Knowledge-based temporal interpolation. J. Exp. Theor. Artif. Intell. **11**(1), 123–144 (1999)

24. Yue, C., Kohnle, U., Hanewinkel, M., Klädtke, J.: Extracting environmentally driven growth trends from diameter increment series based on a multiplicative decomposition model. Can. J. For. Res. **41**(8), 1577–1589 (2011)

Intelligent Modelling of Renewable Energy Resources-Based Hybrid Energy System for Sustainable Power Generation and Monitoring

Priyanka Anand, Mohammad Rizwan, Sarabjeet Kaur Bath, and Gulnar Perveen

Abstract The electrical energy is playing a vital role in the development and sustainability of any country. The demand of electrical energy is rising due to the increased comfort levels, urbanization and technological advancements. Therefore, it is utmost important to invigorate the use of renewable energy resources for bridging the gap and accepting the challenges of increasing electrical energy demands and greenhouse gas emissions. In view of the above, the present research focuses on the optimal design and sizing of hybrid energy system (HES) based on renewable energy resources, including solar photovoltaic (SPV), wind energy system, biomass and biogas with battery to electrify the rural areas of India's Haryana state. Different models of hybrid energy systems have been chosen and optimized using different intelligent approaches such as grey wolf optimization (GWO), harmony search (HS) and particle swarm optimization (PSO) on the MATLAB platform. Finally, the results are compared in view of minimizing net present cost (NPC) and cost of energy (COE) and found the most optimal solution.

Keywords Solar energy · Wind energy · Biomass · Biogas · Optimization

P. Anand (✉)
Department of Electronics and Communication Engineering, B.P.S. Mahila Vishwavidyalaya, Sonipat, Haryana 131305, India
e-mail: anand_priyanka10@yahoo.co.in

M. Rizwan
Department of Electrical Engineering, College of Engineering, Qassim University, Buraydah 52571, Qassim, Saudi Arabia
e-mail: rizwan@dtu.ac.in

Department of Electrical Engineering, Delhi Technological University, Delhi 110042, India

S. K. Bath
Department of Electrical Engineering, Giani Zail Singh Campus College of Engineering and Technology, Bathinda, Punjab 151001, India
e-mail: sjkbath77@gmail.com

G. Perveen
Defence Research and Development Organisation, Metcalfe House Annexe, Delhi, India
e-mail: gulegulnar@gmail.com

© The Author(s), under exclusive license to Springer Nature Singapore Pte Ltd. 2021   217
H. Malik et al. (eds.), *AI and Machine Learning Paradigms for Health Monitoring System*, Studies in Big Data 86,
https://doi.org/10.1007/978-981-33-4412-9_14

1 Introduction

Power generation from renewable energy resources is playing a very significant role for the development and ultimately in achieving the sustainability. As a result, the greenhouse gas (GHG) emission is reduced significantly and may play an important role in the climate change, etc. Due to the volatile nature of renewable energy resources, it is recommended that a set of two or even more renewable energy resources which would form a hybrid energy system (HES) is given substantial focus in the past recent years. Owing to economic and reliability issues, it is further essential to optimize the design and sizing of HES system components. Further, reliable and sustainable energy supply is crucial and inevitable to modern society's endurance, facilitates socio-economic development and is an essential aspect for the enhancement of basic human healthcare services and sanitation. It has been reported that inadequate energy supply, which is omnipresent to lots of developing countries, especially in India, is strongly indicative of poor socio-economic growth. Sometimes, this is predominant in rural areas. In this regard, for many reasons involving global climate change, price variation of fossil fuels, depletion of traditional sources and environmental consequences, renewable energy resources (solar, wind, biomass, biogas, small hydropower, etc.) are being explored extensively. Moreover, renewable energy will increase the scope of power generation and the resilience of the power systems [1, 2].

It is discovered from the literature review that HES incorporating two or more renewable energy resources is more desirable because of intermittent nature, reliance on climate condition, etc. [3, 4]. Various aspects of HES have been studied by the researchers, out of which the most significant is optimal designer sizing of HES components. The size of HES component must be assessed optimally to get a reliable and economical energy system. This problem has been dealt by comprehensive methods such as simulation tools [5–8], graphical construction [9, 10], probabilistic [11–13], iterative [14–16] and artificial intelligence [17–22] have been studied and reported. In recent times, intelligent approaches have been employed extensively to optimize HES with a view of optimizing its economic benefits. In this context, multiple authors exploited intelligent approaches including genetic algorithm (GA), particle swarm optimization (PSO), cuckoo search (CS), harmony search (HS), ant colony optimization (ACO), biogeography-based optimization (BBO), grey wolf optimization (GWO), etc., for optimal sizing of HES, out of which some are discussed in forthcoming paragraphs.

Gupta et al. used GA to develop a standalone solar photovoltaic (SPV) wind HES to generate varying loads in the Rajasthan state district of Jaipur, India. The results show that the algorithm built provides optimal solution, and the developed standalone HES provides power supply at the desired cost [23]. Mostofi and Shayeghi also employed GA to design the hybrid energy systems consisting of solar photovoltaic, wind energy conversion system, fuel cell and small hydro power. The obtained results were compared and found more accurate as compared to hybrid optimization of multiple energy resources platform [24]. Askarzadeh and Leandro dos suggested a

PSO-based optimization model to supply electricity to Kerman's remote location in Iran. The total area inhabited by SPV, the number of batteries and the total swept area of the wind turbine blades were chosen as the decision variables to achieve an optimized model [25]. Mohamed et al. also employed PSO for optimum designing of grid-connected SPV/wind HES to reduce energy costs and facilitate reliability. The optimized HES was compared with the actual power grid in view of cost savings and found more accurate [26]. Using an artificial bee colony (ABC) algorithm, Singh and Kaushik performed optimal sizing for a HES SPV/biomass in grid-linked and off-grid scenarios. Results showed that the grid-linked system is more economical and efficient compared to off grid [27].

Ogunjuyigbe et al. carried out the size optimization of a grid-linked SPV/wind/diesel generator (DG)/battery HES to fulfil the electrical energy demands of a housing complex using GA. The multi-objective problem has been presented in this work by considering two aims: life cycle cost and pollution. Many configurations were examined and it has been discovered that the SPV/wind/DG/battery configuration is better suited to supply the load [28]. Bartolucci et al. explored the role of sizing of HESs on system performance. Two observations were reported, first the FC system influences the stability of the grid, and secondly the proper size of the SPV power plant enables the battery to be used more intelligently and gives less dependence on the energy shared with grid [29]. A modified crow search algorithm (CSA) was developed by Ghaffaria and Askarzadeh to optimize the size of an off-grid HES consisting of a set of SPVs, DG and FC along with electrolysers and hydrogen tanks. Total net present cost (NPC) has been considered an objective function that is optimized under constraints of penetration of renewable energies and loss of power supply probability (LPSP). Results showed that the CSA adaptive AP has found results that are more encouraging and consistent than the original CSA, GA and PSO [30].

Anand et al. used the PSO algorithm to optimally design and size HES for rural area electrification. Eight cases of HES have been optimized and compared. HES, including SPV, biomass, biogas and battery, is found to be better compared with others for the selected region. The optimum HES was also recorded at 5 and 10% unmet load [31]. The same researchers carried out the optimum design of HES consisting of various renewable energy resources in off grid and grid linked using HS algorithm. Integrated and off-grid hybrid systems were considered and configured using HS algorithm. Grid-integrated HES consisting of SPV/wind/biogas/biomass with battery has been found to be most economical for selected area. The findings were compared with the PSO optimization approach and were revealed to be more appropriate [32].

By reviewing the literature, it has been reported that most intelligent approaches have been shown to produce more remarkable results than simulation methods such as HOMER. Therefore, intelligent approaches viz. GWO, HS and PSO have been applied for the sizing and optimization of HES in the present work. These approaches have various advantages such as GWO has good computational efficiency including the qualitative performance and ease of implementation with only a few parameters. HS is capable of handling continuous as well as discrete variables, does not entail initial setting for variables, does not even need differential gradients and is capable of running away from local optima; HS is capable of overcoming the drawbacks of GA's theory of building blocks; PSO has fast convergence speed and efficiency.

The current work has therefore carried out optimum design of SPV/wind/biomass/biogas/battery-based HES to provide continuous electricity to the rural cluster located in Mewat, Haryana state in India. Different models of HES in grid-linked and off-grid mode have been considered and optimized using GWO, HS and PSO algorithms in MATLAB platform. Finally, the obtained results have been compared in view of minimizing NPC and cost of energy (COE) and found the most optimal solution.

2   Site Selection and Data Availability

In this work, a case study has been selected for a total of 638 households of set of four villages namely Silkhoh, Nanuka, Thana alam alias masit and Noorpur located in Mewat district of Haryana state in India. The considered villages are geographically located at the longitude of 76.94° E–77.04° E and latitude of 28.15° N–28.39° N. In the present analysis, three seasons of four months each has been identified due to year-round temperature fluctuations. Summer season makes April–July. Moderate season includes August–November while winter season covers December–March. The study area's daily energy requirement during summer, moderate and winter season has been computed as 3638.955 kWh/day, 2849.355 kWh/day and 1533.149 kWh/day, respectively. An annual energy requirement for selected site is calculated as 977,084.9 kWh/year. In addition, the potential of renewable energy-based resources such as solar irradiance, wind velocity, biomass and biogas has been assessed on the basis of the data obtained. This area's mean solar irradiance has been estimated to be 5.26 kWh/m^2/day [33]. Based on collected data, the identified area has been calculated with a biogas of 236 m^3/day through cattle dung and a biomass of 805 ton/year via crop residues. The selected site has an average annual wind speed of 4.436 m/s with estimated wind power density of 124 W/m^2 [34].

3   Modelling of Renewable Energy Components

The present research focuses on the optimal design of HES that combines the energies of a set of solar, wind, biogas and biomass as depicted in Fig. 1. The DC bus is linked to the SPV panel and the batteries while the wind, biomass and biogas generators are connected to the AC bus, load and grid.

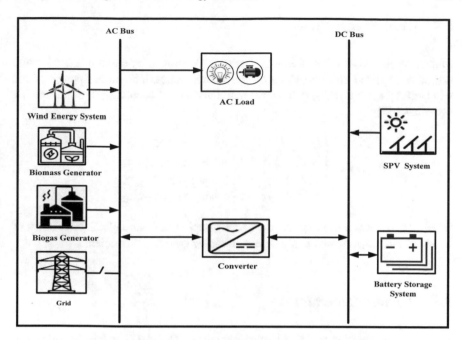

Fig. 1 Schematic diagram of HES

For optimal designing and sizing of HES, mathematical modelling is a key step that offers information about the operation and efficiency of system components under different conditions. Thus, the mathematical expression of each component of HES is presented as follows:

3.1 SPV

The real output power of SPV (P_{SPV} (t)) depends primarily on solar irradiance and ambient temperature and is represented as [31].

$$P_{SPV}(t) = P_{RPV} \times L_F \times \frac{Q_H(t)}{Q_S}(1 + \chi(T_{Cell} - T_{STC}))$$ (1)

L_F symbolizes SPV panel loss factor, Q_H (t) is solar irradiance incident on SPV panel, Q_S is solar irradiance incident under standard test conditions (STC), χ represents temperature coefficient, T_{Cell} denotes SPV cell temperature and T_{STC} is the SPV cell temperature under STC.

3.2 Wind Energy System

Mathematical model of wind energy system is developed by curve fitting of actual power wind speed chart provided by the manufacturer. The output power of the wind energy system (P_{WT}) can be estimated at hour 't' according to the following equations [35]

$$
P_{WT}(t) = \begin{cases}
0 & \text{when} \quad \tau < \tau_{ci} \text{ and } \tau > \tau_{co} \\
x_1\tau^2 + y_1\tau + z_1 & \text{when} \quad \tau_{ci} \leq \tau < \tau_1 \\
x_2\tau^2 + y_2\tau + z_2 & \text{when} \quad \tau_1 \leq \tau < \tau_2 \\
x_3\tau^2 + y_3\tau + z_3 & \text{when} \quad \tau_2 \leq \tau < \tau_{co}
\end{cases}
\tag{2}
$$

where τ symbolizes wind speed. τ_{co} and τ_{ci} depicts cut-out and cut-in velocity of wind turbine, respectively. x, y, z define quadratic equation coefficients.

3.3 Biomass Generator

The output power obtained by biomass generator ($P_{BMS}(t)$) has been evaluated at hour t as [32]:

$$
P_{BMS}(t) = \frac{A_{BM} \times C_{BM} \times \eta_{BMS} \times 1000}{365 \times 860 \times H_{OBM}}
\tag{3}
$$

where A_{BM} indicates biomass availability, C_{BM} is biomass calorific value, η_{BMS} is conversion efficiency (overall) of biomass system and H_{OBM} is the daily number of hours of operation of biomass generator.

3.4 Biogas Generator

The biogas generator output power ($P_{BGS}(t)$) has been measured as [2]:

$$
P_{BGS}(t) = \frac{A_{BG} \times C_{BG} \times \eta_{BGS}}{860 \times H_{OBG}}
\tag{4}
$$

where A_{BG}. symbolizes biogas availability in a day. C_{BG} defines calorific value of biogas and η_{BGS} indicates overall conversion efficiency from biogas to electricity generation. H_{OBG} is biogas generator operating hours in a day.

3.5 Battery

Depending on demand and generation, the battery acts in two states namely charging and discharging. The renewable energy resources-based power generation in charging state is greater than the hourly load demand. However, the hourly load demand is larger than the generation of renewable energy resources during discharging state. During charging and discharging, the battery capacity at hour t has been evaluated in Eqs. (5–8) as:

$$E_{\text{Bat}}^d(t) = E_{\text{Bat}}^d(t-1) + \left[E_{E_{\text{WTS}}}(t) + E_{E_{\text{DMS}}}(t) + E_{E_{\text{BGS}}}(t) + E_{E_{\text{SPVS}}}^d(t) \right] \times \eta_{\text{CH}} \tag{5}$$

where $E_{\text{Bat}}^d(t)$ denotes battery stored energy. $E_{\text{ESPVS}}^d(t)$, and $E_{\text{EBMS}}(t)$ are surplus energy produced by SPV, biogas and biomass generator after satisfying the load demand, respectively, and η_{CH} represents the battery charging efficiency.

$$E_{\text{Bat}}^d(t) = (1 - \gamma) \times E_{\text{Bat}}^d(t-1) - E_{\text{NDD}}(t) \tag{6}$$

$$E_{\text{NDD}}(t) = \frac{E_{\text{NTDM}}(t)}{\eta_{\text{INV}} \times \eta_{\text{DCH}}} \tag{7}$$

$$E_{\text{NTDM}}(t) = E_{\text{DMD}}(t) - \left[E_{\text{WTS}}(t) + E_{\text{BMS}}(t) + E_{\text{BGS}}(t) + E_{\text{SPVS}}^d(t) \times \eta_{\text{INV}} \right] \tag{8}$$

where γ represents battery self-discharging rate at t hour; $E_{\text{NDD}}(t)$ is required energy by demand side in kWh and η_{INV} and η_{DCH} represents inverter efficiency and discharging efficiency of battery, respectively. $E_{\text{NTDM}}(t)$ denotes shortfall or unfulfilled demand not met out by renewable energy resources. $E_{\text{DMD}}(t)$ is hourly load demand.

3.6 Grid

In HES grid-linked scenario, grid may work in two phases. In first phase, it can supply HES with deficit electricity in the event that renewable energy resources along with the battery bank can not satisfy the demand. Electricity that is supplied via the grid can mathematically be modelled as [32]:

$$\begin{aligned} E_{\text{PG}}(t) = E_{\text{DMD}}(t) &- [E_{\text{WTS}}(t) + E_{\text{BMS}}(t) + E_{\text{BGS}}(t) \\ &+ [(E_{\text{SPVS}}^d(t) + (E_{\text{Bat}}^d(t) - E_{\text{Batmin}}) \times \eta_{\text{INV}}]] \end{aligned} \tag{9}$$

where $E_{PG}(t)$ represents the energy to be bought through the grid and E_{Bmin} is battery storage capacity minimum values.

While, in second phase, grid can take surplus electricity if generation exceeds demand and battery banks are completely charged and it is mathematically modelled as:

$$E_{SG}(t) = [E_{WTS}(t) + E_{BMS}(t) + E_{BGS}(t) + [(E_{SPVS}^d(t)$$
$$+ (E_{Batmax} - E_{Bat}^d(t)) \times \eta_{INV}]] - E_{DMD}(t) \qquad (10)$$

where $E_{SG}(t)$ is representing the extra energy required and it must be sold by the grid. E_{Bmax} denotes battery storage capacity maximum values.

4 Optimization Framework

The optimization framework results are provided along with the objective function with associated constraints. The objective of the proposed system is net present cost and cost of energy of the hybrid energy systems. The optimization is carried out considering the various associated constraints including the lower and upper boundaries of components, battery storage capacity limits and unmet load for HES design.

4.1 Objective Function

The total NPC has been considered an economic measure for HES sizing. It constitutes of all expense occurring over the life cycle of the system involving net present capital cost (C_{NV}), replacement cost (RP_{NV}), operational and maintenance (O & M) cost (OM_{NV}), fuel cost (F_{NV}), cost for electricity purchased via utility grid (C_{PG}), etc., and revenue generated in respect of salvage value (SV_{NV}) and sold price of electricity to the utility grid (C_{SG}) that can be represented as:

$$NPC = C_{NV} + OM_{NV} - SV_{NV} + RP_{NV} + F_{NV} - C_{SG} + C_{PG} \qquad (11)$$

4.1.1 C_{NV}

The C_{NV} includes the net present capital cost of each one component of HES and can be evaluated as [32]:

$$C_{NV} = ((N_{SPV} \times \psi_{SPV} \times P_{panel}) + (N_{wT} \times \psi_{wT} \times P_{WT})$$

$$+ (P_{BMS} \times \psi_{BM}) + (P_{BGS} \times \psi_{BG}) + (N_{Bat} \times \psi_{Bat}) + (P_{INV} \times \psi_{INV}))$$
$$(12)$$

where N_{SPV}, N_{WT} and N_{Bat} indicate number of SPV panel, wind turbine and battery, respectively. P_{panel} and P_{WT} symbolize power of individual SPV panel and wind turbine, respectively. P_{BMS}, P_{BGS} and P_{INV} represent power output of biomass and biogas generator and inverter, respectively. Ψ_{SPV}, Ψ_{WT}, Ψ_{BM}, Ψ_{BG}, Ψ_{Bat} and Ψ_{INV} indicate initial cost of SPV panel, wind turbine, biomass generator, biogas generator, battery and inverter, respectively.

4.1.2 OM$_{NV}$

OM$_{NV}$ of HES includes the total O&M costs of each component over the year and has been calculated by Eq. (13) as:

$$
\begin{aligned}
OM_{NV} = {}& ((\varpi_{SPV} \times N_{SPV} \times P_{panel}) + (\varpi_{WT} \times N_{WT} \times P_{WT}) \\
& + (\varpi_{FBM} \times P_{BMS} + \varpi_{VBM} \times P_{ABM}^{W}) \\
& + (\varpi_{FBG} \times P_{BGS} + \varpi_{VBG} \times P_{ABG}^{W}) + (\varpi_{Bat} \times N_{Bat}) \\
& + (\varpi_{INV} \times P_{INV})) \times \sum_{i=1}^{\mu} \left(\frac{1+\zeta}{1+R_i} \right)^{i}
\end{aligned}
$$
$$(13)$$

where ϖ_{SPV}, ϖ_{WT}, ϖ_{Bat} and ϖ_{INV} denote yearly O&M costs of SPV panel, wind turbine and battery and inverter, respectively. ϖ_{FBG} and ϖ_{FBM} indicate annually fixed O&M cost of biogas and biomass generator, respectively. ϖ_{VBG} and ϖ_{VBM} symbolize yearly variable O&M cost of biogas and biomass generator, respectively. P_{ABM}^{W} and P_{ABG}^{W} represent annualy working power of biomass and biogas generator, respectively. ζ is an escalation rate of system components. R_i denotes interest rate. μ is project lifetime.

4.1.3 RP$_{NV}$

In the present analysis, the lifetime of SPV, wind energy system, biomass and biogas have been presumed to be 25 years equal to the project life (25 years). Therefore, there is no need to replace them and thus the cost of replacing these components is not included while determining NPC. The life of battery storage system and the inverter is considered as 5 years and 10 years, respectively, which is less than the life of the project (25 years). Therefore, battery and inverter must be replaced 4 and 2 times over the project's entire lifetime, respectively, and additional investment is required in view of replacement costs that can be calculated as [2]:

$$RP_{NV} = \left(N_{Bat} \times \psi_{Bat} \times \sum_{i=5,10,15,20} \left(\frac{1 + \zeta_{Bat}}{1 + R_i} \right)^i \right)$$
$$+ \left(P_{INV} \times \psi_{INV} \times \sum_{i=10,20} \left(\frac{1 + \zeta_{INV}}{1 + R_i} \right)^i \right) \tag{14}$$

4.1.4 F_{NV}

In the system under consideration, fuels include cattle dung (biogas) and crop residues (biomass) used, respectively, in the biomass and biogas generators. For this purpose, F_{NV} has been calculated by considering the expense of cattle dung and biomass and is presented as follows by Eq. (15) as [2].

$$F_{NV} = (\xi_{BM} \times F_{BMR}) + (\xi_{BG} \times F_{BGR}) \times \sum_{i=1}^{\mu} \left(\frac{1 + \zeta}{1 + R_i} \right)^i \tag{15}$$

where ξ_{BM} and ξ_{BG} are biomass and biogas fuel cost. F_{BMR} and F_{BGR} are yearly biomass and biogas requirement.

4.1.5 SV_{NV}

The SV_{NV} involves the resale value of system components throughout the project lifespan and has been determined as [32]:

$$SV_{NV} = ((\varepsilon_{SPV} \times N_{SPV} \times P_{panel}) + (\varepsilon_{WT} \times N_{WT} \times P_{WT}) + (\varepsilon_{BM} \times P_{BMS})$$
$$+ (\varepsilon_{BG} \times P_{BGS}) + (\varepsilon_{Bat} \times N_{Bat}) + (\varepsilon_{INV} \times P_{INV})) \times \left(\frac{1 + \lambda}{1 + R_i} \right)^{\mu} \tag{16}$$

where ε_{SPV}, ε_{WT}, ε_{BM}, ε_{BG}, ε_{Bat} and ε_{INV} denote the resale price of system components. λ symbolizes inflation rate.

4.1.6 C_{PG} and C_{SG}

In the grid-linked mode, the C_{PG} and C_{SG} have been measured using following Eq. [32]:

$$C_{SG} = \theta_{SG} \times E_{SG} \times \sum_{i=1}^{\mu} \left(\frac{1 + \lambda}{1 + R_i} \right)^i \tag{17}$$

$$C_{PG} = \theta_{PG} \times E_{PG} \times \sum_{i=1}^{\mu} \left(\frac{1 + \lambda}{1 + R_i} \right)^i \qquad (18)$$

where θ_{SG} and θ_{PG} denote unit cost of selling and buying power to or from the grid. Eventually, the COE is determined as:

$$\text{COE} = \frac{\text{NPC} \times C_{RF}}{E_{DMD} + E_{SG}} \qquad (19)$$

where C_{RF} is capital recovery factor which is measured using equation below:

$$C_{RF} = \frac{R_i(1 + R_i)^{\mu}}{R_i(1 + R_i)^{\mu} - 1} \qquad (20)$$

4.2 Design Constraints

In the present study, the selected objective function is optimized subject to the various constrains as discussed below:

4.2.1 HES Components Limits

The sizing of the components, i.e. N_{SPV}, N_{WT}, N_{Bat}, P_{BMS} and P_{BGS}, is according to the load demand. The minimum and maximum boundaries of these components are therefore defined as one of the constraints and given as:

$$N_{SPV} = \text{Integer}, \ N_{SPV}^{min} \le N_{SPV} \le N_{SPV}^{max} \qquad (21)$$

$$N_{WT} = \text{Integer}, \ N_{WT}^{min} \le N_{WT} \le N_{WT}^{max} \qquad (22)$$

$$N_{Bat} = \text{Integer}, \ N_{Bat}^{min} \le N_{Bat} \le N_{Bat}^{max} \qquad (23)$$

$$P_{BGS} = \text{Integer}, \ P_{BGS}^{min} \le P_{BGS} \le P_{BGS}^{max} \qquad (24)$$

$$P_{BMS} = \text{Integer}, \ P_{BMS}^{min} \le P_{BMS} \le P_{BMS}^{max} \qquad (25)$$

4.2.2 Battery Storage Capacity Boundaries

To run the battery in a safe region, the lower and upper limits may be defined for the battery energy storage systems. The description of the same is provided here:

$$E_{\text{Batmin}} \leq E_{\text{Bat}}(t) \leq E_{\text{Batmax}} \tag{26}$$

4.2.3 Unmet Load

Unmet load is presumed as a constraint of power reliability under the present research. If electrical energy demand exceeds the available supply, the user may have not power supply. Therefore, unmet load is estimated by following formula:

$$\text{Unmet load} = \sum_{t=1}^{t=8760} \frac{\text{Unserved load for one year}}{\text{Total load for one year}} \tag{27}$$

Further, the flowchart of the hybrid system optimization in the present work has been illustrated in Fig. 2.

5   GWO

A GWO approach is an evolutionary approach recently established by Mirjalili et al. [36]. This intelligent approach is inspired by grey wolf's social practices and its technique of prey. Grey wolves are known as apex predators, which mean they seem to be at the top of the pyramid. In general, grey wolves have a tendency for living in a crowd or community. Average crowd size ranges from five to twelve. Because of their special interest, they have a rather stringent, social ruling hierarchy [37].

In GWO, the population is classified into various (four) categories such as α, β, δ and ω. α wolves are considered to be supposed to lead wolves, and they are most responsible for making decisions about resting areas, trapping and all other tactics. β wolves are second to α wolves who provide support in supervising or other community tasks. β wolves honour the α wolf but command other wolves that are poor in the leadership structure. Apparently, β wolves perform the position of counsellor to α wolves and discipliner of everyone in the group. Furthermore, δ acts a role of scapegoat. It can seem that δ wolves throughout the whole community are not very significant, but the entire community faces internal struggle and sorrow in the disappearance of δ wolves. α, β and δ wolves provide direction to ω towards enticing search space areas. Furthermore, the chain of command of all the wolves is seen in Fig. 3.

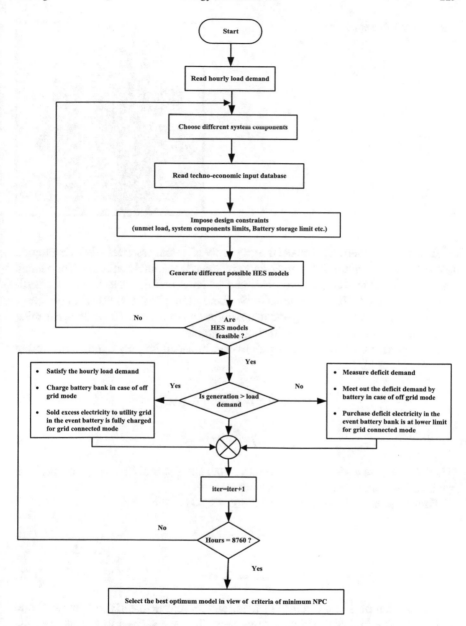

Fig. 2 Flowchart of the hybrid system optimization

Fig. 3 Leadership structure
of grey wolves

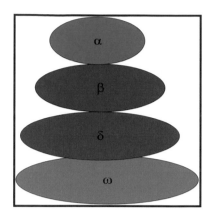

In order to mathematical model the grey wolves' social practices while developing
GWO-based algorithm, α is perceived to be the most suitable solution. The second
and third possible solutions are presumed to be β and δ, respectively. ω constitutes of whatever left candidate solution. Three key phases of searching of prey,
hunting, encircling or trapping and attacking prey are often used while performing
optimization and described in following paragraphs.

Encircling or trapping phase of grey wolves intended for prey throughout hunting
is measured as [37]:

$$\vec{G}_v = \left| \vec{A}_v \cdot \vec{X}_{Py}(t) - \vec{X}_{Gy}(t) \right| \tag{28}$$

$$\vec{X}_{Gy}(t+1) = \vec{X}_{Py}(t) - \vec{e}_v \, \vec{G}_v \tag{29}$$

where G_v, A_v and e_v denotes coefficient vectors and X_{Py} and X_{Gy} represents position
vector of pray and grey wolf, respectively.

Further, e_v and A_v are calculated by Eqs. (30–31) follow as:

$$\vec{e}_v = 2\vec{g} . R_{v1} - \vec{g} \tag{30}$$

$$\vec{A}_v = 2 . \vec{R}_{v2} \tag{31}$$

The portion of g in the course of iterations decreases linearly in between 2 and
0. R_{v1} and R_{v2} indicate random vectors that allow the wolves to get between the
specified points at any location.

A grey wolf can upgrade their location in view of prey's position. By adjusting
the value of e_v and A_v vectors, it is possible to attain the different locations in the
best agent region with reference to the current location. Therefore, by using Eqs. 27
and 28, the position of grey wolf within the space across the prey for any random
place may be modified.

The grey wolves are able to explore their prey. The hunting is normally conducted through α. In hunting, too, β and δ often play a part. There is indeed no knowledge of the prey's location in abstract search space. Therefore, in order to describe the hunting activity mathematically, we presume that α, β and δ wolves are having precise predictions of the possible location of the prey.

The best search agent-based strategy is applied to update their position, and all other search agents should therefore be directed by the first three best solutions. The following Eqs. (32–34) are being used to modify the score and location of α, β and δ wolves as:

$$\vec{F}_\alpha = \left| \vec{A}_{v1}.\vec{X}_\alpha - \vec{X} \right| \tag{32}$$

$$\vec{F}_\beta = \left| \vec{A}_{v2}.\vec{X}_\beta - \vec{X} \right|$$

$$\vec{F}_\beta = \left| \vec{A}_{v2}.\vec{X}_\beta - \vec{X} \right| \tag{33}$$

$$\vec{F}_\delta = \left| \vec{A}_{v3}.\vec{X}_\delta - \vec{X} \right| \tag{34}$$

where A_{v1}, A_{v2}, A_{v3} are random vectors. Further, the prey position vector in relation to the wolves α, β and δ can be determined as:

$$\vec{X}_1 = \vec{X}_\alpha - \vec{e}_{v1}.(\vec{F}_\alpha) \tag{35}$$

$$\vec{X}_2 = \vec{X}_\beta - \vec{e}_{v2}.(\vec{F}_\beta) \tag{36}$$

$$\vec{X}_3 = \vec{X}_\delta - \vec{e}_{v3}.(\vec{F}_\delta) \tag{37}$$

where e_{v1}, e_{v2}, e_{v3} define random vectors.

The best position may be determined by considering average of α, β and δ wolves using Eq. (38) as:

$$\vec{X}(t+1) = \frac{\vec{X}_1 + \vec{X}_2 + \vec{X}_3}{3} \tag{38}$$

Searching for prey implies capability for exploration while targeting the prey is capability for exploitation. e_v is a random value ranges from $+2\,g$ and $-2\,g$; it lessens from 2 to 0 during optimization. When $|e_v|$ is below one, they force grey wolves to strike the prey. When $|e_v|$ is larger than one, population members are forced to stray away from the prey.

To summarize, the search process is initiated in the GWO approach by creating a random grey wolf population (candidate solutions). α, β, δ wolves measure the possible place of the prey during iterations. Each solution for the candidates updates their distance from the prey. Parameter e_v is compressed from 2 to 0 to accentuate exploration and exploitation. Candidate solutions lean to step away from the prey if exceeds one and converges towards the prey if smaller than one. Ultimately, the GWO algorithm ends by accomplishing the final criterion. In addition, the flowchart for the GWO system is illustrated in Fig. 4.

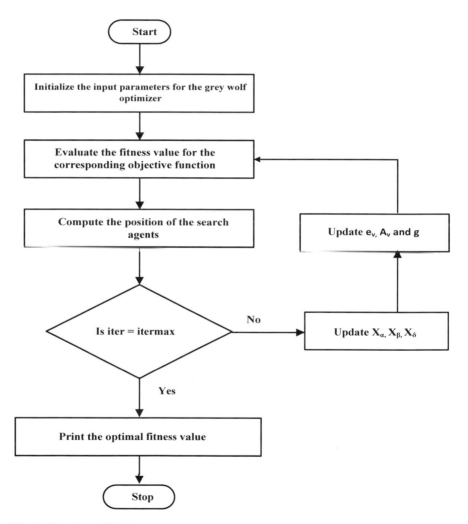

Fig. 4 Flowchart of GWO approach

6 HS

In latest years, HS has gained prominence as an effective algorithm to address complex optimization problems. The stepwise methodology for implementing HS algorithm for optimization is outlined below [38, 39]:

6.1 Formulation of Problem

Firstly, the formulation of problem is carried out. The optimization problem concerning objective function $f(X)$ is described as:
  Min. $f(X)$ subject to

$$x_i^{mn} \leq x_i \leq x_i^{mx}$$

$$(i = 1, 2, 3, 4, \ldots, n)$$

Here, $X = [x_1, x_2, x_3, \ldots x_n]^T$ indicates a series of decision variable; n denotes number of decision variables or problem dimension.

Consequently, different steps for implementing HS code are summarized as:

6.2 HS Parameter Initialization

Initialization of adjustable HS parameters involving harmony memory size (H_{MS}), pitch adjustment rate (P_R), harmony memory consideration rate (H_{MR}) and generation bandwidth (B_H) has been carried out. Further, harmony memory matrix (H_{MM}) is generated by way of solution vectors and H_{MS}. The initialization of H_{MM} elements are achieved using the following equation as:

$$X_{ij} = X_i^{mn} + \text{rand}\,(X_i^{mx} - X_i^{mn}) \tag{39}$$

where $j = 1, 2, 3, 4 \ldots n; i = 1, 2, 3, 4 \ldots H_{MS}$
  X_i^{mx} and X_i^{mn} denote upper and lower limits of decision variable; rand symbolizes a random value that is distributed uniformly between the 0 and 1.
  Mathematically, the H_{MM} is expressed as:

$$H_{\text{MM}} = \begin{bmatrix} x_{11} & x_{12} & x_{13} & \dots x_{1n} \\ x_{21} & x_{22} & x_{23} & \dots x_{2n} \\ x_{31} & x_{32} & x_{33} & \dots x_{3n} \\ \vdots & & & \\ x_{H_{\text{MS}}1} & x_{H_{\text{MS}}2} & x_{H_{\text{MS}}3} & \dots x_{H_{\text{MS}}n} \end{bmatrix}_{H_{\text{MS}} \times n} \tag{40}$$

6.3 New Harmony Development

Changes in new harmony vector depending on past perspective is regarded as improvisation or adjustment of harmony. In order to produce new harmony, i.e. $X_{\text{nw}} = [x_{\text{nw},1}, x_{\text{nw},2}, x_{\text{nw},3}, \dots x_{\text{nw}, n}]$, the following steps are performed with all decision variables:

Stage (i): A new random number (R_{N}) in between 0 and 1 is generated. If $R_{\text{N}} > H_{\text{MR}}$, then the decision variable of X_{ij}^{nw} is generated as:

$$X_{ij}^{\text{nw}} = X_j^{\text{mn}} + \text{rand} \, (X_j^{\text{mx}} - X_j^{\text{mn}}) \tag{41}$$

where $j = 1, 2, 3, 4 \dots n; i = 1, 2, 3, 4 \dots H_{\text{MS}}$

If $R_{\text{N}} \leq H_{\text{MR}}$, on the contrary, then one of the decision variable stored in current harmony memory is randomly selected using following equation:

$$X_{ij}^{\text{nw}} = X_{ij} \tag{42}$$

Stage (ii): HS considers the pitch adjustment mechanism by which the new harmony will shift within possible range to a neighbouring value. A uniformly distributed random number (rand) is generated in the range 0 to 1 after stage (i) to perform pitch adjustment mechanism. If rand $\leq P_{\text{R}}$, then the new harmony uses the following equation to move to a neighbouring value.

$$X_{ij}^{\text{nw}} = X_{ij}^{\text{nw}} + B_H \times (\text{rand} - 0.5) \times (X_j^{\text{mn}} - X_j^{\text{mx}}) \tag{43}$$

In addition, the iteration-wise value of variable P_{R} and B_{H} is determined as [32]:

$$P_{\text{R}}(\text{itr}) = P_{\text{Rmin}} + \frac{(P_{\text{Rmax}} - P_{\text{Rmin}})}{\text{itr}_{\max}} \times (\text{itr}) \tag{44}$$

where itr denotes an iteration index; P_{R} (itr) indicates pitch adjustment rate iterationwise; P_{Rmax} and P_{Rmin} define the limits of the adjustment rate of pitch; Further, bandwidth $(B_{\text{H}}$ (itr)) is measured using the following formula [32]:

$$B_{\text{H}}(\text{itr}) = B_{\text{Hmx}} \exp(a.\text{itr})$$

$$a = \frac{\text{Ln}\left(\frac{B_{\text{Hmn}}}{B_{\text{Hmx}}}\right)}{\text{itr}_{\text{max}}} \tag{45}$$

where B_{Hmn} and B_{Hmx} represent the lower and upper limits of bandwidth.

6.4 Updation

If the newly generated harmony vector (X_{ij}^{nw}) yields better results than that of the worst harmony (X_{ij}^{wst}) in harmony memory, the new harmony vector is considered in harmony memory instead of the current worst harmony and is mathematically defined as:

$$X_{ij}^{\text{wst}} = \left\{ \begin{array}{ll} X_{ij}^{\text{nw}}; & f\left(X_{ij}^{\text{nw}}\right) < f\left(X_{ij}^{\text{wst}}\right) \\ X_{ij}^{\text{wst}}; & \text{Otherwise} \end{array} \right\} \tag{46}$$

Then the best value for objective function is determined on the basis of the obtained solution as:

$$f^{\text{bst}} = \min\left(f_i\right); i \in 1, 2, 3, 4 \ldots H_{\text{MS}} \tag{47}$$

6.5 Check Stopping Criteria

The algorithms will be continued till the best results are obtained. Once the best results are obtained the algorithm should stop and best results may be stored. In case the best results are not achieved then in such case the steps 6.3 and step 6.4 are replicated. The methodology adopted to achieve the best results is also provided here through a flowchart and provided in Fig. 5.

7 PSO

PSO is a metaheuristic approach used with a population (swarm) of quite-called particles to handle complex optimization problems. Every particle composed of m decision variables is represented via a vector and defines a search space position. Particles deal with two sources of knowledge gained through the best individual experience and best experience of the swarm during the iterations, and shift by a

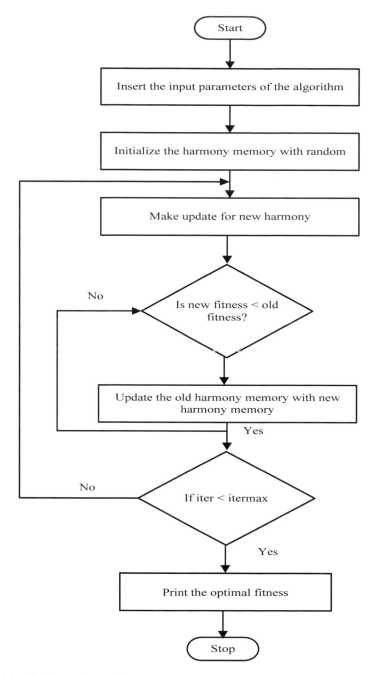

Fig. 5 Flowchart of HS approach

given velocity through the search space. The process continued till the criterion for stoppage is met.

Firstly, in PSO, a population of particles is initialized randomly via a uniform distribution in the search space. Every particle employs its memory to move via the search space to get a better position than its present. A particle recites the best experience discovered on its own (P_{bt}), and the best experience of the group (G_{bt}), in its memory. At each iteration, the updating sequence of particles is as follows [25, 40]:

$$V_j(i+1) = W_F \times V_j(i) + L_{C1} \times r_{a1}\left(P_{btj}(i) - x_j(i)\right) \\ + L_{C2} \times r_{a2}\left(G_{btj}(i) - x_j(i)\right) \tag{48}$$

$$x_j(i+1) = V_j(i+1) + x_j(i) \tag{49}$$

$$i = 1, 2, 3, 4 \ldots, \text{itr}_{\max} \quad j = 1, 2, 3, \ldots, S_{PL}$$

where V_j is velocity of jth particle; x_j is position of jth particle; S_{PL} denotes particles size; L_{C1} and L_{C2} symbolizes learning coefficients; r_{a1} and r_{a2} denote random numbers lies in between 0 and 1 and itr$_{\max}$ represents maximum number of iterations.

W_F, defined as inertia weight factor, is employed to offer a balance between local and global search. A greater value of W_F results in a global search while a lower value leads in local search. The value of W_F is usually varied by using the given formula as [31]:

$$W_F(i) = W_{Fmx} - \frac{W_{Fmx} - W_{Fmn}}{\text{itr}_{\max}} \times i \tag{50}$$

where W_{Fmn} and W_{Fmx} denote initial and final value of inertia weight.

The following steps for implementing the PSO algorithm are further stated as:

7.1 Initialization of the Problem with PSO Parameters

The first step is to do the problem (objective function along with constraints) formulation. Also, the adjustable PSO parameters are defined.

7.2 Initialization of Particles

In the second step, m particles with randomly generated decision vectors have been initialized in the search space. Each particle is initialized using the following equation.

$$x(0) = x_{mn,j} + \text{rand}(x_{mx,j} - x_{mn,j}) \tag{51}$$

where x_{mx} and x_{mn} are initial and final value of x for all the particles.

7.3 Fitness Function Evaluation

The value of an objective function is calculated on the basis of the value of the decision variables associated with each particle.

7.4 Updation

P_{bt} is determined for each particle, and G_{bt} is selected based on the best particle in the population. Further, each particle is allowed to travel to the next new position. More precisely, by employing Eqs. 48 and 49, respectively, the velocity of each particle and its position are updated.

7.5 Stopping Criteria

Whenever the highest number of iterations is accomplished, the algorithm is abandoned and the optimal solution is considered to be G_{bt}. Otherwise, repeat steps 7.2 and 7.4. All the five PSO algorithm steps are demonstrated in Fig. 6

8 Simulation Result and Discussion

In this area of study, it has been worked out to achieve the optimal design and sizing of HES considering the different types of renewable energy resources for the study area. At first, four models of HES in off-grid mode that are considered for the study area have been given as:

1. Model M_1: SPV/Biomass/Biogas/Battery
2. Model M_2 : SPV/Wind/Biomass/Battery
3. Model M_3 : SPV/Wind/Biogas/Battery
4. Model M_4 : SPV/Wind/Biomass/Biogas/Battery.

The hourly simulations of selected off-grid models have been conducted with the GWO, HS and PSO algorithms in MATLAB for one year. In addition, the grid-integrated model of SPV/wind/biomass/biogas/battery has been considered and optimized using all three algorithms. At the end, a comparison between grid-integrated

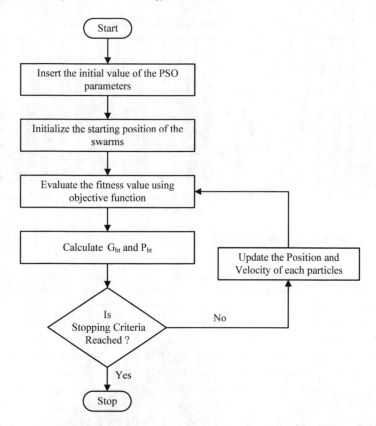

Fig. 6 Flowchart of PSO approach

and off-grid hybrid models has been done in respect of technical and economic concerns and the optimal solution has been found. The results of the optimization were obtained on the basis of various techno-economic parameters as shown in Table 1 [2]. Additionally, selected site's hourly load demand, solar irradiance, wind speed and ambient temperature are shown in Figs. 7, 8, 9 and 10. Biogenerators are also scheduled to operate in each season at peak load hours, and are demonstrated in Table 2.

Table 1 Economical database of HES components

System	Capital cost ($)	O&M cost ($)	Salvage value ($)	Fuel cost
Solar photovoltaic system (0.235 kW)	166.4	3.328	16.64	–
Wind generator (3.3 kW)	3033.33	60.67	910	–
Biomass generator (1 kW)	895.27	44.76	268.58	13$/ton
Biogas generator (1 kW)	572	28.6	171.6	6.93 $/ton

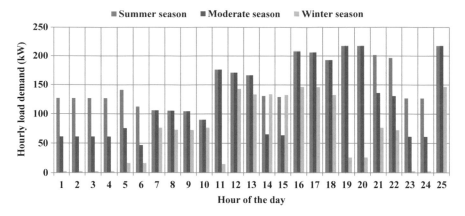

Fig. 7 Load demand on hourly basis of the selected site

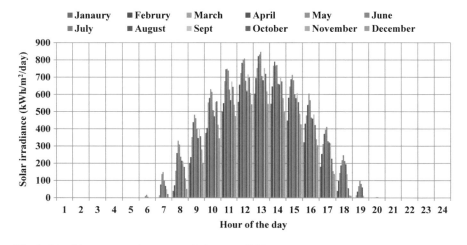

Fig. 8 Monthly average solar energy of given area [33]

An annual rate of real interest, inflation and escalation were fixed at 0.11, 0.05 and 0.075, respectively. The parameters of the algorithms GWO, HS and PSO are as follows: GWO: $itr_{max} = 100$, Run = 30; HS: $itr_{max} = 100$; $H_{MS} = 5$; $H_{MR} = 0.95$; $P_R = 0.1$; $P_{Rmax} = 1$, $P_{Rmin} = 0.1$; PSO: m = 5, $L_{C1} = 2$, $L_{C2} = 2$, $S_{PL} = 30$, $itr_{max} = 100$. The optimization results acquired for selected off-grid models after hourly simulation along with their size are presented in Table 3.

From Table 3, it is noted that the GWO algorithm gives the lowest NPC of model M_2 with minimal COE. The GWO algorithm estimates 235 kW SPV array, 259 kW biomass, 13.2 kW wind energy system, 3397 kWh battery bank storage and 100 kW converter resulting in NPC of $1.334 * 10^6$ and COE of $0.162/kWh. The

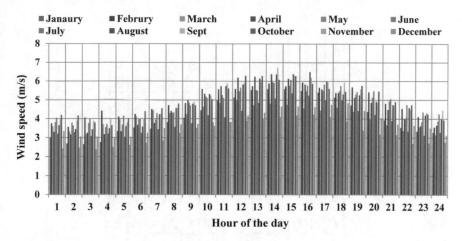

Fig. 9 Monthly average wind energy of given area [34]

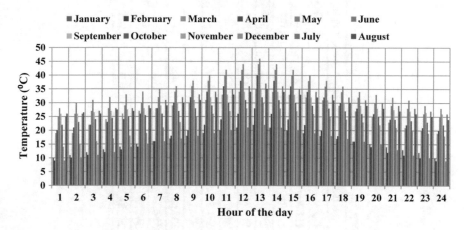

Fig. 10 Monthly average ambient temperature for given area [33]

Table 2 Scheduling of biogas and biomass generator for selected region

Biogenerator	Summer season	Moderate season	Winter season
Biogas generator	15.00 pm to 24.00 am	11.00 am to 20.00 pm	13.00 pm to 22.00 pm
Biomass generator	05.00 am to 14.00 pm	01.00 am to 10.00 am	07.00 am to 12.00 pm

optimizing results acquired using the above-mentioned algorithms for grid-linked SPV/Wind/Biomass/Biogas/Battery HES are further illustrated in Table 4.

From Tables 3 and 4, it is revealed that the grid-linked HES model is more economical than off-grid models. In addition, there is a smaller number of batteries used in grid-connected model in comparison with off-grid models. Based on the achieved

Table 3 Result of off-grid hybrid models using GWO, HS and PSO algorithms

Model	Algorithm	N_{SPV}	N_{Bat}	N_{WT}	P_{SPV} (kW)	E_{Bat} (kWh)	P_{WT} (kW)	P_{BMS} (kW)	P_{BGS} (kW)	NPC (10^6 \$)	COE (\$/kWh)
M_1	GWO	1800	1007	–	423	2417.8	–	177	31	1.558	0.190
	HS	1753	1041	–	411.96	2498.4	–	188	27	1.600	0.195
	PSO	1778	1060	–	417.83	2544	–	191	25	1.627	0.197
M_2	GWO	1000	1415	4	235	3397	13.2	259	–	1.334	0.162
	HS	499	689	6	117.27	1653.6	19.8	331	–	1.560	0.189
	PSO	397	643	21	93.29	1543.2	69.3	336	–	1.573	0.192
M_3	GWO	2500	1415	117	587.5	3397	382.8	–	32	1.967	0.243
	HS	2461	1480	159	578.33	3552	524.7	–	26	2.174	0.263
	PSO	2288	1681	156	537.68	4034.4	514.8	–	22	2.320	0.282
M_4	GWO	1500	1047	7	352.5	2512.8	23.?	213	31	1.697	0.206
	HS	1452	1178	41	341.22	2827.2	135.4	232	15	1.940	0.236
	PSO	1229	1248	11	288.81	2995.2	36.?	245	25	1.941	0.236

Table 4 Result of grid-linked HES using GWO, HS and PSO algorithms

Algorithm	P_{SPV} (kW)	P_{WT} (kW)	P_{BMS} (kW)	P_{BGS} (kW)	E_{Bat} (kWh)	NPC (10^5 \$)	COE (\$/kWh)
GWO	235	49.5	10	27	24	6.78	0.0778
HS	230.77	108.9	12	24	97	6.83	0.0779
PSO	215.27	99	21	31	129.7	7.12	0.0822

findings, grid-connected HES comprising of SPV, wind, biogas, biomass and battery is proposed for given site. The most optimal model includes a 235 kW SPV array, a 49.5 kW wind energy system, a 27 kW biogas generator, a 10 kW biomass generator, a 24 kWh battery bank storage and a 100 kW converter that have NPC and COE of \$6.78 * 10^5 and \$0.0778/kWh, respectively.

It is also revealed that the GWO performance is superior compared with HS and PSO. Likewise, PSO, HS and GWO convergence curve for NPC is also given in Fig. 11. It is found that GWO converges faster than PSO and HS and provides the optimal solution before 10 iterations. Further, the results pertaining to proposed grid-linked model are discussed in following paragraphs.

The proportion of each renewable energy resources of proposed HES in annual electricity generation is given in Fig. 12. It shows that the highest portion of electricity production arises from 448,740 kWh /year (68%) SPV panels led by 94,900 kWh/year (14%) biogas, 82,081 kWh/year (13%) wind energy system and 31,770 kWh/year (5%) biomass, respectively.

The costwise bifurcation of NPC is demonstrated in Table 5 in light of various forms of costs and revenues. It is revealed that the cost of buying power is largest among all. Also, Fig. 13 shows the bifurcation of NPC in sight of system components

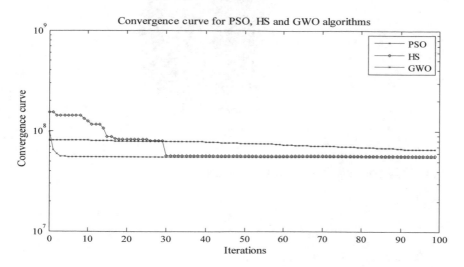

Fig. 11 PSO, HS and GWO convergence curve in context of NPC

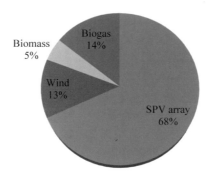

Fig. 12 Proportion of different renewable energy resources in yearly energy generation

Table 5 Proportion of various costs in NPC

S. No.	Indicator	Value ($)
1	C_{NV}	121,093.1
2	OM_{NV}	76,030.75
3	F_{NV}	64,490.67
4	SV_{NV}	9462.067
5	C_{SG}	67,448.09
6	C_{PG}	501,026.7

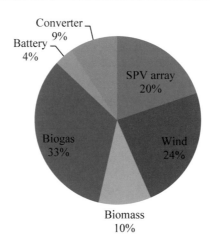

Fig. 13 Bifurcation of NPC in terms of HES components

Table 6 Seasonal variation in purchased/sold electrical energy from/to utility grid

Description of season	Energy purchase from the grid (kWh)	Energy sold to the grid (kWh)
Summer	234,440	21,777
Moderate	151,140	5220.4
Winter	47,839	29,040
Total purchased and sold energy (kWh/year)	432,419	55,927

Table 7 Seasonal variability in battery energy

Season	Battery input power (kWh)	Battery output power (kWh)
Summer season	25,417	235,430
Moderate season	9885.4	152,480
Winter season	37,030	48,874
Total (kWh/year)	72,204	437,784

and finds that wind energy system has a maximum share of 24% compared SPV array, biomass, converter and battery of 33%, 20%, 10%, 9% and 4%, respectively.

Additionally, the total energy bought and sold for each season to the power grid is listed in Table 6. Owing to high demand, the biggest electricity purchased in the summer season has been experienced. In the opposite, buying and selling the grid is less than other seasons due to less demand for electricity. Moreover, the electricity sold on the grid is higher in winter season than in other seasons due to reduced demand for energy. The annual purchase and selling of electricity by utility grid is measured as 432,419 kWh/year and 55,927 kWh/year, respectively.

The seasonal variability in the input and output capacity of the batteries is indicated in Table 7. Battery input power has been reported to be higher while output power is lower in winter season. On the opposite, the power of the battery output is larger and the input power is smaller in summer season.

9 Conclusion

In the present study, optimal design and sizing of renewable energy resources-based hybrid energy systems based on the available renewable energy resources is developed and presented for rural locations in Haryana state (India). The proposed model is analysed for various scenarios like in off-grid and grid-linked mode using GWO, HS and PSO algorithms. Here, both the stand-alone and grid-connected system are utilized. The composition of the grid-connected model is made up of SPV/wind/biomass/biogas/battery confirmed to be the optimum for area under considered in this study. The optimum size of the proposed grid-linked HES for the selected site is mainly having the ratings of 235 kW solar photovoltaic system, 24 kWh battery-based energy storage, 49.5 kW wind energy conversion system, 27 kW biogas, 10 kW biomass and 100 kVA size of the converter. The calculated NPC and COE is, respectively, $6.78 * 10^5$ and $0.0778/kWh.

In the current research, all efforts have been made to develop most optimal solution for selected site in terms of least cost. Further, more intelligent approaches or hybrid optimization methods can be explored, such as ant lion optimizer (ALO), moth flame optimizer (MFO), school of fish, random search, hybrid PSO-GWO and hybrid HS-random search.

Form this research, the people of remote areas would be benefitted and have the societal impacts as well would be helpful in the government planning and providing power to all. Through this, we would be able to exploit more and more renewable energy resources and reduces the conventional fuels as a result the environments pollution and GHG emissions would be reduced significantly. Finally, it is observed that the proposed solution will not only provide the electricity to the remote areas but also environment friendly. Moreover, there is a great opportunity to enhance the employment in the emerging area.

References

1. Akinyele, D.: Techno-economic design and performance analysis of nanogrid systems for households in energy-poor villages. Sustain. Cities Soc. **34**, 335–357 (2017). https://doi.org/10.1016/j.scs.2017.07.004
2. Anand, P., Rizwan, M., Bath, S.K.: Sizing of renewable energy based hybrid system for rural electrification using grey wolf optimization approach. IET Energy Syst. Integr. 1:158–172 (2019). https://doi.org/10.1049/iet-esi.2018.0053
3. Bagen, B.R.: Evaluation of different operating strategies in small stand-alone power systems. IEEE Trans Energy Convers. **20**, 654–60 (2005). https://doi.org/10.1109/tec.2005.847996
4. Himri, Y., BoudgheneStambouli, A., Draoui, B., Himri, S.: Techno-economical study of hybrid power system for a remote village in Algeria. Energy **33**, 1128–1136 (2008). https://doi.org/10.1016/j.energy.2008.01.016
5. Razmjoo, A.D.: Developing various hybrid energy systems for residential application as an appropriate and reliable way to achieve energy sustainability. Energy Sources, Part A: Recovery, Utilization, Environ. Eff. **41**(10), 1180–1193 (2019). https://doi.org/10.1080/15567036.2018.1544996
6. Murugaperumala, K., Ajay, P., Vimal Ra, D.: Feasibility design and techno-economic analysis of hybrid renewable energy system for rural electrification. Sol. Energy **188**, 1068–1083 (2019). https://doi.org/10.1016/j.solener.2019.07.008
7. Anayochukwu, V., Nnene, E.A.: Simulation and optimization of photovoltaic/diesel hybrid power generation systems for health service facilities in rural environments. Electron J Energy Environ **1**(1), 5770–5775 (2013). https://doi.org/10.7770/ejee-v1n1-art485
8. Anand, P., Bath, S.K., Rizwan, M.: Design and development of stand-alone renewable energy based hybrid power system for remote base transceiver station. Int. J. Comput. Appl. **169**, 34–41 (2017). https://doi.org/10.5120/ijca2017914776
9. Borowy, B.S., Salameh, Z.M.: Methodology for optimally sizing the combination of a battery bank and PV array in a wind/PV hybrid system. IEEE Trans. Energy Convers. **11**(2), 367–375 (1996). https://doi.org/10.1109/60.507648

10. Markvart, T., Fragaki, A., Ross, J.: PV system sizing using observed time series of solar radiation. Sol. Energy **80**(1), 46–50 (2006). https://doi.org/10.1016/j.solener.2005.08.011
11. Karaki, S., Chedid, R., Ramadan, R.: Probabilistic performance assessment of autonomous solar-wind energy conversion systems. IEEE Trans. Energy Convers. **14**(3), 766–772 (1999). https://doi.org/10.1109/60.790949
12. Tina, G., Gagliano, S., Raiti, S.: Hybrid solar/wind power system probabilistic modelling for long-term performance assessment. Sol. Energy **80**(5), 578–588 (2006). https://doi.org/10.1016/j.solener.2005.03.013
13. Lujano-Rojas, J.M., Dufo-López, R., Bernal-Agustín, J.L.: Probabilistic modelling and analysis of stand-alone hybrid power systems. Energy **63**, 19–27 (2013). https://doi.org/10.1016/j.energy.2013.10.003
14. Kellogg, W., Nehrir, M., Venkataramanan, G., Gerez, V.: Generation unit sizing and cost analysis for stand-alone wind, photovoltaic, and hybrid wind/PV systems. IEEE Trans. Energy Convers. **13**(1), 70–75 (1998). https://doi.org/10.1109/60.658206
15. Ekren, B.Y., Ekren, O.: Simulation based size optimization of a PV/wind hybrid energy conversion system with battery storage under various load and auxiliary energy conditions. Appl. Energy **86**(9), 1387–1394 (2009). https://doi.org/10.1016/j.apenergy.2008.12.015
16. Zhang, X., Tan, S.C., Li, G., Li, J., Fang, Z.: Components sizing of hybrid energy systems via the optimization of power dispatch simulations. Energy **52**, 165–172 (2013). https://doi.org/10.1016/j.energy.2013.01.013
17. Tong, W., Zhang, H., Shang, L.: Optimal sizing of a grid-connected hybrid renewable energy systems considering hydroelectric storage. Energy Sources, Part A: Recov. Utilization, and Environ. Eff. 1–17 2020. https://doi.org/10.1080/15567036.2020.1731018
18. Sadeghi, D., Naghshbandy, A.H., Bahramara, S.: Optimal sizing of hybrid renewable energy systems in presence of electric vehicles using multi-objective particle swarm optimization. Energy **209**(118471), 1–17 (2020). https://doi.org/10.1016/j.energy.2020.118471
19. Lu, X., Wang, H.: Optimal sizing and energy management for cost-effective pev hybrid energy storage systems. IEEE Trans. Ind Inf. **16**(5), 3407–3416 (2020). https://doi.org/10.1109/tii.2019.2957297
20. Koutroulis, E., Kolokotsa, D., Potirakis, A., Kalaitzakis, K.: Methodology for optimal sizing of stand-alone photovoltaic/wind-generator systems using genetic algorithms. Sol. Energy **80**(9), 1072–1088 (2006). https://doi.org/10.1016/j.solener.2005.11.002
21. Askarzadeh, A.: A discrete chaotic harmony search-based simulated annealing algorithm for optimum design of pv/wind hybrid system. Sol. Energy, **97**, 93–101 (2013). https://doi.org/10.1016/j.solener.2013.08.014
22. Kumar, R., Gupta, R.A., Bansal, A.K.: Economic analysis and power management of a stand-alone wind/photovoltaic hybrid energy system using biogeography based optimization algorithm. Swarm Evol. Comput. **8**, 33–43 (2013). https://doi.org/10.1016/j.swevo.2012.08.002
23. Gupta, R.A., Kumar, R., Bansal, A.K.: Economic nalysis and design of stand-alone wind/photovoltaic hybrid energy system using genetic algorithm. In: International Conference on Computing, Communication and Applications (ICCCA), Dindigul, Tamilnadu, India, 1–6 (2012). https://doi.org/10.1109/iccca.2012.6179189
24. Mostofi, F., Shayeghi, H.: Feasibility and optimal reliable design of renewable hybrid energy system for rural electrification in Iran. Int. J. Renew. Energy Res. **2**(4), 574–582 (2012). https://doi.org/10.1.1.462.8025
25. Askarzadeh, S.C., dos, L.: A novel framework for optimization of a grid independent hybrid renewable energy system: a case study of Iran. Sol. Energy **112**(1), 383–396 (2015). https://doi.org/10.1016/j.solener.2014.12.013
26. Mohamed, M.A., Eltamaly, A.M., Alolah, A.I.: Swarm intelligence-based optimization of grid-dependent hybrid renewable energy systems. Renew. Sustain. Energy Rev. **77**, 515–524 (2017). https://doi.org/10.1016/j.rser.2017.04.048
27. Singh, S., Kaushik, S.C.: Optimal sizing of grid integrated hybrid pv-biomass energy system using artificial bee colony algorithm. IET Renew. Power Gener. **10**(5), 642–650 (2016). https://doi.org/10.1049/iet-rpg.2015.0298

28. Ogunjuyigbe, S.O., Ayodele, T.R., Akinola, O.A.: Optimal allocation and sizing of pv/wind/split-diesel/battery hybrid energy system for minimizing life cycle cost, carbon emission and dump energy of remote residential building. Appl. Energy **171**, 153–171 (2016). https://doi.org/10.1016/j.apenergy.2016.03.051

29. Bartolucci, L., Cordiner, S., Mulone, V., Rocco, V., Rossi, J.L.: Hybrid renewable energy systems for renewable integration in microgrids: influence of sizing on performance. Energy **152**, 744–758 (2018). https://doi.org/10.1016/j.energy.2018.03.165

30. Ghaffaria, A., Askarzadeh, A.: Design optimization of a hybrid system subject to reliability level and renewable energy penetration. Energy **193**, 116754 (2020). https://doi.org/10.1016/j.energy.2019.116754

31. Anand, P., Bath, S.K., Rizwan, M.: Renewable energy based hybrid model for rural electrification. Int. J. Energy Technol. Policy **15**(1), 86–113, (2019). https://doi.org/10.1504/ijetp.2019.096633

32. Anand, P., Bath, S.K., Rizwan, M.: Size optimization of res based grid connected hybrid power system using harmony search algorithm. Int. J. Energy Technol. Policy **16**(3), 238–276 (2020). https://doi.org/10.1504/ijetp.2020.107035

33. Solar irradiance data and ambient temperature of study area: NASA. Surface meteorology and solar energy: a renewable energy resource website: Accessed on 04 June 2020 at https://eosweb.larc.nasa.gov/sse/

34. Wind energy data of study area: National Institute of Wind Energy. Ministry of New and Renewable Energy, Government of India; 2020, Accessed on 04 June 2020 at http://niwe.res.in/department_wra_est.php

35. Chauhan, A., Saini, R.P.: Discrete harmony search based size optimization of integrated renewable energy system for remote rural areas of uttarakhand state in India. Renew. Energy **94**, 587–604 (2016). https://doi.org/10.1016/j.renene.2016.03.079

36. Mirjalili, S., Mirjalili, S.M., Lewis, A.: Grey wolf optimizer. Adv. Eng. Softw. **69**, 46–61 (2014). https://doi.org/10.1016/j.advengsoft.2013.12.007

37. Kamboj, V.K., Bath, S.K., Dhillon, J.S.: Solution of non-convex economic load dispatch problem using grey wolf optimizer. Neural Comput. Appl. **27**(5), 1301–1316 (2016). https://doi.org/10.1007/s00521-015-1934-8

38. Askarzadeh, A.: Developing a discrete harmony search algorithm for size optimization of wind-photovoltaic hybrid energy system. Solar Energy **98**, 190–195 (2013). https://doi.org/10.1016/j.solener.2013.10.008

39. Kamboj, V., Bath, S.K., Dhillon, J.S.: Implementation of hybrid harmony search/random search algorithm for single area unit commitment problem. Electr. Power Energy Syst. **77**, 228–249 (2016). https://doi.org/10.1016/j.ijepes.2015.11.045

40. Mahesh, K.S.S.: Optimal sizing of a grid-connected pv/wind/battery system using particle swarm optimization. Iran. J. Sci. Technol. Trans. Electr. Eng. **43**, 107–121 (2019). https://doi.org/10.1007/s40998-018-0083-3

Economic Load Dispatch Monitoring and Optimization for Emission Control Using Flower Pollination Algorithm: A Case Study

Deepesh Mali, D. Saxena, and Rajeev Kumar Chauhan

Abstract An attempt has been made in this chapter to decipher highly nonlinear power system economic load and emission dispatch (EELD) problems, using optimization algorithm, called flower pollination algorithm (FPA). The electrical energy market has historically not been that complex, and focus was put solely on optimizing the energy dispatch costs. Since last few years, environmental pollution is the eye-catching issue, and government is making tough regulations to control it. Reducing the toxic pollution generated by the operations of thermal-based power generation plants becomes equally important. In view of the above, both single- and multi-objective problems, with various power system constraints, are solved using the proposed algorithm. The probability switching and Levy flight distribution phenomenon help the algorithm to find the global optima in an efficient manner. This algorithm's ability to outperform both traditional and modern algorithms is exploited effectively to achieve various objectives associated with power system problems associated with economic load dispatch (ELD). The results of the simulation demonstrate the competence of the FPA with regard to its efficiency and robustness.

Keywords Flower pollination algorithm · Emission · Multi-objective optimization · Weighted-sum approach · Valve-point loading · Prohibited operating zone

D. Mali · D. Saxena (✉)
Department of Electrical Engineering, MNIT, Jaipur, Rajasthan 302017, India
e-mail: dsaxena.ee@mnit.ac.in

D. Mali
e-mail: deepesh130698@gmail.com

R. K. Chauhan
Department of EN, IMS Engineering College, Ghaziabad, UP 201009, India
e-mail: mmmec.rkc@gmail.com

1 Introduction

The economic load dispatch (ELD) refers to the correspondence between the load demands and the assignment of the demands to generating units in such a way that their service entails minimum generation costs and other constraints in the power systems [1]. In contrast to the modern ones, the activity of the conventional energy market was very simple. Prior to the 1980s, the main concern of the power systems operator was to optimize the cumulative operating costs of the power system [2]. But after the 1980s, due to the country's changing atmosphere resulting from the emission of greenhouse gases such as NO_x, Co_x and SO_x from thermal generating units, governments of the respective countries imposed some tough regulations to control the same. Therefore, the situation has changed in the new power system and the operators pay attention in minimizing the emission together with the operating cost [2]. Concentrating solely on minimizing the generating cost may increase the environmental emission and vice versa which cannot be the desirable criterion. Therefore, in order to incorporate both the objective of minimum emission and minimum fuel cost, the theory of emission and load dispatch (EELD) comes into existence [3, 4]. The EELD problem is intended to preserve the balance between emissions and fuel costs. Therefore, the issue of multi-objective economic emission and load dispatch is established as the EELD. Many methods are suggested in [2] to lower the environmental emission.

By considering the importance of fuel costs and emissions as an objective feature, several authors have addressed the ELD. In [4], Granelli considered emission as constraints and solve the dynamic dispatch problem. Abido, using the metamorphic algorithm, solved the EELD problem in [5, 6] and compared the results with the non-influenced genetic sorting algorithm (NSGA). Malik et al. consider a more complicated cost-curve, i.e. cost with valve-point effect in order to solve the economic load dispatch problem [7]. In [8], Varadrajan solved the multi-objective optimization problem using a multi-objective evolution algorithm. They have not only taken cost and emission as multi-objective, but also loss and cost, loss and voltage deviations are also considered as multi-objective optimal problems. Some researchers also tried to get solutions of multi-objective optimization through hybrid algorithms. Novel foraging bacteria combined with Nelder–Mead and shuffled frog leaping with Nelder–Mead algorithms and implement to solve environmental/economic load dispatch problems were presented in [9, 10]. Basu in [11] has also solved multi-objective optimization problem taking emission and economic cost as an objective function, using differential evolution method. Hotta et al. [12] provide an interactive fuzzy tool for dispatching economic loads. The weighted-sum approach charged model algorithm and gravitational search algorithms addressed multi-objective optimization in [13, 14]. Jadid et al. used load flow analysis in [15] to analyse transmission losses and solve mutual economic and emission dispatches and used fuzzy decision-making technique to announce a reasonable solution. The real coded chemical reaction algorithm [16] was first utilized to solve the problem of economic emission dispatch. Many other authors have applied nature-based optimization techniques to solve EELD problems. Mabu et al. [17], Srinivasa Rao et al. [18], Duman et al. [19] and Shaw et al. [20] have solved EELD problems using time-varying acceleration coefficient PSO, colonial selection algorithm, seeker-optimization technique and particle-swarm GSA respectively. Solmaz et al. [21] have solved multi-objective power flow exploiting PSO and evolutionary programming, and GA. Mishra et al. [22] have solved ELD problems with constraints, such as the valve-point effect using the genetic algorithm inspired by Chemo. Prithwish Chakraborty et al. changed the algorithm for harmony search by changing mutation operator to differential mutation operator. In view of the above algorithms and their implementation in solving both single- and multi-objective power system problems, current authors have also tried to take advantage of the newly developed flower pollination algorithm (FPA) optimizer to solve both single- and multi-objective EELD problems. To the best of authors' knowledge, FPA is not implemented to date to solve multi-objective EELD problems. This algorithm is based on the process of reproduction of flowering plants. Pollination is used to reproduce in flowering plants. It is the process of transporting pollens from anther to stigma between the flowers of same plant or to the other plant. When it is transferred within the flowers of the same plant, then it is called as self-pollination and when it is transferred to other plant then this process is called as cross-pollination [23]. This process of self-and cross-pollination exhibits the process of exploitation and exploration, respectively. Xin-She-Yang has developed this algorithm in the year 2012. Since then many engineering problems have been solved which brings FPA to compete with several other algorithms. In [24], Yang et al. also developed the multi-objective FPA and demonstrated its efficacy in solving multi-objective optimization problems. Some multi-objective problems are given [25–27], which are helpful for better understanding.

2 Problem Formulation

The ELD and emission dispatch problems of power system are very basic, but at the same time, a vital problem of power system as they are related to the economy of power industries, and its impact on the environment, respectively. From [3–5], it is found that the nature of fuel cost curve and emissions curve is different. Hence, economic load dispatch and emission dispatch problem can mathematically be modelled as a multi-objective optimization problem. In this project, both multi-objective and single-objective problems are considered.

2.1 Single Objective

2.1.1 Minimization of Quadratic Fuel Cost

The generator's fuel cost function is a quadratic power output function. In the problem of economic load dispatch (ELD), this fuel cost must be minimized to satisfy all constraints of equality and inequalities of power systems. The total fuel cost of the generating units can be expressed as follows:

$$F^{cost} = \sum_{k=1}^{N_g} (\alpha_k P_k + \beta_k P_k + \gamma_k) \tag{1}$$

where α_k, β_k, γ_k are cost function coefficient for kth generation, and N_g is number of units.

2.1.2 Minimization of Fuel Cost with Valve-Point Loading Effect

Many steam valves control the power output of the generators, either by opening or closing them. The gradual closing or opening of these valves, along with the wire drawing effects, has a nonlinear behaviour and is responsible for causing random or abrupt losses, thereby rendering the generator's power output nonlinear. This nonlinear variation of power must be taken into account in calculating the total fuel cost of all generating systems. Instead of a quadratic curve known as the valve-point loading effect, a ribbed line was therefore used to represent the practical total fuel cost. This valve-point loading effect thus makes the total cost function of the generator more nonlinear and makes it extremely nonlinear and discontinuous. A sinusoidal function is added to the principal objective function to incorporate the loading effects of the valve point. This sinusoidal function changes the fuel cost by incorporating quadratic and sinusoidal functions (2): provides a pictorial illustration of overall fuel costs with loading impact from valve point:

$$F^{cost} = \sum_{k=1}^{N_g} (\alpha_k P_k + \beta_k P_k + \gamma_k) + e_k \sin\{h_k(P_{kmin} - P_k)\} \tag{2}$$

where e_k and h_k are constants and represent valve-point loading effect of the kth unit.

2.1.3 Minimization of Economic Emission Dispatch

In the modern power generation industry, generator emission mainly comprises of $S O_x$ and $N O_x$ gases. The EED problem is mathematically modelled as (3).

$$F^{\text{emission}} = \sum_{k=1}^{N_g} (a_k + b_k P_k + c_k P_k \exp(d_k P_k)) \tag{3}$$

where a_k, b_k, c_k and d_k are the quadratic and exponential coefficients of the emission of kth generator.

2.2 Multi-objective Problems

A mathematical framework for optimizing more than one and overlapping objective functions is the multi-objective optimization technique [6]. This technique has been an eye-catching tool in the recent past for solving problems of optimization.

This technique gives a set of optimal solutions unlike single-objective technique. Multiple optimal solutions make the user more flexible to select the best optimal solution among other reasonable solutions. Such optimal solution is known as pareto-optimal solution [13]. Economic load dispatch and economic emission dispatch are seen as competing objective functions in power systems because the economic load dispatch variables that reduce the total cost of generation deviate the economic emission dispatch from its optimum value and thus suffer from economic emission dispatch. Similarly, the economic emission–dispatch minimizes the emission but deviates the economic load dispatch from its optimum value. Thus, it became a thought-provoking issue to hit a right balance between the economy of power systems and environmental hazards. Multi-objective optimization thus emerges as an effective method for achieving a compromised solution that gives both the power industry and environmental emission problems a win-win situation [6]. ELD and EED are modelled as multi-objective optimization in the present work, keeping in mind the above information. In this paper, weighted-sum approach is considered as one multi-objective function modelling the two separate conflicting single-objective function (ELD and EED). The weighted-sum method uses the weight factor (w) to transform multiple objective functions into a single-objective function [15]. EELD problems formulated using weight factor can be represented as:

$$F(\cos t, \text{emission}) = w F^{\text{cost}}_{\text{normalized}} + (1 - w) F^{\text{emission}}_{\text{normalized}} \tag{4}$$

Here w is the weight factor having range [0 1] and $\sum_{i=1}^{t} w_i = 1$ where t is total number of objectives in multi-objective function. In this case, there are two objective functions: $F^{\text{cost}}_{\text{normalized}} = $ the normalized value of fuel cost and $F^{\text{emission}}_{\text{normalized}} = $ the normalized value of emission.

2.3   Decision-Making

In general practice, solutions with weight factor 0.5 are declared as compromised solution. The fact behind declaring the solutions corresponding to weight factor 0.5, as compromised solution is that, it gives equal weight, i.e. 50% to both of the objective functions.

Several literature published various strategies designed to announce the best compromise solution. In recent years, techniques such as the fuzzy approach [15] and the partial weight vector [8] have become common. The present work used fuzzy membership approach (FMA) to declare the best solution. In this, the objective function's imprecise target is accomplished using the fuzzy function in the range [0 1]. This range of function from 0 to 1 defines the capability in increasing order, i.e. 0 means incapable and 1 means fully capable. The membership function μ_i^k can be defined as:

$$\mu_i^m = \begin{array}{ll} 1 & f_i \leq f_i^{\min} \\ \frac{f_i^{\max}}{f_i^{\max}} & f_i^{\min} \leq f_i \leq f_i^{\max} \\ 0 & f_i \geq f_i^{\max} \end{array} \tag{5}$$

Here, i is number of objective functions and m is the solution in given pareto fronts. $f_i^{\min}$ and $f_i^{\max}$ are minimum and maximum value of objective function. For each compromised solution k, normalized function can be calculated as:

$$\mu^k = \frac{\sum_{i=1}^m \mu_i^k}{\sum_{k=1}^n \sum_{i=1}^m \mu_i^k} \tag{6}$$

where, m is total number of objective functions, and n is number of all compromised solutions. The solution corresponds to maximum μ and can be declared as the best compromised solution.

2.4   Constraints

Both inequality and equality constraints are considered in the emission cost ELD problem. Active power equation is taken as equality constraints in the present work, covering total output power generation, total load demand and actual power loss in transmission lines. The inequality constraints consist of power limits for the generator output and limits for the ramp.

2.4.1   Equality Constraint

Real power balance equation: Both load demand (P_D) and complete loss of transmission (P_L) should be balanced by the real power generation. Then, the constraint equation is:

$$\sum_{k=1}^{N_g} P_k - P_D - P_L = 0 \tag{7}$$

where the load demand is P_D and P_L represents the total real power loss and P_k represents kth unit output power. Here, George's formula is used for line loss calculations. The total real power loss is calculated using conventional B-loss matrices and the loss coefficient. It may be defined as:

$$P_L = \sum_{k=1}^{N_g} \sum_{l=1}^{N_g} P_k B_{kl} P_l + \sum_{k=1}^{N_g} B_{0k} P_k + B_{00} P_L \tag{8}$$

where the loss coefficient constants are B_{00}, B_{0k} is kth element in the vector of loss coefficient, and B_{kl} is element of loss coefficient matrix.

2.4.2   Generators Inequality Constraint

Power Limits

The generator is expected to operate within a given range of power output due to the thermal limitations of the boiler. This range sets the upper and lower power limits for the kth generating unit as follows:

$$P_{k\min} \leq P_k \leq P_{k\max} \tag{9}$$

where $P_{k\min}$ and $P_{k\max}$ represent the lower and upper limits for real power generation of kth unit.

Prohibited Zone

As steam input to the generating units is controlled, this causes vibration in the generator shaft with sufficiently high vibrational frequencies, which force the generator into subsynchronous resonance to satisfy some precise load demand. Therefore, there is a need to restrict the generator power output into certain zones, thereby preventing such catastrophic event. These particular zones are known as prohibited zones of operation in input-output performance curve of the generating unit and it is defined as:

$$P_n^{\min} \leq P_n \leq P_{n,1}^z \tag{10}$$

$$P_{n,l}^u \leq P_n \leq P_{n,l}^z \tag{11}$$

$$P_{n,PZ}^u \leq P_n \leq P_n^{\max} \tag{12}$$

for $k = 1, 2, 3, \ldots, N_G$

Where $P_{n,1}^z$, $P_{n,l}^u$ are lower and upper limits of real power generation of the prohibited zone for nth generating unit, and $P_{n,1}^z$ is prohibited zone number for nth generating unit.

Generator Ramp Rate Limit

Steam valve openings and closing are continuously adjusted to meet the varying load demand, but such changes do not immediately change the power output of the generator, due to the massive inertia of the synchronous generators. A limit is set on generators output power to understand the actual operation of the generating unit. This limit is called ramp limit. There are two limits: up ramp rate limit and the down ramp rate limit. This limit determines the various intermediate limits of output power in its range for a particular generating unit.

$$\max(P_k^{\min}, P_k^0 - DR_k) \leq P_k \leq \min(P_k^{\max}, P_k^0 + UR_k) \tag{13}$$

where UR_k and DR_k represent the ramp-up and ramp-down limits.

3 Flower Pollination Description

Flowers are the responsible part of a plant as they are actively involved in the reproduction process. The process of reproduction in plants is carried out using a system, called pollination. In this process, pollens of the flowers are moved to other flowers through natural carriers like insects, bees, bats, wind, etc. sometimes also called pollinators. These organisms get the nectar from flowers exploiting minimum resources and learning with utmost reproduction in plants. This wonderful phenomenon of reproduction in flowers and the behaviour of pollinators to develop constancy towards certain flower motivated Xin-She Yang to develop an efficient optimizer. In view of this, Yang studied very deeply about the reproduction process of flowers and finally in the year 2012, he came up with a very wise optimization tool, called flower pollination algorithm or simply flower algorithm [23].

Yang has defined some basic rules. There are four basic rules [23].

1. Biotics or cross-pollination can be seen as process of global pollination, in which all pollinators fly in a way that fits Levy's flights.
2. Local pollination is achieved with abiotic pollination or self-pollination.
3. Flower constancy can be accomplished by pollinators such as insects and is equal to the possibility of reproduction directly linked to the resemblance between two flowers.
4. Local pollination activity and switching can be regulated with a switching probability p [0, 1], which is favourable for local one.

Mathematical modelling is performed based on these laws. We can mathematically interpret the combination of Rule No. 1 and Rule No. 3 as:

$$z_i^{n+1} = z_i^n + \gamma L(\lambda)(g * -z_i^n) \tag{14}$$

where z_i^n is ith pollen or pollen vector at nth iteration, $g*$ represents the current best solution present among all the solutions at current iteration, and γ is scaling factor that controls the step size. $L(\lambda)$ is step-size parameter for observing the Levy's flights, which represents the pollination strength. Levy's flights can be used to represent the travelling insects over large distances with different distance steps, i.e. for $L > 0$, L is drawn from a Levy's distribution as [23].

$$L \sim \left[\frac{(\lambda \Gamma(\lambda) \sin(\frac{\pi \lambda}{2}))(1)}{\pi (s^{(1+\lambda)})} \right] (s >> s_o >> 0) \tag{15}$$

where $\Gamma(\lambda)$ is simple distribution of gamma function and valid only for large steps. The method used here to generate pseudo-random step sizes $s > 0$. The Muktangan algorithm is used to draw step sizes using the following transformations, using two Gaussian distributions U and V [23].

$$s = \left[\frac{U}{|V|^{1/\lambda}} \right] U \sim N(0, \sigma^2), V \sim N(0, 1) \tag{16}$$

where $U \sim N(0, \sigma^2)$ represents the samples of a Gaussian normal distribution having a mean value zero and variance σ^2. σ^2 can be calculated by using the formula:

$$\sigma^2 = \left[\frac{\Gamma(1 + \lambda)}{\lambda \Gamma((1 + \lambda)/2)} \cdot \frac{\sin(\pi \lambda / 2)}{2^{(\lambda - 1)/2}} \right]^{1/\lambda} \tag{17}$$

Rule 2 and rule 3 are used for the local pollination and represented as:

$$z_i^{t+1} = z_i^t + \varepsilon(z_j^t - z_k^t) \tag{18}$$

where z_i^t and z_k^t are pollen from different flowers of a single plant. It basically reflects the constancy of the flowers in a restricted area. ε is a random number and uniformly distributed between [0, 1].

4 Test Systems and Results

To demonstrate the degree of competition, reliability and robustness of the FPA algorithm, it is implemented on different benchmark power system test systems, such as 6 unit, 13 unit and 15 unit systems. The results were compared with several algorithms published in the literature and statistical analysis was performed on each method to check the accuracy of the algorithm FPA. Table 8 represents the statistical analysis (deviation) for the first four case study. FPA is written in the MATLAB environment and has been tested on Intel i-5 processor, 4 GB Ram system.

4.1 Case Study 1: Optimization of Fuel Cost with Valve-Point Loading Effect Considering Losses

In this case, the system takes 30-bus with 6 units. The total demand for the system was 283.4 MW. The data needed for the simulation is extracted from [19]. FPA's exploitation and discovery property is used effectively for solving this case study. The results found are then compared with different algorithms available in the literatures, like GA [19], GA-APO [19], NSOA [19], PSO [19], MSGHP [19] and FPSOGSA [19]. The best control variable settings and comparison with existing methods are given in Tables 1 and 2. From Table 1, it can be seen that the optimal cost obtained from proposed algorithm is 924.8844 $/h, which is 7.1436%, 16.0334%, 6.097%, 0.0944%, 0.0817% and 0.0571% less than GA, GA-APO, NSOA, PSO, MSGHP and FPSOGSA respectively.

4.2 Case Study 2: Fuel Cost Optimization with Prohibited Zone and Ramp Limits

For this case, IEEE 6-unit system with a load demand of 1248 MW is considered with different nonlinear constraints. Prohibited zone and ramp limits data is taken from [13]. Results observed by FPA algorithm are also compared with several other executed algorithms in this field. The optimal cost obtained by FPA is found to be 1544.8095$/h, which is 0.0271%, 0.0853%, 0.0989%, 0.0588%,0.0275% and 0.0040% less than PSO [13], GA [13], SA [13], TS [13], MTS [13] and CSS [13], respectively. A comparison table is shown in Tables 3 and 4, respectively. It can

Table 1 Control variables optimal setting for case study 1

Power (MW)	GA [19]	GA-APO [19]	NSOA [19]	PSO [19]	MSG-HP [19]	FPSOGSA [19]	FPA (Proposed)
P1	150.7	133.9	182.4	197.8	199.6	19.5	199.6
P1	60.8	37.2	48.3	50.33	20	20	20.0
P3	30.8	37.7	19.8	15	23.7	23.9	24.1
P4	14.2	28.3	17.1	10	18.3	18.84	19.3
P5	19.4	18.7	13.6	10	17.1	18.21	17.7
P6	15.9	38.0	12.3	12	15.6	13.8	13.4
Total power	292.1	294.1	293.8	295.2	294.5	294.5	294.3
Cost ($/h)	996.0	1101.4	984.9	925.7	925.6	925.4	**924.8**
Loss	8.7	10.7	10.4	11.8	11.183	11.1	10.9

Bold represents that our proposed method is better than the existing methods

Table 2 Comparison table for case study 1

Method	Cost ($/h)
MSG-HS [29]	925.641
GA [29]	996.0369
GAAPO [29]	996.03689
NSOA [29]	984.93649
DE [29]	963.001
PSO [29]	925.75809
ABC [29]	928.437
EP [29]	955.508
IEP [29]	953.573
SADE ALM [29]	944.031
TS [29]	956.498
TS-SA [29]	959.563
ITS [29]	969.109
FPSOGSA [19]	925.4135
FPA (Proposed)	**924.8844**

Bold represents that our proposed method is better than the existing methods

be seen that FPA has attained its optimum functional value, i.e. fuel cost in just 30 iterations.

Table 3 Control variables optimal setting for case study 2

Power (MW)	PSO [13]	GA [13]	SA [13]	TS [13]	MTS [13]	CSS [13]	FPA (proposed)
P1	447.497	474.8066	478.1258	459.0753	448.1287	447.1763	**446.3778**
P1	173.3221	178.6363	163.0249	185.0675	172.8082	173.393	**168.0908**
P3	263.4745	262.2089	261.7143	264.2094	262.5932	263.504	**265**
P4	139.0594	134.2826	125.7665	138.122	136.9605	138.684	**150**
P5	165.4761	151.9039	153.7056	154.4716	168.2031	165.408	**149.7235**
P6	87.128	74.1812	93.7965	74.99	87.3304	86.9499	**95.8338**
Total power	1276.01	1276.03	1276.134	1275.94	1276.023	1275.115	**1275.0259**
Cost ($/h)	15450	15459	15461.1	15454.89	15450.06	15446.43	**15445.8095**
Loss	12.9584	13.0217	13.1317	12.9422	13.0205	12.203	**12.1208**

Bold represents that our proposed method is better than the existing methods

Table 4 Comparison table for case 2

Methods	Cost ($/h)
SA [30]	15461.1
GA [30]	15457.96
TS [30]	15454.89
PSO [30]	15450.14
MTS [30]	15450.06
New MPS [31]	15447
SOH-PSO [31]	15446.019
PSO-LRS [31]	15450.001
NPSO [31]	15450.001
NPSO-LRS [31]	15450
CSS [32]	15446.42
HAS [32]	15449
TSA [32]	15451.63
SAPSO [33]	15455
APSO [33]	15449.99
CPSO1 [34]	15447
CPSO2 [34]	15446
BFO [35]	15443.85
SGA [35]	15447
SOH_PSO [35]	15446.02
DE [35]	15449.766
FPA	**15445.81**

Bold represents that our proposed method is better than the existing methods

4.3 Case Study 2: Optimization of Cost Function with Prohibited Zone and Ramp Limits

In this case, standard IEEE 15-unit system, with high level of nonlinearity (i.e. prohibited operation zone and ramp limits) and a load demand of 2630 MW is considered. Similar to above two cases, in this case also pertain to the optimization of fuel cost of generating units. The fuel cost coefficient, prohibited zone and ramp limit data are given in [28]. The optimized fuel cost is found to be 32,366.71 $/h and compared with PSOCFIWA [28] and others shown in Tables 5 and 6. The result obtained by algorithm is observed to be 0.2720% lower than PSOCFIWA's.

Table 5 Comparison table for case 3

Methods	Cost ($/h)
PSO [34]	32858
GA [34]	33113
CPSO1 [34]	32835
CPSO2 [34]	32834
HHS [34]	32692.857
AIS [36]	32854
APSO [36]	32742
SA-PSO [36]	32708
ABC [36]	32707
IPSO [37]	32706
ESO [37]	32568.54
IDE [37]	32418.79
CA [37]	32854
BF [37]	32784.5
CE [37]	32588.87
SOH-PSO [37]	32751.39
MTS [37]	32716.87
CSO [37]	32588.92
BSA-EV [37]	32604.49
QPSO-DM [37]	32652.58
DEPSO [37]	32588.81
FPA	**32366.71**

Bold represents that our proposed method is better than the existing methods

Table 6 Control variables optimized solution for case study 3

Power (MW)	PSO [28]	PSOCFA [28]	PSOIWA [28]	PSOCFIWA [28]	FPA (proposed)
P1	455	409.1917	449.3242	408.7283	**454.9973**
P1	455	455	453.3263	389.0564	**380**
P3	130	129.9769	130	125.2584	**130**
P4	130	130	130	127.1344	**129.9994**
P5	269.8497	168.9652	169.2737	161.9051	**170**
P6	459.9985	440.4041	459.176	441.0358	**460**
P7	465	465	465	428.077	**430**
P8	60	60	69.1907	73.452	**72.02637**
P9	25.0039	37.7333	25	101.7855	**27.97911**
P10	25.0009	118.7288	96.6216	151.324	**160**
P11	44.043	80	55.2023	75.0901	**80**
P12	56.1041	80	64.1294	79.995	**79.99269**
P13	25	25	25	27.6989	**25.0009**
P14	15	15	23.7557	24.259	**15.00422**
P15	15	15	15	15	**15**
Total power	2630	2630	2630	2630	**2630**
Cost ($/h)	32257	32320	32306	32455	**32366.71**

Bold represents that our proposed method is better than the existing methods

4.4   Case Study 4: Multi-objective Fuel Cost and Emission Optimization Without Losses

The FPA is being tested on the IEEE 6-generator 30-bus system to solve the emission-restricted ELD problem. As the problem demanded, the minimization of both total fuel costs and emission, the objective function was formulated as multi-objective consisting of emission and total fuel cost. In order to solve the multi-objective functions, a weighted-sum approach is used. All other required data is collected from [13]. Membership function for fuzzy environment implementation is given in Table 7. The optimum emission and fuel cost obtained is 0.1862 ton/h and 600.1114 $/h at $w = 0$ and $w = 1$, respectively. The convergence plot for the best fuel cost at $w = 1$ and the best emission at $w = 0$ is shown in Tables 8 and 9, respectively. From Table 10, it can be seen that with equal weightage approach, i.e. $w = 0.5$, emission and total fuel costs is obtained as 0.1942 ton/h and 607.3650 $/h, respectively. At weight $w = 0.5$, it is found that the value of membership is maximum in fuzzy membership approach. Hence, corresponding values are the solutions, i.e. 608.9980 $/h and 0.1930 ton/h as fuel cost and emission. The details of controlling variable setting and comparisons from other consulted literatures are given in Tables 8 and 9. From Table 9, it can be concluded that FPA surpasses the several algorithms in terms of converging time and efficient searching of global optima.

Table 7 Membership function table for fuzzy environment implementation of case study 4

Pareto points (k)	Cost ($/h)	Emission (ton/h)	μ_1^m	μ_2^m	μ^m	W
1	633.3389	0.18621	0	1.0000	0.0745	0.0
2	626.2424	0.1870	0.2136	0.9584	0.0873	0.1
3	619.0217	0.1890	0.4309	0.8531	0.0957	0.2
4	611.9947	0.1915	0.6424	0.7214	0.1016	0.3
5	609.9980	0.1930	0.7326	0.6424	0.1025	0.4
6	607.3650	0.1942	0.7818	0.5793	0.1014	0.5
7	605.6858	0.1966	0.8323	0.4529	0.0958	0.6
8	604.6912	0.1978	0.8622	0.3897	0.0933	0.7
9	603.6862	0.1993	0.8925	0.3107	0.0897	0.8
10	601.5835	0.2020	0.9558	0.1685	0.0838	0.9
11	600.114	0.2052	1.0000	0	0.0746	1.0

Bold represents that our proposed method is better than the existing methods

Table 8 Power generation, total fuel costs and emission for selected values for w for case study 4

w	P1	P2	P3	P4	P5	P6	Total fuel costs ($/h)	Total emission (ton/h)
1.0	10.970	29.975	52.429	101.61	52.433	35.972	600.11	0.20
0.9	20.366	30.147	52.377	99.806	46.926	33.775	601.18	0.20
0.8	9.3943	42.319	59.992	85.953	50.540	35.200	603.68	0.19
0.7	16.171	33.165	42.708	81.401	69.276	40.678	604.69	0.19
0.6	19.824	35.658	49.642	88.221	38.285	51.767	605.68	0.19
0.5	**25.061**	**44.716**	**55.448**	**83.179**	**40.600**	**34.393**	**607.36**	**0.19**
0.4	28.054	37.811	52.532	71.909	63.670	29.419	609.99	0.19
0.3	35.116	40.888	55.638	76.043	39.552	36.160	611.99	0.19
0.2	29.697	40.569	66.135	56.813	44.252	45.933	619.02	0.18
0.1	40.856	47.355	43.855	55.505	52.630	43.196	626.24	0.18
0	39.067	49.281	58.285	45.247	50.286	49.232	633.33	0.18

Bold represents that our proposed method is better than the existing methods

4.5 Case Study 4: Multi-objective Fuel Cost and Emission Optimization with Losses

This case study is the extension of case study 3, which includes the losses in the system. Rest of the other parameters are same as considered in case study 4. The system data required for simulation is given in [13]. The extreme solution for total cost and emission at weights 1 and 0 are found to be 605.7700 $/h and 0.1861 ton/h,

Table 9 Comparison of FPA with other reported algorithms for case study 4

	Case	SPEA [15]	NGSA [15]	NGSA-II [15]	NPGA [15]	FCPSO [15]	EC [15]	FPA
Best fuel cost	P1	0.1062	0.1567	0.1059	0.108	0.107	0.1097	0.10971
	P2	0.2897	0.28	0.3177	0.3284	0.2897	0.2998	0.29975
	P3	0.5289	0.4671	0.5216	0.5386	0.525	0.5243	0.52429
	P4	1.0025	1.0467	1.0146	1.0067	1.015	1.0162	1.01619
	P5	0.5402	0.5037	0.5159	0.4949	0.53	0.5243	0.24335
	P6	0.3664	0.3729	0.3583	0.3574	0.3673	0.3597	0.35972
	Costs ($/h)	600.15	600.572	600.155	600.529	600.132	600.111	600.111
	Emission_(ton/h)	00.2214	0.22281	0.22189	00.2116	00.2223	0.2221	0.2052
Best emission	P1	0.4116	0.4394	0.7074	0.4002	0.4097	0.406	0.39067
	P2	0.4532	0.4155	0.4577	0.4474	0.455	0.459	0.49028
	P3	0.5329	0.515	0.5389	0.5166	0.5363	0.5379	0.58285
	P4	0.3832	0.3871	0.3837	0.3688	0.3842	0.383	0.45275
	P5	0.5383	0.555	0.5352	0.5751	0.5348	0.538	0.50286
	P6	0.5148	0.4905	0.511	0.5259	0.514	0.51	0.49232
	Emissions (ton/h)	0.1942	0.19436	0.1942	0.19433	0.1942	0.1942	0.1862
	Cost ($/h)	638.51	639.231	638.269	6339.18	638.358	638.27	633.339

Bold represents that our proposed method is better than the existing methods

and corresponding emission and cost are 0.2044 ton/h and 641.2894 $/h, respectively. The results from both the approaches are shown in Tables 10 and 11. A compromised solution is obtained for $w = 0.5$, which is 0.1913 ton/h and 619.2636 $/h as the total emissions and total fuel costs, respectively. From fuzzy approach, 616.2122 $/h and 0.1924 ton/h is declared as the best compromised solution. The comparison is shown in Table 11 with numerous other available algorithms.

5   Conclusion and Future Scope

This chapter uses a metaheuristic algorithm called the flower pollination algorithm (FPA) which is motivated by nature to strive for economics and environmental welfare. FPA is tested on many standard IEEE bus systems to address single as well as multi-objective (EELD) power system-related issues. The idea of the frequency of switching between self-pollination (exploitation) and cross-pollination (exploration) makes the algorithm flexible for searching in the search space for the global optimum. Results obtained by FPA on various IEEE systems dominate many other known algorithms used to solve ELD and EELD problems.

Table 10 Unit power generation, fuel cost and emission for selected values for w for case study 5

W	P1	P2	P3	P4	P5	P6	Total fuel cost ($/h)	Total emission (ton/h)	Losses (ton/h)
1.0	12.080	28.489	58.143	99.293	52.630	35.219	605.77	0.204	2.46
0.9	16.466	24.606	63.899	87.264	52.556	40.810	607.64	0.200	2.20
0.8	11.635	34.699	57.736	83.115	48.665	50.120	610.31	0.197	2.57
0.7	21.332	38.685	59.978	76.876	58.924	29.957	611.75	0.194	2.35
0.6	19.839	35.918	44.027	77.010	68.483	40.851	612.56	0.195	2.72
0.5	**17.087**	**37.426**	**45.627**	**74.945**	**64.427**	**46.643**	**613.44**	**0.194**	**2.75**
0.4	25.864	28.801	52.296	68.295	64.746	45.922	616.21	0.192	2.52
0.3	21.456	39.768	54.087	70.137	43.608	57.118	619.26	0.191	2.76
0.2	28.224	42.073	69.375	61.526	50.165	34.465	621.07	0.190	2.42
0.1	31.431	52.045	39.856	66.591	49.332	47.596	627.08	0.188	3.39
0	39.687	49.818	50.742	45.983	50.846	49.793	641.28	0.186	3.44

Bold represents that our proposed method is better than the existing methods

Table 11 Comparison of FPA with other reported algorithms for case study 5

	Case	SPEA [15]	NGSA [15]	NGSA-II [15]	NPGA [15]	FCPSO [15]	EC [15]	FPA
Best fuel cost	P1	0.10866	0.1186	0.1182	0.1245	0.113	0.1076	0.1208
	P2	0.3056	0.3156	0.3148	0.2792	0.3145	0.3012	0.28495
	P3	0.5818	0.5441	0.591	0.6284	0.5826	0.597	0.58143
	P4	0.9846	0.9447	0.9701	1.0264	0.986	0.9897	0.99293
	P5	0.5288	0.5498	0.5172	0.4693	0.5264	0.512	0.5263
	P6	0.3584	0.3694	0.3548	0.3993	0.345	0.3511	0.3522
	Costs ($/h)	607.807	608.245	607.801	608.147	607.7862	605.836	**605.77**
	Emission (ton/h)	00.2201	00.21664	00.21891	00.2364	00.2201	00.2208	00.2044
Best emission	P1	0.4043	0.4113	0.4141	0.3923	0.4063	0.4102	0.39687
	P2	0.4525	0.4591	0.4602	0.47	0.4586	0.4633	0.49189
	P3	0.5525	0.5117	0.5429	0.5565	0.551	0.5447	0.50742
	P4	0.4079	0.3724	0.4011	0.3695	0.4084	0.3921	0.45983
	P5	0.5468	0.581	0.5422	0.5599	0.5432	0.5447	0.50846
	P6	0.5005	0.5304	0.5045	0.5163	0.4974	0.5152	0.49793
	Emissions (ton/h)	00.19422	00.19432	00.19419	00.19424	00.1942	00.1942	**0.1861**
	Cost ($/h)	642.603	647.251	644.133	645.984	624.896	646.22	641.289

Bold represents that our proposed method is better than the existing methods

Due to its higher ability to solve complex goals, the above-listed algorithm can also be evaluated for several other problems of power system optimization. In addition to other optimization problems in power systems, this algorithm can be expanded as system complexity increases with increasing load demands and the use of electronically controlled loads, as the suggested algorithm solves multi-objective issues with greater performance.

References

1. Wood, J., Wollenberg, B.F.: Power Generation Operation and Control, 2nd edn. Wiley (1996)
2. Keib, E., Ma, H., Hart, J.: Economic dispatch in view of the clean air act of 1990. IEEE Trans. Power Syst. **9**(2), 972–978 (1994)
3. Talaq, J., Hawary, F.E., Hawary, M.E.: A summary of environmental/economic dispatch algorithms. IEEE Trans. Power Syst. **9**(3), 1508–1516 (1994)
4. Granelli, G., Montagna, M., Pasini, G., Marannino, P.: Emission constrained dynamic dispatch. Electr. Power Syst. Res. **24**(1), 55–64 (1992)
5. Abido, M.: Environmental/economic power dispatch using multi-objective evolutionary algorithms. IEEE Trans. Power Syst. **18**(4), 1529–1537 (2003)

6. Abido, M.: A novel multi-objective evolutionary algorithm for environmental economic power dispatch. Electr. Power Syst. Res. **65**(1) (2003)
7. Malik, T.N., Asar, A.U., Wyne, M.F., Akhtar, S.: A new hybrid approach for the solution of nonconvex economic dispatch problem with valve-point effects. Electr. Power Syst. Res. **80**, 1128–1136 (2010)
8. Varadarajan, M., Swarup, K.S.: Solving multi-objective optimal power flow using differential evolution. IET GenerTransmDistrib (2008)
9. Panigrahi, B.K., Pandi, V.R.: Bacterial foraging optimization: Nelder-Mead hybrid algorithm for economic load dispatch. IET Gener. Transm. Distrib. **2**(4), 556–565 (2008)
10. Khorsandi, A., Alimardani, B., Vahidi, Hosseinian, S.H.: Hybrid shuffled frog leaping algorithm and Nelder–Mead simplex search for optimal reactive power dispatch. IET Gener. Transm. Distrib. **5**(2), 249–56 (2010)
11. Basu, M.: Economic environmental dispatch using multi-objective differential evalution. Appl. Soft comput. **11**(2) (2011)
12. Hota, P.K., Chakrabarti, R., Chattopadhyay, P.K.: Economic emission load dispatch through an interactive fuzzy satisfying method. EPSR, **54**(3) (2000)
13. Ozyon, S., Temurtas, H., Durmus, B., Kuvat, G.: Charged system algorithm for emission constrained economic power dispatch problem. Energy **46**(1) (2012)
14. Mondal, S., Bhattacharya, A., Dey, S.H.N.: Multi-objective economic load dispatch solution using gravitational search algorithm and considering wind power penetration. Int. J. Power Energy Syst **44**, 282–292 (2013)
15. Vahidinasab, V., Jadid, S.: Joint economic and emission dispatch in energy market: a Multi-objective programming approach. Energy **35**, 1497–1504 (2010)
16. Bhattacharjee, K., Bhattacharya, A., Dey, S.H.N.: Solution of economic emission load dispatch problems of power systems by real coded chemical reaction algorithm
17. Subhani, T.M., Babu, C.S., Reddy, A.S.V.: Particle swarm optimization with time varying acceleration coefficients for economic dispatch considering valve point loading effects. Comput. Commun. Networking Technol. (ICCCNT), IEEE (2012)
18. Rao, B.S., Vaisakh, K.: Multi-objective adaptive Clonal selection algorithm for solving environmental/economic dispatch and OPF problems with load uncertainty. Electr. Power Energ. Syst. **53**, 390–408 (2013)
19. Duman, S., Yorukeren, N., Altas, I.H.: A novel modified hybrid PSOGSA based on fuzzy logic for non-convex economic dispatch problem with valve-point effect. Electr. Power Energ. Syst. **64**, 121–135 (2015)
20. Shaw, B., Mukherjee, V., Ghoshal, S.P.: Solution of economic dispatch problems by seeker optimization algorithm. Expert Syst. Appl. **39**, 508–519 (2012)
21. Kahourzade, S., Mahmoudi, A., Mokhlis, H.B.: A comparative study of multi-objective optimal power flow based on particle swarm, evolutionary programming, and genetic algorithm. Springer, Electrical Engineering (2015)
22. Mishra, R., Das, K.N.: A novel chemo-inspired genetic algorithm for economic load dispatch with valve point loading effect. In: Proceedings of fourth international conference on soft computing for problem solving advances in intelligent systems and computing. Springer, vol. 335, pp. 443–460 (2015)
23. Yang, X.S.: Flower pollination algorithm for global optimization. In: Unconventional Computation and Natural Computation" Lecture Notes in Computer Science, vol. 7445, pp. 240–249 (2012)
24. Yang, X.S., Karamanoglu, M., He, X.: Flower pollination algorithm: a novel approach for multiobjective optimization. Eng. Optim. **46**(9), 1222–1237 (2014)
25. Iqbal, A., et al.: Metaheurestic algorithm based hybrid model for identification of building sale prices. In: Springer Nature Book: Metaheuristic and Evolutionary Computation: Algorithms and Applications, under book series "Studies in Computational Intelligence", (2020). https://doi.org/10.1007/978-981-15-7571-6_32
26. Nandan, N.K., et al.: Solving Nonconvex economic thermal power dispatch problem with multiple fuel system and valve point loading effect using fuzzy reinforcement learning. J. Intell. Fuzzy Syst. **35**(5), 4921–4931 (2018). https://doi.org/10.3233/jifs-169776

27. Minai, F., et al.: Metaheuristics paradigms for renewable energy systems: advances in optimization algorithms. In: Springer Nature Book: Metaheuristic and Evolutionary Computation: Algorithms and Applications, under book series "Studies in Computational Intelligence" (2020). https://doi.org/10.1007/978-981-15-7571-6_2

28. Oasgupta, K., Banerjee, S.: An Analysis of economic load dispatch with prohibited zone and ramp-rate limit constraints using different algorithms. In: 2014 Power and Energy Systems: Towards Sustainable Energy, PESTSE (2014)

29. Aydin, D., Ozyon, S.: Solution to non-convex economic dispatch problem with valve point effects by incremental artificial bee colony with local search. Appl. Soft Comput. **13**, 2456–2466 (2013)

30. Pothiya, S., Ngamroo, I., Kongprawechnon, W.: Application of multiple tabu search algorithm to solve dynamic economic dispatch considering generator constraints. Energy Convers. Manage. **49**, 506–516 (2008)

31. Bhattacharya, A., Chattopadhyay, P.K.: Biogeography-based optimization for different economic load dispatch problems. IEEE Trans. Power Syst. **25**(2) (2010)

32. Jeddi, B., Vahidinasab, V.: A modified harmony search method for environmental/economic load dispatch of real-world power systems. Energ. Convers. Manage. **78**, 661–675 (2014)

33. Hosseinnezhad, V., Babaei, E.: Economic load dispatch using h-PSO. Electr. Power Energ. Syst. **49**, 160–169 (2013)

34. Pandi, V.R., Panigrahi, B.K., Bansal, R.C., Das, S., Mohapatra, A.: Economic load dispatch using hybrid swarm intelligence based harmony search algorithm. Electr. Power Compon. Syst. **39**(8), 751–767 (2010)

35. Dalvand, M.M., Ivatloo, B.M., Najafi, A., Rabiee, A.: Continuous quick group search optimizer for solving non-convex economic dispatch problems. Electr. Power Syst. Res. **93**, 93–105 (2012)

36. Hemamalini, S., Simon, S.P.: Artificial bee colony algorithm for economic load dispatch problem with non-smooth cost functions. Electr. Power Compon. Syst. **38**(7), 786–803 (2009)

37. Sayah, S., Hamouda, A.: A hybrid differential evolution algorithm based on particle swarm optimization for nonconvex economic dispatch problems. Appl. Soft Comput. **13**, 1608–1619 (2013)

Planning and Monitoring of EV Fast-Charging Stations Including DG in Distribution System Using Particle Swarm Optimization

Dhiraj Kumar Singh and Aashish Kumar Bohre

Abstract Today the electric vehicles (EVs) market in India is increasing very fast but the availability of efficient charging infrastructure for the EVs is still a big issue. The adoption of EVs is more advantageous and cost-efficient than the internal combustion (IC) engine-based vehicles due to the problem of depletion of convention fuel sources and increasing pollution and offering social as well as technical benefits. Therefore, the adoption of EVs is the alternate source of transportation and efficient replacement in transportation as they emit zero carbon emission, energy-efficient and are economical. For the expansion of EV market, the charging station infrastructure is very important to provide efficient energy for various EVs. This work presents innovative method for the optimal planning of charging stations with distributed generations (DGs) to establish an efficient charging infrastructure by considering the novel parameters such as power losses, voltage, reliability, and economic parameters in the proposed modified radial distribution network of study area. Furthermore, the innovative proposed multi-objective function is utilized for the optimal planning of distributed generations and the electric vehicle charging stations considering the network performance parameters as objectives variables. The minimum value of multi-objective function decides based on the system performance indices as power loss, charging cost, voltage deviation, and reliability indices. The objective function is minimized using particle swarm optimization to obtain the optimal allocation of the EV charging station as well as the placement of DG in the modified IEEE 33-bus radial distribution system. In this work, the case study for Durgapur, WB, India, is presented for particular network section in city center area with modified IEEE 33-bus radial distribution system. The MATLAB/MATPOWER tool is used to solve the power flow through backward and forward method. This work concludes that

D. K. Singh (✉) · A. K. Bohre
Electrical Engineering Department, National Institute of Technology (NIT) Durgapur, Durgapur, WB 713209, India
e-mail: dhirajklrsingh100@gmail.com

A. K. Bohre
e-mail: aashishkumar.bohre@ee.nitdgp.ac.in

minimization of power losses, charging cost, voltage deviation, and improved reliability of the system is increased leading to secure and stable EV charging stations with DGs.

Keywords Electric Vehicles (EVs) · EV fast charging stations · Distributed Generation (DG) · Distribution System · Particle Swarm Optimization (PSO)

1 Introduction

Concern of global warming, climate change, urban air pollution, and dependence on ambiguous and costly supplies of foreign oil have advanced research and policy-makers management to explore alternatives [1, 2]. Electric operated vehicles have the lowest or negligible greenhouse gases and urban air pollutant [3, 4]. Two environmental impacts are accounted for traveling from one place to another is air pollution and greenhouse gases (GHGs) emission. The greenhouse gases are carbon dioxide (CO_2), methane (CH_4), nitrous oxide (N_2O), and sulfur hexafluoride (SF_6) which have green house gases impact weighing coefficient relative to CO_2 of 1, 21, 310, and 24,900, respectively [5, 6]. Air pollutants like carbon monoxide (CO), nitrogen oxides (NO_x), sulfur oxides (SO_x), and volatile organic compounds (VOCs) impact weighing coefficient 0.017, 1, 1.3, and 0.64, respectively. Of the major industries that have to adapt and redesign to meet the present requirement for sustainable development, vehicle assembling is one of the most important requirements. With the availability the electric vehicle in the present scenario, the overall requirement of electrical power increases with a large ratio [7]. To overcome this problem, power generation must be increased in the same ratio. Power generation dependence should also decrease from thermal to other conventional source to meet the objective of the implementation EVs that is air pollution and GHGs.

The pie chart in Fig. 1 represents that the dependence of power generation in India on fossil fuel should change completely before the implementation EVs, because the objective will not meet the requirement [8–10]. It will only reduce the pollution of certain cities but globally the scenario remains the same. After the major change, the next step milestone is the life cycle of the batteries of EVs, the cost of the EVs manufacturing, and anxiety of charging station as well as the charging [11, 12]. All the above-mentioned challenges are the areas of research these days. In this work, focus is on the charging station and the charging time that is allocation of fast-charging station (FCS) and also deal with present scenario of the power system configuration to handle the requirement of power by EVs [13].

Depending upon the power level, there are four different modes of charging time and charging speed are as [1–3, 8–10]:

- Mode 1:- This is simply an extension cord that plugs into a standard domestic 16 A socket. Max power is limited to 16 A/2 kW. Actively discouraged as no safety protection for the socket or user.

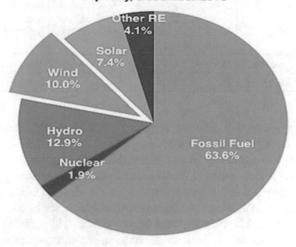

Technology-wise share in India's installed capacity, December 2018

Fig. 1 Pie chart of power generation in India [14, 15]

- Mode 2:- Charging is a smart extension cord that has electronics in line to communicate with the car under charge and associated safety features. Better than Mode 1, but still very limited charging capacity for larger batteries. For example, a Tesla X with a 100 kW battery will take about 3 days to fully charge using a Mode 2 charger.
- Mode 3:- Mode 3 is single or three-phase AC fast charging up to 22 kW. This mode having protection circuit between vehicle and ac supply.
- Mode 4:- DC Fast or fast chargers. They are also the most expensive.

This case study configures the IEEE 33-bus distribution system [1, 16–18] to be capable to handle the load increased in the system due to the rising EVs load in the power system and the IEEE system is modified for considered work. Zones are created depending range anxiety. Different zones have specific areas where there is a need of charging station. But due to economical consideration, we cannot place charging station randomly at different places. So, this work allocates the optimum location depending upon the requirement of specific zone having a specific fast-charging station which ultimately overcomes range anxiety.

As Table 1 represents the technical and economical characteristics for conventional and EVs, the table completely expresses the advantages as well as the disadvantage in broad point of view. Despite the major disadvantages like initial cost and battery replacement cost, one of the major concerns of motivation toward EV is the running cost that is fuel cost. Fuel cost of EV is almost one-third of the conventional vehicle. Another anxiety of pursuing EV is the availability of charging station because the table represents the driving range of the EV. In this work, our major concern deals with the driving range anxiety. The driving range anxiety can

Table 1 Comparison of conventional vehicle and EV

Vehicle type	Fuel	Initial cost (k$)	Battery replacement cost, life cycle 10 years (k$)	Specific fuel consumption (MJ/100 km)	Specific fuel cost (k$/100 km)	Range of driving (km)
Conventional	Gasoline	15.3	1 * 0.1	236.8	2.94	540
Electric	Electricity	42	2 * 15.4	67.2	0.901	164

be decreased by increasing the charging stations in the specified range limits as we are having the conventional gasoline station.

Usually, load demand is served by national or central generation, transmission and distribution systems, whereas from decades, small and medium generating units are being implemented in the power system and these are termed as distribution generation (DG). This unit is power through renewable source or combined heat and power unit (CHP), or like usually diesel or gas turbine. This unit has its advantage as it reduces the power loss in the system, enhances the voltage profile, improves the reliability, and improves the power quality of the power system. However, it is having disadvantages too like improper planning can lead to a reduction in reliability; voltage stability and can also increase the power losses of the system. As mentioned above, the EVs are encouraged because it reduces environmental pollution as well as it has energy-efficient benefits. But, EVs enhance the upstream emission in fuel production that is generation, transmission, and distribution of electric power. Upstream emission analysis became a major concern after the introduction of EV was viewed as an option [19, 20].

As it is stated above that the most important that coal used for the power industry leads to enhance GHGs emissions. The reduction of GHGs emissions can only be achieved by shifting the coal-based power plant with renewable or nuclear-based power plants. However, with a certain mixer of feedstock of coal, renewable and natural gases, the USA could have achieved only 20–50%. The reduction up to 90% can be achieved only when all EVs are operated through renewable and nuclear power-based power plant. In this work, we have considered only renewable DGs. Distribution generation has similar advantages as the EV station as it decreases the emission of carbon dioxide and NOX, and it also rectifies the voltage profile and voltage stability in the distribution system. It intensifies the reliability and power quality of the distribution feeder. But, inappropriate planning of DGs will not meet the above-mentioned advantages related to the power system that is voltage stability, reliability, and other safety issues. So, to meet the demand DGs optimal sizing must be considered [21–24].

The microgrid is a localized generating unit that is centralized with the national grid and able to operate after localizing the network which means it can be able to operate independently. DGs are the part of the microgrid which can be able to operate independently as well as with the central grid. Independent operation means if the EV stations are being in operation at its full load of EV charging whereas if the EV station is on underloaded condition then the extra power can be transmitted to the

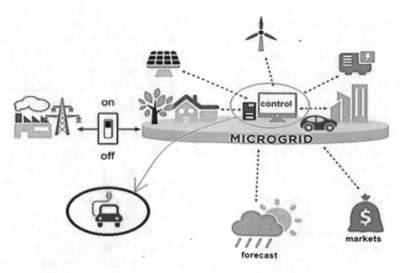

Fig. 2 Microgrid structure

central grid. Figure 2 represents that the controller will decide the direction of power flow as per the condition mentioned in above paragraph. This figure represents DG like solar, wind, and diesel operate DGs which is connected to the grid with a switch and the power flow to EV station as well the grid is being calculated by the controller [1–5, 14, 25, 26]. The main reason of presenting the problem of EV charging station planning in Indian scenario is because of rapid growing demand for EVs day by day. Already in Durgapur city more than 300 E-rickshaw and more that 100 small EV two wheelers are present also very few EV car came in the market. Therefore, this study presents the attention on current situation of EV charging infrastructure which is essential nowadays due to fast growing EV scenario globally.

2 Recent Scenario and Motivation

The recent scenario and development in this section includes the literature review which specifically deals with the EV stations impact on the power system and implementing DGs at that EV station. Nowadays as the trends are shift on EV the requirement of power is being increased which impacts the existing power system. These impacts on the power system are economical, quality of power, and reliability of the system. In [1], considered parameters are charging cost of EV, penalty function of voltage and power. They represented economical aspect and used the objective function in terms of power loss and cost of charging, and for quality aspect, the objective function in terms of voltage deviation is used and also the considered assumption and setting are being introduced here. In [2], a reliability calculation-based method for integrated transportation and electrical power systems incorporating electric vehicle are presented by considering the case studies based on RBTS system using optimal control strategy and practical validation also performed for same. The model for battery switching station for electric buses is proposed through the optimal scheduling of battery charging using an efficient algorithm in [3]. The EV station development cost which includes equipment, installation, operation, and maintenance cost is presented in [4]. They considered the optimal placing and sizing of the fast-charging stations as main objective. The detailed idea about the renewables and battery storage system to manage the energy are described including a case study of off-grid system using PSO are discussed in [5]. Rani et al. [6] considered different parameters such as power loss, voltage, and economic factor that includes installation, operation, and maintenance and also pondered the objective that is determining optimal size and placement of renewable DG considering variation of load. The economic and environmental comparison and different prospective while considering the impact of electric vehicle and charging infrastructure are presented in [7–9]. In [10], multi-types of charging facilities for the electric vehicle charging are optimal planned using a new optimization model which minimizes the annual social cost of entire EV charging infrastructure. The charging stations for the electric vehicles based on GIS and multi-objectives particles swarms optimization and a mathematically optimal model are developed to analyze the relationship between upfront investments and operating costs and service coverage of charging station system is planned in [11]. Battapothula et al. [12] implemented the multi-objective for optimal planning of EV and DG station simultaneously by including the effect of cost of station development.

The potential benefits of plug-in hybrid electric vehicles and battery electric vehicles with configured dispersed energy storage acting in a vehicle-to-building (V2B) operating mode are explored in [27]. The estimation of reliability impact due to EVs with battery exchange operation using the behavior analysis of EVs as well as extraction method is described in [13]. MATPOWER provides the best tool to handle power system analysis with the different cases of numerous distribution and transmission systems in [16]. The third parameter that is reliability and power loss also reported the index in terms of energy not supplied (ENS) for the calculation of reliability in [17]. The optimal planning and allocation of storage devices and different types of DGs in the distribution systems using different approaches and methodologies are presented in [18, 19]. In [20], the DG installation, operation, and maintenance cost by using the particle swarm optimization for sizing and placement of DGs from DG owner's and distribution company's viewpoint are specified. In [21–24], the optimization technique that is the PSO, butterfly-PSO, and GA to solve the problem of different DGs allocations including system performance indices including power loss, reliability, and ENS is used. The detailed idea about the total installed capacity of different renewable, conventional, and other sources is described in [14]. The mathematical models for powers systems reliability and its applications in various fields are reported in [15]. The comprehensive idea and detailed modeling with numerous example and case studies are presented in [25, 26]. The EV charging infrastructure development in view of low emissions in the UK for the future prospective are presented in [28] and also the comprehensive reviews on EVs recent trends, challenges, status, and scopes are explored in [29]. The multi-objective approach to manage EVs charging and discharging strategy is utilized in [30]. The development of EVs charging stations for different systems and with distinct objectives is planned by considering the optimal size and site [31, 32]. Some other examples are given in [33–35] for better understanding of recent advancement of PSO and it applications.

The above literature review for recent scenario motivates to plan optimally EVs charging infrastructure and DGs in microgrid and distributions systems by considering Indian scenario of EVs. The world's concern on renewable energy is increasing day by day which leads to motivating the use of EV, but the ultimate goal of EV is not achieved if proper planning is not implemented on power generation and utilization. This work is fulfilling the above criterion that is renewable power generation in terms of DG and utilization of power through EV. EV requires power in which in India is completely dependent on thermal energy. So, first of all, we should have our concern on renewable sources of energy like solar power, wind power, biogas, biomass, small hydro. These sources have their limitation which must be considered. Distribution generation is the process of implementation of renewable energy by decentralizing the energy requirements which would impact the grid with the increase of EV loads. The microgrid is also a modern grid that connects the small-scale generating units to the national grid and can be disconnected from the central grid when required. DG is the part of microgrid whenever required connected and disconnected from the central grid. Now, after the implementation of the DG the fast-charging station is also required to motivate the EV users and also to enhance and maintain system reliability and sustainability. The anxiety of the EV user is the EV charging station allocation and the charging time. So, to achieve our motivation, we must have a planned allocation of FCS over a city. Planning of FCS has own complication like voltage deviation and power loss reliability which is being to be taken care off. This work tries a bit to reduce the world's concern on global warming, climate change, and urban air pollution.

3 Station Development

Mainly the development of EV charging and DG station is considered in this case study, which is explained below.

3.1 EV Station

Economical aspects of EV station are also the important content of concern for the EV station owner. Equipment related to charging station has their certain cost and

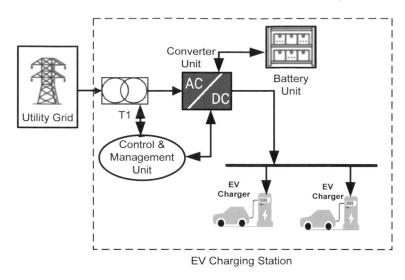

EV Charging Station

Fig. 3 General structure of EV charging station

requirements must be observed before the implementation. This chapter has considered the different requirements including land requirements. Electrical equipment includes the bus bars, transformers, etc. The infrastructure of FCS consists of a substation via a dedicated overhead line. Substation consists of LV and HV bus bar and has two parallel transformers [1–3]. Station infrastructure development requires equipment and land area. The linear variation of equipment cost is considered which has a dependence on the capacity and number of the connector to be installed. Each connector requires at least 9 feet width and 18 feet in length. And clearance between each connector is considered to be 3 feet. Area required for each connector to be assumed being 25 m^2. Figure 3 shows the general structure of EV station [14, 25, 26].

For station, the infrastructure cost (SIC$_i$) is then calculated as:

$$SIC_i = C_{ini} + 25 * C_{land} * S_i + RP * C_{con} * (S_i - 1) \qquad (1)$$

where

RP   connector rated power, kW;
C_{con} connector infrastructure cost, $/kW;
C_{ini} fixed cost, $;
C_{land} rental cost of land per annum, $/m^2; and
S_i number of connectors

The capacity of station (in KW) SC$_i$:

$$SC_i = RP * S_i \qquad (2)$$

3.2   DG Station

The cost of DG depends largely upon the MW rating. Before implementation, we have optimized the size of the DG at the EV station. Similarly, as the EV stations we have to consider the economical aspects of the DG before being into operation. The size of the DG is used in the optimization technique which reduces the cost as well achieved the objective that is voltage stability, reduced power losses, improved reliability, and enhanced voltage profile. The cost of DG station depends on the parameter that is investment cost, operational cost, and maintenance cost [18–21]. The considered parameters for DG station cost are given in Table 2.

4   Defining Problem and Methodology

This chapter attempts to configure EV zones with uniform distribution of EV in each zone and also tries to maintain the minimum distance of two consecutive EV station is within the anxiety limit of the EV user. Therefore, this work presents innovative method for the optimal planning of charging stations with distributed generations (DGs) to establish an efficient charging infrastructure by considering the novel parameters such as power losses, voltage, reliability, and economic parameters in the proposed modified radial distribution network of study area. Furthermore, the innovative proposed multi-objective function is utilized for the optimal planning of distributed generations and the electric vehicle charging stations considering the network performance parameters as objective variables. The minimum value of multi-objective function decides based on the system performance indices as power loss, charging cost, voltage deviation, and reliability indices. Also, calculate the objective function and index functions for the optimization of the EV station at a particular location with minimum power loss and voltage deviation and maximization of reliability. From the DG point of view, the cost of DG is to be minimized through the optimization technique. In this work, we have used the size of DG for the economical consideration for the EV station owner. Size of the DG is used in the optimization technique which reduces the cost as well achieved the objective that is voltage stability, reduced power losses, improved reliability, and enhanced voltage profile.

Table 2 DG station cost

Parameter	Unit	Value
Investment cost	$/MW	15,900
Operational cost	$/MW	29
Maintenance cost	$/MW	7

4.1 Without DGs

The main objective here is to locate the EV charging station; there must be a charging station of EV considering the technical and economical aspects. This work tries to find a fast-charging station in all the four zones distribution system (IEEE 33). Considering the Durgapur map having 33-bus configurations as shown in Fig. 4, where four different FCS are to be placed in different zones and also the IEEE 33-bus system is given in Fig. 5, Evaluation is done by considering the area in four different zones as Z_1, Z_2, Z_3, and Z_4. Each zone has a uniformly distributed EV population as:

- Z_1 have bus number 19, 20, 21, and 22.
- Z_2 have bus number 23, 24, and 25
- Z_3 have bus number 27, 28, 29, 30, 31, 32, and 33
- Z_4 have bus number 9–18.

Finally, the goal is to place the fast-charging stations (FCS) where the power loss is minimum which reduces the cost and also the voltage deviation. We have also considered the reliability parameter which is to be maximized.

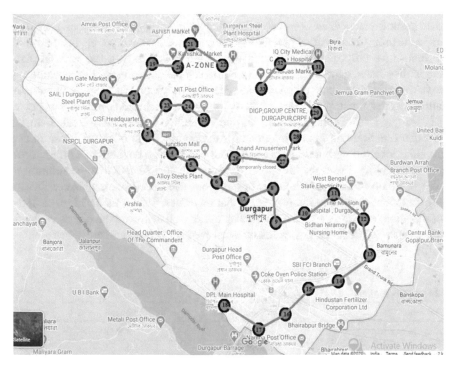

Fig. 4 Durgapur with the placement FCS

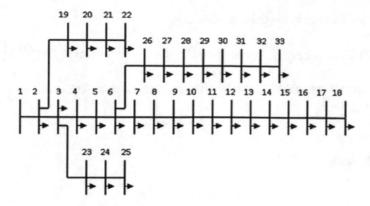

Fig. 5 IEEE 33-bus distribution system

Decision Variable

Locating the fast-charging stations in all the four zones, consider the variable as mentioned above.

Objective Function

As mentioned before, the optimization problem consists of cost as well as the power loss of the system including the EV station.

$$Z_{1i} = \min\{(PL + S_1 + S_2 + S_3 + S_\$) * pri\} \tag{3}$$

where

P_{loss} power loss of overall system
S_1 EV charging station no. 1
S_2 EV charging station no. 2
S_3 EV charging station no. 3
S_4 EV charging station no. 4
Pri   Cost of charging.

Constraints:

The constraints are the voltage deviation which considers the stability of the bus voltage. Due to the increase in demand, these parameters are disturbed throughout the area. These constraints are as follows:

$$V_i^{\min} \leq V_i^t \leq V_i^{\max} \tag{4}$$

where $\forall i \varepsilon \{1, 2, \ldots N_b\}$

Penalty function in the objective function:

$$\text{PVC}_i = \left[\max(V_{i,t}, V, \max) - V_i^{\max}\right] + \left[V_i^{\min} - \min\left(V_{i,t}, V_i^{\min}\right)\right] \quad (5)$$

The second constraint is the reliability which must be maximized.

$$Z_{2i} = 1/\text{Reliability} \quad (6)$$

Index function

$$\text{Index}_{1i} = Z_1/Z_{10} \quad (7)$$

$$\text{Index}_{2i} = \max(\text{PVC})/\max(\text{PVC}_0) \quad (8)$$

$$\text{Index}_{3i} = Z_{20}/Z_2 \quad (9)$$

The overall objective function is:

$$O_i = \min\{a * (\text{Index}_{1i}) + b * (\text{Index}_{2i}) + c * (\text{Index}_{3i})\} \quad (10)$$

where

a coefficient of cost and power loss (0.4)
b coefficient of penalty factor (0.3)
c coefficient of reliability (0.3)
i "denotes the function with EV station only"
0 "denotes the initial condition that is without EV and DG station (specific in second term underlined like Z_{20})."

The numerical value of the coefficient is considered as per the experimental point of view or can be termed as the priority of the overall three objective functions.

4.2 With DGs

The location obtained after the optimization is implemented with DGs. The location is being fixed now the size is to be calculated (through PSO optimization) with a similar objective function as above the only difference in Eq. 3 that is:

Objective Function

As mentioned before, the optimization problem consists of cost as well as the power loss of the system including the EV station.

$$Z_{1i} = \min\{(PL + S_1 + S_2 + S_3 + S_4 + DG_1 + DG_2 + DG_3 + DG_4) * pri\} \quad (11)$$

where

P_{loss} power loss of overall system
S_1 EV charging station no. 1
S_2 EV charging station no. 2
S_3 EV charging station no. 3
S_4 EV charging station no. 4
Pri   Cost of charging
DG_1 EV charging station cum DG station no. 1
DG_2 EV charging station cum DG station no. 2
DG_3 EV charging station cum DG station no. 3
DG_4 EV charging station cum DG station no. 4.

Constraints:

The constraints are the voltage deviation which considers the stability of the bus voltage. Due to the increase in demand, these parameters are disturbed throughout the area. These constraints are as follows:

$$V_f^{\min} \leq V_f^t \leq V_f^{\max} \tag{12}$$

Penalty function in the objective function:

$$PVC_f = \left[\max\left(V_{f,t}, V, \max\right) - V_f^{\max}\right] + \left[V_f^{\min} - \min\left(V_{f,t}, V_f^{\min}\right)\right] \tag{13}$$

The second constraint is the reliability which must be maximized.

$$Z_{2f} = 1/\text{Reliability} \tag{14}$$

Index function:

$$\text{Index}_{1f} = Z_1/Z_{11} \tag{15}$$

$$\text{Index}_{2f} = \max(PVC)/\max(PVC_1) \tag{16}$$

$$\text{Index}_{3f} = Z_{21}/Z_2 \tag{17}$$

The overall objective function is:

$$O_f = \min\{a * (\text{Index}_{1f}) + b * (\text{Index}_{2f}) + c * (\text{Index}_{3f})\} \tag{18}$$

where

a coefficient of cost and power loss (0.4)
b coefficient of penalty factor (0.3)
c coefficient of reliability (0.3)
f "denotes the function with EV station and DG station both"
1 "denotes the initial condition that is without EV and DG station (specific in second term underlined like Z_{21})."

The numerical value of the coefficient is considered as per the experimental point of view or can be termed as the priority of the overall three objective functions.

4.3 System Parameters

The presented work mainly deals with the three parameters of power system which are voltage profile, power losses, and reliability.

Voltage profile:

Quality of power depends upon two factors that are frequency and voltage. If voltage deviation is within the limits, then power is considered as good quality of power. All equipment is designed to operate smoothly on a certain voltage or with a variation of 5%. Considering the example of this work, EV load is implemented on the IEEE 33-bus system without DGs, and the below graph explains the impact of the voltage deviation. The improvement of voltage profile of system is targeted base on Eqs. (5) and (13) for both cases.

Power Losses:

Active power loss:

$$PL = \sum_{i=1}^{N_{br}} |I_i|^2 * R_i \tag{19}$$

Reactive power loss:

$$QL = \sum_{i=1}^{N_{br}} |I_{br}|^2 * X_{br} \tag{20}$$

where

R resistance of the line
X inductance of the branch.
I_i bus current
I_{br} branch current.

As the load is increased in the system, the value of current is increased in the system which leads to the increase in power losses. With the implementation of DG, the generation of power is localized which reduces the power losses in the system. The flowchart of presented work for optimal planning of EV stations with DGs is given in Fig. 6.

Reliability:

The primary objective of the power system is to provide its customer uninterrupted power supply. System ability to satisfy consumer power demand is termed as power system reliability. Power outage has several factors like load condition, worst weather, environment state, failed equipment, and improper planning. The outage has a major

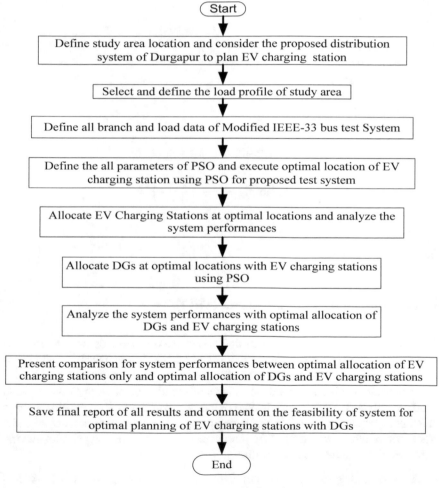

Start

Define study area location and consider the proposed distribution system of Durgapur to plan EV charging station

Select and define the load profile of study area

Define all branch and load data of Modified IEEE-33 bus test System

Define the all parameters of PSO and execute optimal location of EV charging station using PSO for proposed test system

Allocate EV Charging Stations at optimal locations and analyze the system performances

Allocate DGs at optimal locations with EV charging stations using PSO

Analyze the system performances with optimal allocation of DGs and EV charging stations

Present comparison for system performances between optimal allocation of EV charging stations only and optimal allocation of DGs and EV charging stations

Save final report of all results and comment on the feasibility of system for optimal planning of EV charging stations with DGs

End

Fig. 6 Flowchart of presented work for optimal planning of EV stations with DGs

impact on the economical aspect for the power sector as well as the power consumer. The importance of reliability came into existence after the large-scale blackout. Now reliability is the part of the power system for designing and planning points of view. It is also considered for the operation and maintenance of the power system. For calculation point of view, there are a lot of indices to measures reliability like energy not supplied (ENS), loss of load probability (LOLP), expected frequency of load curtailment (EFLC), expected duration of load curtailment (EDLC), and loss of load expectation (LOLE). In this work, we are using the index that is ENS. ENS mathematical formula can be given as:

$$\text{ENS} = \beta \mu \sum_{i=1}^{N_{br}} \gamma_i |I_{ik}| * V_{rated} \tag{21}$$

where

N_{br} number of branch or line
β load factor
μ Repair duration
γ_i failure rate of kth bus
I_{ik} peak load branch current
V_{rated} rated voltage.

Mathematical formula for reliability can be given as:

$$\text{Reliability} = 1 - \left(\frac{\text{ENS}}{\text{PD}}\right) \tag{22}$$

Where

PD   total power demand

5   Particle Swarm Optimization (PSO)

The particle swarm optimization was firstly suggested in 1995 by experts Eberhart Russell and Kennedy James, which was basically driven through the birds and fishes social behavior. It is an optimization technique based on the movement and intelligence of swarms [21–24]. It uses the concept of social interaction to search for food (problem-solving). Each swarm is considered as a particle in N-dimensional space which changes its speed and flying technique as per own experience and also the experience of other swarms [21, 22]. It uses the number of swarms (particle) moving in the search space for the best solution.

- Each swarm keeps the record of its solution space which helps to obtain the fitness (best solution) that has obtained till now. This is termed as personal best (pbest)

- PSO keeps the track of another best value obtained till now by any swarm (particle) in the neighborhood of that swarm. This is termed as global best (gbest)
- PSO basic concept lies in accelerating each particle toward its personal best (pbest) and global best (gbest) locations, with a random weighted factor in every step time.

The basic two equations for updated values of velocity and population for ith iteration are given as:

$$V_i^{t+1} = V_i^t + c_1 U_1^t \left(pb_i^t - p_i^t\right) + c_2 U_2^t \left(gb_i^t - p_i^t\right) \tag{23}$$

$$p_i^{t+1} = p_i^t + V_i^t \tag{24}$$

where

V_i	inertia of the particle
p_i	position of the particle
pb_i	personal best solution
gb_i	global best solution
c_1 & c_2	random weighted factor
$t + 1$	updated value.

The different PSO parameters considered for case study are such as $c_1 = c_2 = 2$, inertia weight (w) rage 0.95 to 0.4, and the random variables in the range of 0 to 1. Also, the total number of trials and number of iterations considered in the presented study are 30 and 50 respectively. The detailed graphical representation by flow chart for presented work using PSO is given in Figs. 7 and 8.

5.1 PSO Algorithm for EV FCS Allocation Optimization

STEP 1:- Read input data of IEEE 33-bus system.
STEP 2:- Execute power flow and calculate all the system parameter without EV FCS station.
STEP 3:- Updating of some parameter in the test system.
STEP 4:- Initialization of the EV FCS location of all the four zone.
STEP 5:- Execute power flow and calculate all the system parameters.
STEP 6:- Evaluating initial fitness function using multi-objective function
STEP 7:- Compute local best and global best.
STEP 8:- Update swarm velocity and swarm position.
STEP 9:- Update EV FCS station location based on the swarm and updated system data.
STEP 10:- Calculate fitness using multi-objective function.

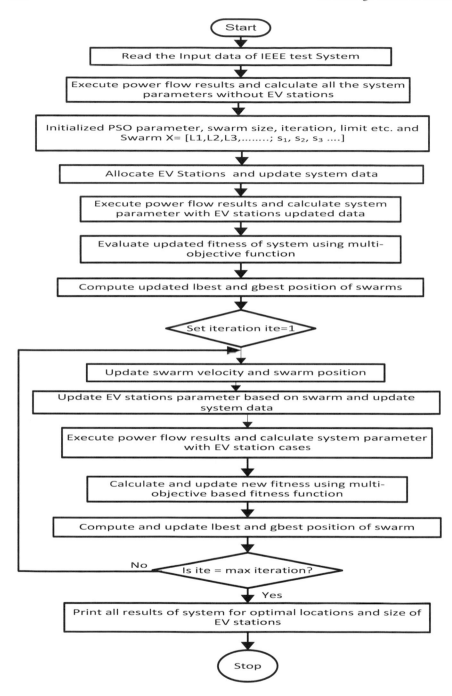

Fig. 7 PSO flowchart algorithm with EV station only

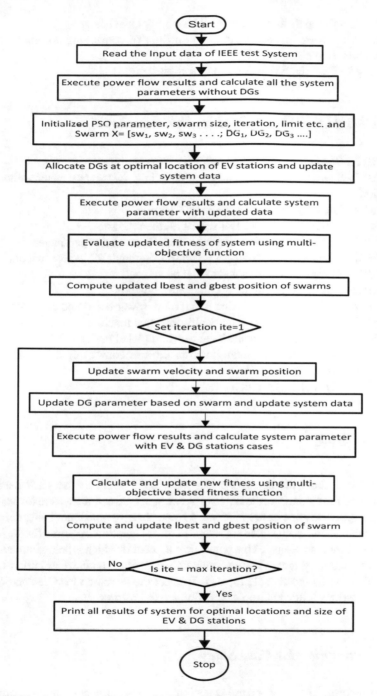

Fig. 8 PSO implementation flowchart with EV and DG station

STEP 11:- Compute and update local best and global best.
STEP 12:- Check for maximum iteration limit or converging criteria if exceed move next step *else go to STEP 7*
STEP 13:- Print the EV FCS station location.

5.2 PSO Algorithm for DG Size Optimization

STEP 1:- Read input data system with EV FCS station.
STEP 2:- Execute power flow and calculate all the system parameter without DG station.
STEP 3:- Locating DG station at EV FCS station.
STEP 4:- Initialization of the DG size of all the four zone.
STEP 5:- Execute power flow and calculate all the system parameters.
STEP 6:- Evaluating initial fitness function using multi-objective function
STEP 7:- Compute local best and global best.
STEP 8:- Update swarm velocity and swarm position.
STEP 9:- Update DG size location based on the swarm and updated system data.
STEP 10:- Calculate fitness using multi-objective function.
STEP 11:- Compute and update local best and global best.
STEP 12:- Check for maximum iteration limit or converging criteria if exceed move next step *else go to STEP 7*.
STEP 13:- Print the DG station size.

6 Case Study

As mentioned about the cases, consider the case 1 where the only EV station is connected to the system. As the EV load may impact the overall system to overcome such an impact we must have to introduce some changes which are being described in this chapter. This chapter also considers all the assumptions required for the implementation. This also discusses the power flow algorithm which is being implemented in the distribution system as we are completely concerned on the distribution system of the IEEE 33-bus system [1, 15, 20,]. To meet the increased load demand of EV, charging stations following implementation are to be done:

6.1 Assumption for Case Study

1. The requirement of fast-charging station (FCS) is being considered at different locations before implementations of optimization.

2. Although it does not make difference any difference in the solution, we are considering the Tesla Model S (released in 2014) having an efficiency of 92% and having a battery capacity of 85kWh.
3. In this study three charging stations are considered in which each charging station can charge at least 20 EV at a time whereas the overall system can charge 60 EV.
4. Considered the Durgapur map having 33 bus configurations as shown in Fig. 4, where four different FCS is to be placed in different zones.
5. EV station location obtained by the optimization technique is used to place the DG at that particular location.
6. For the reliability calculation, consider the energy not supplied (ENS) equation.

6.2 Electrical Distribution System

The IEEE 33-bus system is modified system considered for presented case study. The overall load of the system is raised from 3.75 to 11.1 MW. So, we raised the active load as well the reactive load in the same ratio that is 11.1/3.75 and to meet the demand, we have to alter different parameters like the overall voltage of the system is raised from 12 to 20 kV. As well as the parameter like resistance and inductance of the line to be reduced with a factor that is (2/3). Maximum and minimum voltage deviation is maintained from 1.05 to 0.95 p.u. It is assumed that initially the EV charging station is considered at the bus number 18, 12, 33, and 28. As we are using the distribution system which has high R/X ratio as well as an unbalanced load, then we cannot use the Newton–Rapson or Guass-Shield method of power flow studies. For the distribution system, we usually the help of forward and backward sweep method of load flow study.

Load flow—forward and backward sweep method steps as:

STEP 1:- Initialization current $= 0$ and initialization voltage $= V_0$
STEP 2:- Compute node current I_b using node model
STEP 3:- Backward compute branch current using link model and KCL
STEP 4:- Forward update $V_{K+1} = V_k$ based on I_b over link model
STEP 5:- Check the convergence $d(s) <$ error limit stop or go to Step 2.

Table 3 is implemented in this work after certain modifications which are mentioned in earlier section. Resistance and inductance of the line are reduced by a factor of 2/3.

7 Results and Discussions

The results are presented in this section for the considered system for both cases namely with EV only and with EV and DG cases.

Table 3 Electrical parameters of the test system

Bus/parameters		Initial		Modified	
Start bus i	End bus j	R_{ij} (in Ω)	X_{ij} (in Ω)	R_{ij} (in Ω)	X_{ij} (in Ω)
1	2	0.05752591	0.02932449	0.038350608	0.019549659
2	3	0.30759517	0.15666764	0.205063445	0.104445093
3	4	0.22835666	0.11629967	0.152237771	0.077533116
4	5	0.23777793	0.1211039	0.158518619	0.080735933
5	6	0.51099481	0.44111518	0.340663207	0.294076786
6	7	0.11679881	0.38608497	0.077865876	0.257389979
7	8	0.44386045	0.14668484	0.295906967	0.09778989
8	9	0.64264305	0.46170471	0.428428698	0.307803143
9	10	0.651378	0.46170471	0.434252001	0.307803143
10	11	0.12266371	0.04055514	0.081775808	0.027036763
11	12	0.23359763	0.07724195	0.155731752	0.051494634
12	13	0.91592232	0.72063371	0.610614883	0.480422472
13	14	0.33791794	0.44479634	0.225278624	0.296530892
14	15	0.36873985	0.3281847	0.245826564	0.218789801
15	16	0.46563544	0.34003928	0.310423629	0.226692855
16	17	0.8042397	1.07377542	0.536159798	0.715850281
17	18	0.45671331	0.35813312	0.304475541	0.238755411
2	19	0.10232375	0.09764431	0.068215831	0.065096205
19	20	0.93850842	0.84566834	0.625672279	0.563778891
20	21	0.25549741	0.29848586	0.170331604	0.198990572
21	22	0.44230064	0.58480517	0.294867091	0.389870115
3	23	0.28151509	0.19235617	0.187676727	0.128237445
23	24	0.56028491	0.44242542	0.373523273	0.294950281
24	25	0.55903706	0.43743402	0.372691373	0.29162268
6	26	0.12665683	0.06451388	0.084437889	0.04300925
26	27	0.17731957	0.09028199	0.118213045	0.060187993
27	28	0.66073688	0.58255904	0.440491254	0.388372695
28	29	0.50176072	0.43712206	0.334507145	0.291414705
29	30	0.31664208	0.16128469	0.211094723	0.107523125
30	31	0.6079528	0.60084005	0.405301867	0.400560035
31	32	0.1937288	0.22579856	0.129152535	0.150532375
32	33	0.21275852	0.33080519	0.141839015	0.220536792
21	8	1.24785058	1.24785058	0.831900385	0.831900385
9	15	1.24785058	1.24785058	0.831900385	0.831900385
12	22	1.24785058	1.24785058	0.831900385	0.831900385
18	33	0.31196264	0.31196264	0.207975096	0.207975096

(continued)

Table 3 (continued)

Bus/parameters		Initial		Modified	
Start bus i	End bus j	R_{ij} (in Ω)	X_{ij} (in Ω)	R_{ij} (in Ω)	X_{ij} (in Ω)
25	29	0.31196264	0.31196264	0.207975096	0.207975096

7.1 Case-1: With EV Station only

To evaluate the PSO algorithm, we have used the 30 trial and 50 iterations for evaluating the accuracy of the result. Best trial having a minimum value of the objective function is considered as the result. Below table represents the minimum value of the objective function that is about 4.92644 and the EV FCS location obtained are 9, 28, 25 and 22 buses, respectively, which are illustrated in Table 4.

As Fig. 4 displayed the overall bus configuration in Durgapur City which has four different zones such as $Z_1, Z_2, Z_3,$ and Z_4, each zone has a uniformly distributed EV population as discussed in previous section.

Results of different zones are as follow:

- Z_1 FCS is 22.
- Z_2 FCS is 25.
- Z_3 FCS is 28.
- Z_4 FCS is 9.

Zone 1 has its EV FCS at bus number 22 from the collection set of bus sets that is 19, 20, 21, and 22. Zone 2 has its EV FCS at bus number 25 from the collection set of buses that is 23, 24, and 25. Zone 3 has its EV FCS at bus number 28 from the collection set that is 26, 27, 28, 29, 30, 31, 32, and 33. Zone 4 has its EV FCS at bus number 9 from the collection set that is from bus number 9 to 18 buses. Figure 9 represents that the fitness function converges at 23rd iteration of the best trial. And the best fitness value obtained is about 4.9244 which is the lowest value of all the ten trials executed in the program.

Fitness value is obtained by the objective function as mentioned in Eq. 10 of previous section. It is obtained by three index function minimization having appropriate coefficient value as mentioned in chapter. Each index function is related to the electrical parameters like power losses, voltage deviation, and reliability. The voltage profile is shown in Fig. 10 for different buses, as we know that voltage deteriorates

Table 4 EV FCS location

Objective function	4.926440795
EV station no. 1 location	9th bus
EV station no. 2 location	28th bus
EV station no. 3 location	25th bus
EV station no. 4 location	22nd bus

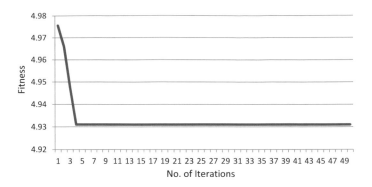

Fig. 9 Fitness function convergence with EV station only

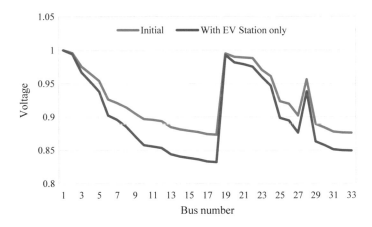

Fig. 10 Voltage graph with EV station only

with the increased load. EV load changes the voltage profile as shown in the figure below. Figure 10 represents the voltage profile of all the two cases that are initial and with EV only. With the increased load, the lowest voltage is observed at bus number 18. With the increased load, reliability of the system must be decreased, but the objective function is designed in such a manner that the reliability improves. As mentioned above for the calculation of reliability, we have considered the energy not supplied (ENS) index. The objective function is designed to maximize the reliability and also considering the appropriate value of objective function coefficient for the reliability index.

Figure 11 represents the reliability of the system of the initial (case 1) and the system connected with EVs (case 2), respectively. The reliability of the system increases by 1.63 percentage after the implementation of FCS in the system. As the load increases then the reliability should decrease but the objective function is

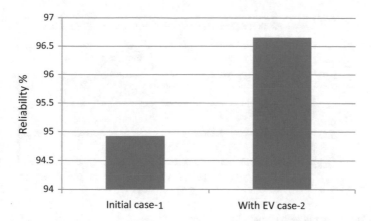

Fig. 11 Reliability with EV station only

designed in such a manner that it improves the reliability because of higher dependence on the weightage factor of the reliability index. The station development cost with EV FCS station only is obtained from Eqs. 1 and 2 combined and the station development cost (SDC) without DGs is 1,391,600 $.

7.2 Case-2: EV Station with DGs

The PSO algorithm has used to evaluate by considering Eq. 18 for the 30 trial and 50 iterations to obtain the results under EV station with DG case. Figure 12 shows that the fitness function converges at 26th iteration of the best trial and the best fitness value obtained is about 3.5618 which is the lowest value of all the ten trials executed in the program. Fitness value is obtained by the objective function as mentioned in Eq. 18 of previous section. It is obtained by three index function minimization

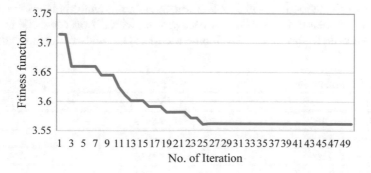

Fig. 12 Fitness function convergence with EV and DG station

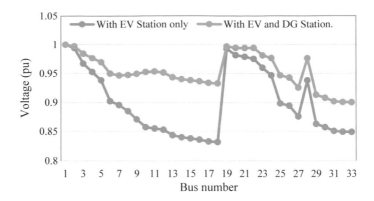

Fig. 13 Voltage graph with EV and DG station

having appropriate coefficient value as mentioned. Each index function is related to the electrical parameters like power losses, voltage deviation, and reliability. Voltage profile is shown on different buses, as we know that the voltage profile improves with the increased generation. DG generation changes the voltage profile as shown in the figure below. Figure 13 represents the voltage profile of all the two cases that is with EV station only and with EV & DG station. With the increased load as well as generation, lowest voltage is observed at bus number 33 which is 0.9 p.u. The cost of DG depends largely upon the MW rating. Before implementation, we have optimized the size of the DG at the EV station. The size of the DG is used in the optimization technique which reduces the cost as well achieved the objective that is voltage stability, reduced power losses, improved reliability, and enhanced voltage profile.

As Table 5 represents the DG station size which is located in the different EV station that is bus number 9, 28, 25, and 22, respectively, each EV station will have its generating unit of different size obtained after optimization is 0.001 MW, 4.183 MW, 3.7992 MW, and 2.951 MW, respectively. Station development cost of DG station is calculated from the data mentioned in Table 2. And the station development cost (SDC) of DG station is 1,356,300 $. The overall result analysis is also presented based on the comparative analysis of base system, with EV only and EV with DG. Therefore overall, the station development cost (SDC) with EV station and DGs

Table 5 DG station size

Parameters	Values (MW)
Objective function	3.5618
DG station no. 1 size	0.001
DG station no. 2 size	4.1830
DG station no. 3 size	3.7992
DG station no. 4 size	2.9510

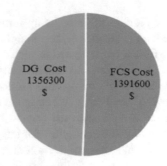

Fig. 14 Pie chart of components cost

is 2,747,900 $. Figure 14 represents that the cost of EV station and DG station is 1,391,600 $ and 1,356,300 $, respectively.

Voltage profile of the system in the arrangement of minimum and maximum value of all the bus voltages is depicted in Fig. 15. Voltage profile is shown on different buses, as we know that the voltage profile improves with the increased generation. DG generation changes the voltage profile as shown in the figure below. As we know that voltage deteriorates with the increased load, EV load changes the voltage profile as shown in the figure below. Both EV and DG stations combined and have a positive impact on voltage profile. Minimum voltage is 0.9 p.u. at the extreme end bus number 33, which is better than the initially considered test system that is the modified IEEE 33-bus system.

In Fig. 15, the voltage profile of all the three cases is initial, with EV only and with EV and DG, respectively. As the figure represents the improved voltage profile after the implementation of DGs, voltage profile which was having a negative impact after

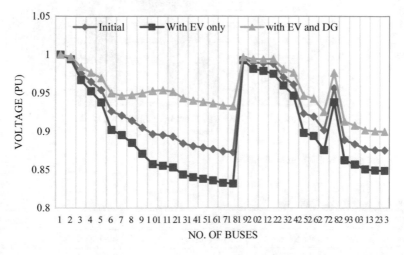

Fig. 15 Comparative voltage profile of different cases of system

the implementation of EV station only is also being improved better than the base case test system. When the load is increased, the reliability of the system should be decreased, but the objective function is designed in such a manner that the reliability improves and optimal solution of EV and DG station obtained for higher reliability using PSO optimization. As mentioned in previous section, the calculation of reliability considered on the basis of the energy not supplied (ENS) in the system. The objective function is designed to maximize the reliability an also considering the appropriate value of objective function coefficient for the reliability index. The reliability of the system with EVs and DGs connection is improved to approximately up to 99.60%. The comparative analysis of reliability for different cases is shown in Table 6. Also, Fig. 16 represents that the reliability of the system initial was 94.93% which improved to 99.60% after the implementation of EV as well as DG station simultaneously.

As the load is increased in the system, the value of current is increased in the system which leads to the increase in power losses. With the implementation of the DG, the generation of power is localized which reduces the power losses in the system. The comparison of active and reactive power losses for different cases is given in Table 7. In Fig. 17, the conical graph represents the impact of power losses

Table 6 Reliability comparison for different cases

Parameters	Initial	With EV station only	With EV and DG station
ENS	0.3658	0.4396	0.01154
Reliability	0.9493	0.9665	0.996035
Reliability (%)	94.93	96.65	99.6035

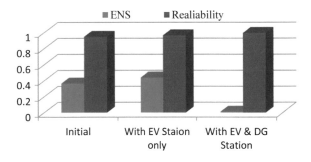

Fig. 16 Bar graph of ENS and reliability

Table 7 Power loss comparison

Losses	Initial	With EV station only	With EV and DG station
P loss (in MW)	0.667867	1.139965624	0.418907724
Q loss (in Mvar)	0.445989	0.760827628	0.280953995

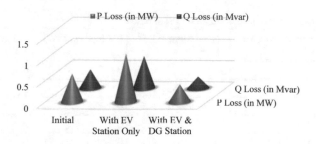

Fig. 17 Real and reactive power losses

in the system. The P and Q losses of the system are represented below with all the three cases that are initial, with EV only and with EV and DG, respectively. It clearly shows that for case 3 (i.e., with EV and DG) the losses are reduced.

Table 8 represents the initial load on each bus that is the initial modified system load only, EV load at bus obtained after optimal EV station placement by optimization and each EV FCS station has capacity of 0.93 MW and DG generation size obtained after optimization on the same EV FCS stations. The representation is shown in Fig. 18 where each bus has their defined system P load and Q load, EV load and DG generation unit. Figure 19 shows the modified IEEE 33-bus system for case study with optimal allocations of EV load and DGs.

8 Conclusion

This work allocated the optimum location fast-charging station (FCS) in different four zones of the Durgapur city which covers the overall requirements of the EV distribution in the city. A particle swarm optimization technique is used to allocate the best location FCS in the city. The electrical parameter mentioned above is improved from the initial condition that is the test system. Finally, PSO is used for minimization of cost by minimizing the power losses, minimization of voltage deviation, and maximizing the reliability of the system. Also, the station infrastructure cost (SIC), which is fixed as per the land area requirement as well as the electrical equipment like connector, transformer, etc., are calculated. And the station development cost (SDC) of EV FCS station without DGs is 1,391,600 $. The placement of FCS at different location is bus number 9, 22, 25 and 28. Each location FCS is the best location as per the concern of this work which depends on cost, voltage, and reliability.

After the allocation of EV FCS station, DGs are also placed at that particular location by the FCS station owner. DGs optimal size (in MW) is calculated by PSO. Each FCS station is having the DG station of different sizes that is 1 kW, 2.591 MW, 3.7992 MW, and 4.183 MW at bus number 9, 28, 25, and 22, respectively. Calculation of the DG station cost which includes investment cost, operational cost, and maintenance cost. The station development cost (SDC) of DGs is 1,356,300

Table 8 EV load and DG generation on different buses

Bus no.	P load (demand) in MW	Q load (demand) in Mvar	EV load (in MW)	DG generation (in MW)
1	0	0	0	0
2	0.194074306	0.150444152	0	0
3	0.174666875	0.100296101	0	0
4	0.232889167	0.200592202	0	0
5	0.116444583	0.075222076	0	0
6	0.116444583	0.050148051	0	0
7	0.388148611	0.250740253	0	0
8	0.388148611	0.250740253	0	0
9	0.116444583	0.050148051	0.93	0.001
10	0.116444583	0.050148051	0	0
11	0.087333438	0.075222076	0	0
12	0.116444583	0.087759089	0	0
13	0.116444583	0.087759089	0	0
14	0.232889167	0.200592202	0	0
15	0.116444583	0.025074025	0	0
16	0.116444583	0.050148051	0	0
17	0.116444583	0.050148051	0	0
18	0.174666875	0.100296101	0	0
19	0.174666875	0.100296101	0	0
20	0.174666875	0.100296101	0	0
21	0.174666875	0.100296101	0	0
22	0.174666875	0.100296101	0.93	2.951
23	0.174666875	0.125370126	0	0
24	0.815112083	0.501480506	0	0
25	0.116444583	0.062685063	0.93	3.7992
26	0.116444583	0.062685063	0	0
27	0.116444583	0.050148051	0	0
28	0.815112083	0.501480506	0.93	4.183
29	0.232889167	0.175518177	0	0
30	0.388148611	1.504441517	0	0
31	0.291111458	0.175518177	0	0
32	0.407556042	0.250740253	0	0
33	0.116444583	0.100296101	0	0
Total	7.209860451	5.767025817	3.72	10.9342

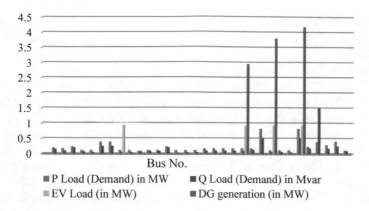

Fig. 18 Load demand and DG generation bar graph

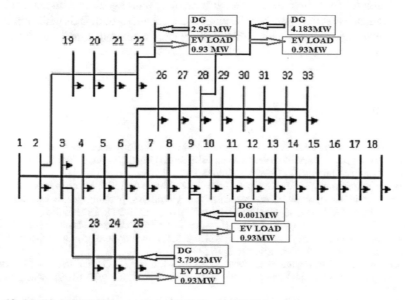

Fig. 19 Modified IEEE 33-bus system with EV load and DG generation

$. The electrical parameter mentioned above is improved from the initial condition that is the test system as well as the system having EV station. The reliability of the system is improved to approximately 99.60% after the implementation of DG station on the same FCS station. Voltage profile which was having a negative impact after the implementation of EV station only is also being improved better than the test system. As the load is increased in the system, the value of current is increased in the system which leads to the increase in power losses. With the implementation of the DG, the generation of power is localized which reduces the power losses in the system. Power loss which increased after the implementation of EV station only also changes positively with the implementation of DG station on the same system having FCS station. All the electrical parameter mentioned that is power losses, voltage deviation, and reliability of the system is improved after the implementation of DG and EV FCS simultaneously. Power losses are reduced by approximately 37% of the initial test system. Reliability is improved by about 6% of the initial test system and the voltage deviation reduced and its minimum valve is maintained at 0.9 per unit. The reported study is validated with the software platform and based on that all results are included for case study, because the experimental setup at instant requires a lot of investment, land area, and other limitation also in real-time or online environment. Moreover, for online or real-time planning, the assessment real-time data is required and based on that actual real-time data, the power flow required at each instant and after that the behavior of EVs also required to implement as whole at each instant, which create more complexity in analysis. Therefore, offline analysis of case study is done based on the software platform implementation and the investigation recommends the solution for study area for EV charging station planning. The result and analysis clearly indicate that the system performances are enhanced with DGs while planning the EV charging station and also offer technical and economic benefits as discussed in result section.

References

1. Amiris, S.S., Jadids, S.: Optimal charging schedule of electrics vehicles at battery swapping stations in a smart distribution network. In: IEEE Smart Grid Conferences (SGC) 2017, pp. 1–8 (2017). https://doi.org/10.1109/SGC.2017.8308875
2. Hou, K., Xu, X., Jia, H., Yu, X., Jiang, T., Zhang, K., Shu, B.: A reliability assessment approach for integrated transportation and electrical power systems incorporating electric vehicles. IEEE Trans. Smart Grid 9(1), 88–100 (2016). https://doi.org/10.1109/TSG.2016.2545113
3. You, P., Yang, Z., Zhang, Y., Low, S.H., Sun, Y.: Optimal charging schedule for a battery switching station serving electric buses. IEEE Trans. Power Syst. 31(5), 3473–3483 (2015). https://doi.org/10.1109/TPWRS.2015.2487273
4. Sadeghi-Barzani, P., Rajabi-Ghahnavieh, A., Kazemi-Karegar, H.: Optimal fast charging station placing and sizing. Appl. Ener. 125, 289–299 (2014). https://doi.org/10.1016/j.apenergy.2014.03.077
5. Sawle, Y., Gupta, S.C., Bohre, A.K.: Review of hybrid renewable energy systems with comparative analysis of off-grid hybrid system. Renew. Sustain. Energ. Rev. 81, 2217–2235 (2018). https://doi.org/10.1016/j.rser.2017.06.033
6. Rani, K.S., Sannigrahi, S., Acharjee, P., Bohre, A.K.: Determining optimal size and placement of renewable DG considering variation of load. Int. J. Recent Technol. Eng. (IJRTE), 8(2S7), 310–315 (2019). https://doi.org/10.35940/ijrte.B1117.0782S719
7. Granovskii, M., Dincer, I., Rosen, M.A.: Economic and environmental comparison of conventional, hybrid, electric and hydrogen fuel cell vehicles. J. Power Sources 159(2), 1186–1193 (2006). https://doi.org/10.1016/j.jpowsour.2005.11.086
8. Ren, X., Zhang, H., Ruohan, H., Qiu, Y.: Location of electric vehicle charging stations: a perspective using the grey decision-making model. Energy 173(2019), 548–553 (2019). https://doi.org/10.1016/j.energy.2019.02.015
9. Liu, Z., Wen, F., Ledwich, G.: Optimal planning of electric-vehicle charging stations in distribution systems. IEEE Trans. Power Del. 28(1), 102–110. (2012). https://doi.org/10.1109/TPWRD.2012.2223489

10. Luo, L., Gu, W., Zhou, S., Huang, H., Gao, S., Han, J., Wu, Z., Dou, X.: Optimal planning of electric vehicle charging stations comprising multi-types of charging facilities. Appl. Energ. **226**, 1087–1099 (2018). https://doi.org/10.1016/j.apenergy.2018.06.014

11. Zhang, Y., Zhang, Q., Farnoosh, A., Chen, S., Li, Y.: GIS-based multi-objective particle swarm optimization of charging stations for electric vehicles. Energy **169**, 844–853 (2019). https://doi.org/10.1016/j.energy.2018.12.062

12. Battapothula, G., Yammani, C., Maheswarapu, S.: Multi-objective simultaneous optimal planning of electrical vehicle fast charging stations and DGs in distribution system. J. Mod. Power Syst. Clean Energ. **7**(4), 923–934 (2019). https://doi.org/10.1007/s40565-018-0493-2

13. Cheng, L., Chang, Y., Lin, J., Singh, C.: Power system reliability assessment with electric vehicle integration using battery exchange mode. IEEE Trans. Sustain. Energ. **4**(4), 1034–1042 (2013). https://doi.org/10.1109/TSTE.2013.2265703

14. Chadha, M.: India's wind capacity crosses 10% share in overall installed base. Clean Technica, 30 July 2019. https://www.cleantechnica.com/2019/01/21/indias-wind-capacity-crosses-10-share-in-overall-installed-base/

15. Medjoudj, R., Bediaf, H., Aissani, D.: Power system reliability: mathematical models and applications. Syst. Reliabil. **279** (2017) https://www.intechopen.com/books/system-reliability/power-system-reliability-mathematical-models-and-applications

16. Zimmerman, R.D., Murillo-Sánchez, C.: MATPOWER User's Manual. http://www.pserc.cornell.edu/matpower/

17. Bohre, A.K., Agnihotri, G., Dubey, M.: Optimal sizing and sitting of DG with load models using soft computing techniques in practical distribution system. IET Gener. Trans. Distrib. **10**(11), 2606–2621 (2016). https://doi.org/10.1049/iet-gtd.2015.1034

18. Kalambe, S., Agnihotri, G., Bohre, A.K.: An analytical approach for multiple dg allocation in distribution system. Elect and Electron Engg: An Inter. J. (ELELIJ), **2**(3), 39–48 (2013). https://wireilla.com/engg/eeeij/papers/2313elelij04.pdf

19. Sedghi, M., Ahmadian, A., Aliakbar-Golkar, M.: Optimal storage planning in active distribution network considering uncertainty of wind power distributed generation. IEEE Trans. Power Syst. **31**(1), 304–316 (2015). https://doi.org/10.1109/TPWRS.2015.2404533

20. Ameli, A., Bahrami, S., Khazaeli, F., Haghifam, M.R.: A multiobjective particle swarm optimization for sizing and placement of DGs from DG owner's and distribution company's viewpoints. IEEE Trans. Power Del. **29**(4), 1831–1840 (2014). https://doi.org/10.1109/TPWRD.2014.2300845

21. Bohre, A., Agnihotri, G., Dubey, M.: The optimal distributed generation placement and sizing using novel optimization technique. Middle-East J. Sci. Res. 10, 1228–1236 (2015). https://doi.org/10.5829/idosi.mejsr.2015.23.06.22275

22. Bohre, A.K., Agnihotri, G., Dubey, M.: Impact of the load model on Optimal sizing and siting of distributed generation in distribution system. World Appl. Sci. J. **33**(7), 1197–1205 (2015). https://doi.org/10.5829/idosi.wasj.2015.33.07.238

23. Bohre, A. K., Agnihotri, G., Dubey, M.: The OPF and butterfly-PSO (BF-PSO) technique based optimal location and sizing of distributed generation in mesh system. Electr. Electron. Eng.: An Int. J. **4**(2), 127–141 (2015). https://doi.org/10.14810/elelij.2015.4211

24. Bohre, A.K., Agnihotri, G., Dubey, M.: The butterfly-particle swarm optimization (butterfly-PSO/BF-PSO) technique and its variables. Int. J. Soft Comput. Math. Control (IJSCMC) **4**(3), 23–39 (2015). https://doi.org/10.14810/ijscmc.2015.4302

25. Pistoia, G. (Ed.).: Electric and Hybrid Vehicles: Power Sources, Models, Sustainability, Infrastructure and the Market. Elsevier (2010). https://www.elsevier.com/books/electric-and-hybrid-vehicles/pistoia/978-0-444-53565-8

26. Larminie, J., Lowry, J.: Electric Vehicle Technology Explained, pp. 340. Wiley-Blackwell (2012). https://www.wiley.com/en-in/Electric+Vehicle+Technology+Explained%2C+2nd+Edition-p-9781119942733

27. Pang, C., Dutta, P., Kezunovic, M.: BEVs/PHEVs as dispersed energy storage for V2B uses in the smart grid. IEEE Trans. Smart Grid **3**(1), 473–482 (2011). https://doi.org/10.1109/TSG.2011.2172228

28. Chen, T., Zhang, X.-P., Wang, J., Li, J., Cong, W., Mingzhu, H., Bian, H.: A review on electric vehicle charging infrastructure development in the UK. IEEE J. Mod. Power Syst. Clean Energ. **8**(2), 193–205 (2020). https://doi.org/10.35833/MPCE.2018.000374

29. Arias, N.B., Hashemi, S., Andersen, P.B., Træholt, C., Romero, R.: Distribution system services provided by electric vehicles: recent status, challenges, and future prospects. IEEE Trans. Intell. Trans. Syst. **20**(12), 4277–4296 (2019). https://doi.org/10.1109/TITS.2018.2889439

30. Kasturi, K., Nayak, C.K., Nayak, M.R.: Electric vehicles management enabling G2V and V2G in smart distribution system for maximizing profits using MOMVO. Wiley, Int. Trans. Electr. Energ. Syst. **29**(6), e12013. (2019). https://doi.org/10.1002/2050-7038.12013

31. AbuElrub, A., Hamed, F., Saadeh, O.: Microgrid integrated electric vehicle charging algorithm with photovoltaic generation, J. Energ. Storage, **32**(101858), 1–11 (2020). https://doi.org/10.1016/j.est.2020.101858

32. Bouguerra, S., Layeb, S.B.: Determining optimal deployment of electric vehicles charging stations: Case of Tunis City, Tunisia. Case Stud. Trans. Policy, **7**(3), 628–642 (2019). https://doi.org/10.1016/j.cstp.2019.06.003

33. Iqbal, A., et al.: Metaheurestic algorithm based hybrid model for identification of building sale prices. In Springer Nature Book: Metaheuristic and Evolutionary Computation: Algorithms and Applications, under book series "Studies in Computational Intelligence" (2020). https://doi.org/10.1007/978-981-15-7571-6_32

34. Fatema, N., et al.: Data-driven occupancy detection hybrid model using particle swarm optimization based artificial neural network. In: Springer Nature Book: Metaheuristic and Evolutionary Computation: Algorithms and Applications, under book series "Studies in Computational Intelligence" (2020). https://doi.org/10.1007/978-981-15-7571-6_13

35. Minai, F., et al.: Metaheuristics paradigms for renewable energy systems: advances in optimization algorithms. In: Springer Nature Book: Metaheuristic and Evolutionary Computation: Algorithms and Applications, under book series "Studies in Computational Intelligence" (2020). https://doi.org/10.1007/978-981-15-7571-6_2

IoT-Based LPG Leakage Detection System with Prevention Compensation

Mohammad Abas Malik, Magray Abrar Hassan, and Adnan Shafi

Abstract Safety apparatus for the use of LPG gas connections in common households and industries against hazardous conditions such as gas leak, fire and explosion of compressed gas cylinders should be provided. Our aim of this research is to give security to all the people around the world from LP gas leakage by equipping them with an economical and effective alarming system which not only can detect this menace threat but also can automatically control it by its safety line of action. The module consists of a gas sensor MQ6 which has a high sensitivity to gases such as propane and butane which in combination constitutes the LPG. The aim behind our research is to implement a mechanism by automatically disabling the gas supply from the source instantly once the leakage of gas is detected, followed by rapid closure of regulator valve along with triggering an sounding alarm and alerted Wi-Fi display that too without any manual dependence.

Keywords Liquid petroleum gas · Gas sensor · Wi-Fi module · Servo motor

1 Introduction

Liquefied petroleum gas is seeking its sole importance for use in industrial, agricultural, horticultural, manufacturing, and commercial applications. There is a drastic increase in the demand of LP gas due to its ecofriendly nature as energy surfed from it is free of pollution and is being extracted from the fossil fuels. It has an ease in its installation process that is the reason for its wide market demand. It even powers cogeneration plants but at the same time it is one of the common reasons for fire breakouts causing terrible accidents particularly in closed buildings by its leakage in the vicinity. The content energy source in LPG includes 60% of butane ($C4H10$) and 40% of propane ($C3H8$), which is highly flammable and an odorless gas. In case of the leakage of such gas takes place, then it mingles with the air and replaces oxygen

M. A. Malik (✉) · M. A. Hassan · A. Shafi
Department of Electronics and Communication Engineering, BGSB University, Rajouri, J&K, India
e-mail: abasmalik@bgsbu.ac.in

© The Author(s), under exclusive license to Springer Nature Singapore Pte Ltd. 2021 303
H. Malik et al. (eds.), *AI and Machine Learning Paradigms for Health Monitoring System*, Studies in Big Data 86,
https://doi.org/10.1007/978-981-33-4412-9_17

instantly causing suffocation and ignition, resulting in the terrible fire eruption and explosions due to the rupturing of the gas cylinders.

The LPG gas cylinder is designed to withstand a pressure of up to 25 kg per square cm. That is like a 25 kg weight put on an area of your fingernail. That is a massive pressure to control. Usually inside the cylinder, the gas stays at a pressure of about 5–7 kg/cm^2 (almost 1/3rd of the maximum pressure). But occasionally, people indulge in unsafe practices of heating the cylinder or throwing the cylinder which damages the welding and/or body of the cylinder. This damage can lead to leakage of gas which can catch fire and this cylinder then starts getting heated up in the fire caused. The fire raises the temperature and leads to massive increase of pressure inside. Once it goes beyond the maximum limit, the metal of the cylinder fractures and explodes.

The tendency of LP gas ignition is when it forms almost 2 and 10% of a vapor/air mixture. Also, as a colorless liquid, LP gas constitutes around 0.4% of its vapor volume, but still is about half of the density of water and can easily float on water before vaporizing. Uncontrolled fire eruption of LP gas may lead to devastating fires along with explosions. An already flame of fire available at some distance from the source of LP gas leak can rapidly direct toward it resulting in the overheating and bursting of cylinder exhibiting gaseous volume violently (Fig. 1).

Apart from being colorless, LP gas is odorless and to compose it to an odorant gas, we manually add ethyl mercaptan so as to be smelled and sensed. Being heavier than air, these gases do not disperse easily and tend to settle the down surfaces. It may lead to suffocation when inhaled but in case there is the absence of any human resources at the spot to perceive the smelling signals, then it is unaffordable to depend on this

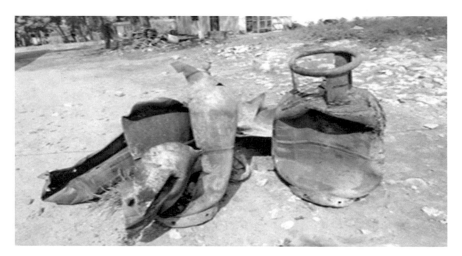

Fig. 1 Shows an exploded cooking gas cylinder at a house of Shyamala Buchamma, 60, at Veerannagutta Hyderabad, India, [1] where she was staying along with her son Raju, daughter-in-law 'Rani'

inbuilt precautionary mechanism. Also, some people have a weakened sensation of smelling and thus are too feeble to detect any surrounding odor.

So to avoid this problem, there is a need for developing a system which will detect the leakage of LPG in domestic and commercial premises in its early stages and would also facilitate the safety measures to eliminate the accidental possibility. Our research has successfully fulfilled these demands and is efficient enough to operate in any surrounding circumstances.

Some of the recent hazardous accidents due to domestic LPG cylinder blasts are mentioned below:

1. **At Banihal (Jammu and Kashmir)**
   On Friday *November 30, 2019,* a woman, resident of Ballot, identified as Darshana Devi along with six others, including three of her daughters, got killed after the explosion of *LPG gas cylinder* at her house in district Ramban of Jammu and Kashmir [2].
2. **Duo of Mother and Son Got Killed. Also, 32 Injured After LPG Cylinder Blast (Giaspora, India)**
   On *April 27, 2018,* at 7 am in the house of Sunita and her son, the leaking LPG cylinder bursted to flames after the electricity supply to the area was restored. Sunita and her son Raj Yadav succumbed to their injuries at CMC Hospital Ludhiana in the evening [3].
3. **Five Got Killed by the LPG Cylinder Blast at Dibrugarh/Assam**
   On Saturday October 19, 2019, four from a family and five others lost their lives after LPG cylinder blast at their residence caught fire followed by numerous more explosions. The victims include Krishna Sunar (husband), Maya Sunar (wife), Vishal Sunar (younger son), Sankar Sunar (grandson), and 50-year-old Nunu, (house keeper) [4].
4. **At Indian Labortory, A Researcher Got Killed Due to LP Gas Explosion**
   On Wednesday December 5, 2018, one researcher 'Manoj Kumar' 32 years old was flung 20 feet above ground and died instantly after explosion of LP gas at the Laboratory of the Indian Institute of Science known as Hypersonic and Shock Wave Research lab, in Bangalore/India [5].
   Following mentioned are the details of total number of accidents across India reported by IndiaStat [6] due to LPG and deaths reported. Since now continuous efforts are being made to overcome the issue of LPG leakage, many systems of LPG detection and alert system have been proposed in the literature to identify potentially hazardous gas leaks by means of various sensors.

Our project entitled 'IoT-based LPG Leakage Detection System with Prevention Compensation,' will impart its role to surf for safety of people and impart prevention from any danger to be caused by the leakage of LPG.

We use a gas sensor MQ6, which has a rapid response time to examine the LPG leakage when it exceeds the threshold value. Apart from informing the authorized person via a display connected to the Wi-Fi module and activating a sounding buzzer, the system owns the capability to trigger the valve using servo motor to turn off the gas flow from the source and to avoid any mishap in advanced form (Fig. 2).

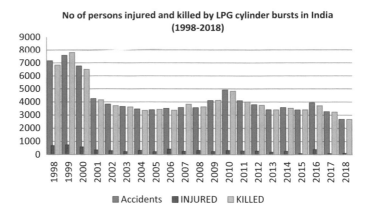

Fig. 2 No. of persons injured and killed by LPG cylinder burst in India (1998–2018)

2   System Designing

2.1   Electronic Part of the System

The designing of our proposed LPG gas leakage detection system with prevention compensation consists of a microcontroller board (ATmega328P) called as Arduino Uno, a MQ-6 gas sensor which continuously senses the surrounding atmosphere and owns a threshold value of 200 ppm, a piezo buzzer is being used, and ESP8266 Wi-Fi module and LEDs as accessory circuitry for sensitivity adjustment.

It is battery operated and hence portable. The information about the leakage has to be informed to the user. For this purpose, a piezo buzzer generates a steep sound with red LED blinking simultaneously and Esp8266 Wi-Fi module displays a warning status on to the display.

The required simulation for the system designing is fulfilled by an open-source Arduino software (IDE), which manufactures an easy code for uploading to the panel.

2.2   Mechanical Part of the System

The kit exhibits the integration of a 'servo motor' tied with the knob of the gas tank 'Regulator.' Since servo motor in itself is an electronic part but exhibits mechanical action, it is encoded by Arduino software (IDE) to rotate on precise angle or in the direction opposite to ON rotation cycle at the instant of gas leakage which is being detected by MQ-6 gas sensor. The rotation is from 90° to 0° so as to turn the knob and consequently the gas regulator to the OFF state, thus ensuring the automatic closure of the gas source.

The servo motor which is programmed to rotate at precise angle after the gas leakage detection being perceived can be directly connected to the knob of the regulator as there are no threats in the production of electrical sparks. So the adjustment of the project is done in such a way that electronic parts are kept at a distance for prevention purposes and servo motor is tied directly with the gas regulator.

3 Functional Block Diagram of the Developed System

The LPG gas sensor is directly connected with the Arduino Uno and is being programmed by the software Arduino IDE. The buzzer is also integrated with Arduino and its operational function is being programmed as well. The Wi-Fi module is connected with any of the electronic gadget that may be either the computer or the mobile phone or a tablet to enable the displaying medium for the representation of the schematic working of the project. Also, for its working, there is no need of Internet connection. It can view the 'ensuring message' as well as a 'warning message,' so as to satisfy the user on behalf of the working procedure of system. The servo motor that is connected with the Arduino by means of jumper wires is in turn directly tied with the knob of gas regulator by a tensile thread so as to control the rotating valve positions of this regulator and acquire control over the supply of LP gas from proceeding further (Fig. 3).

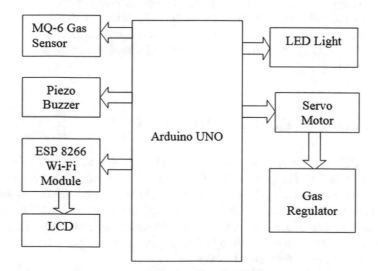

Fig. 3 Block diagram of LPG leakage detection system with prevention compensation

4   System Operation

After feeding this IoT-based system with DC power source of 9 v, it is preferred to place the Mq6 gas sensor to the ground level from the gas platform as the vapor of LP gas is denser and heavier than air and tends to settle at low areas such as cellars, drains, and other depressions [7].

The detection power of gases by the gas sensor depends on the chemiresistor acting as integrated nosal part of Mq6 gas sensor to promote current. Tin dioxide (SnO_2) is the most commonly used chemiresistor which is n-type semiconductor thus having free electrons. Since the atmosphere in normal conditions contains more oxygen than that of combustible gases, the free electrons are attracted by oxygen particles available in SnO_2 that pushes them toward the surface of the SnO_2. As soon as the sensor is kept in the combustible or toxic gaseous environment, it leads to the reaction with the adsorbed particles of oxygen and ultimately breaks the chemical bond between oxygen and free electrons which results in the conduction of current, and consequently this conduction will always be proportional to the amount of free electrons available in SnO_2.

In normal situations when LPG is proceeding through proper encased pipelines, the status of the display which is connected to the Wi-Fi module follows statement 'Gas Connection Normal.' Also, the green LED glows to provide visual satisfaction to the user.

But in the conditions of LPG leakage, the gas sensor induces an emergency situation in IoT system exactly as per programmed, by enabling the buzzer sound 'ON,' blinking of red LED and the servo motor turns the knob of the gas regulator to 'OFF' state to terminate the LPG supply and avoid any disastrous condition. The display which is connected to the Wi-Fi module follows statement as 'Leakage at Plug Detected.'

5   Schematic Connections in the System

We use a DC battery and connect it with Arduino board with the help of a jack to turn the system ON. The green LED of Arduino blinks, confirming the connection status is established. The components to be used in this project are integrated with the Arduino board and the program is being compiled using Arduino IDE software.

On the interface of Arduino, we connect Mq6 gas sensor first with 5 v pin and other with gnd terminal of Arduino board, and its output as per program is being taken at digital Pin 3 of Arduino board.

Then we take ESP8266 Wi-Fi module and integrate it with Arduino board. It is connected with 3.3 v pin and gnd pin. The TX of Wi-Fi module as per program is connected with Pin 10 and Rx with Pin 11.

The connection of buzzer and red led is same, that is Anode with Pin 12 and other terminal is grounded.

The green LED is connected with Pin 13 of Arduino board. Then, we take servo motor and connect with 5 v pin and gnd pin, and its output is derived from digital Pin 4. The rotation of the servo motor is precise and tested well. It triggers the knob of the gas regulator by means of a tensile thread so that it rotates automatically to turn the knob off and demands deliberate manual effort to turn the knob back to On position (Fig. 4).

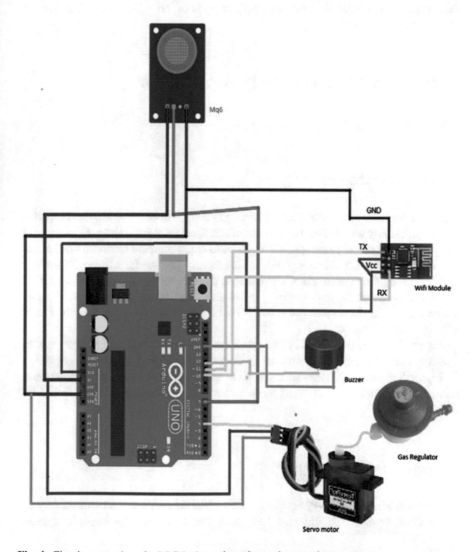

Fig. 4 Circuit connections for LPG leakage detection and prevention system

6 The Arduino IDE Sketch

Once the circuit has been established, we upload the program also known as a sketch which is a set of instructions that directing the board of what particular functions it needs to execute.

The code that we have used for establishing the functional working procedure of this project after controlling the input/output ports of the Arduino board follows in sequence as (Fig. 5).

7 Data Flow Diagram of the Proposed System

See Fig. 6.

8 Tests and the Results

We use a 'lighter' as a replicate of a LPG gas source in order to check the system function. Initially we imitate low-level concentration from the lighter and then gradually brought it closer to the gas sensor so as to expel high concentration of LP gas, and we found that the detector provides satisfactory results. Excellent performance was shown by the system when we repeated the test several times. The sensor has an immediate response to the fuming gases once the leakage is perceived. As soon as the gas concentration reduced below 25% of the monetary value, then the buzzer goes off automatically.

Figure 7 shows the system state when no gas is detected and follows up the statement as shown in Fig. 9. State of servo motor is 90° and green LED is ON.

Figure 8 shows the system state when LP gas is detected and it follows the statement as shown in Fig. 10. State of servo motor is shifted to 0 degree and RED LED is ON (Table 1).

9 Future Scope of the Project

1. The overall cost of the system is Rs. 350 which is very less and affordable.
2. Notices butane leak and also LPG leak and any such combustible gaseous material.
3. Produces sound alarm when gas fume is perceived.
4. Can also be updated to transmit the SMS alert to the owner.
5. Displaying the gas flow status which signifies whether the gas is in normal stage or not.

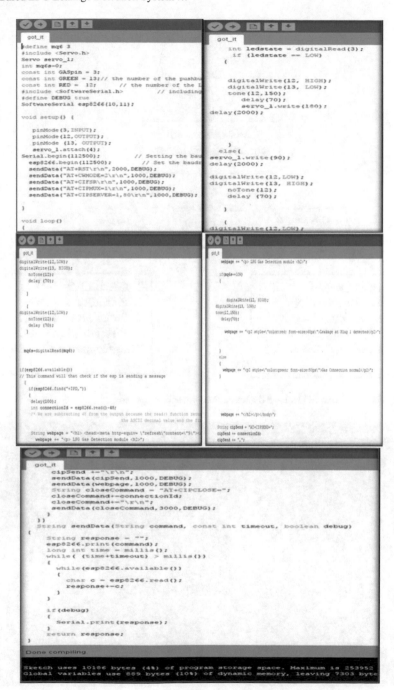

Fig. 5 Compiled Arduino code for LPG leakage detection and prevention method

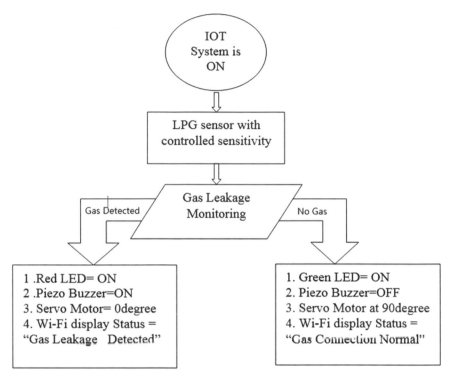

Fig. 6 Flowchart of LPG leakage detection and prevention system

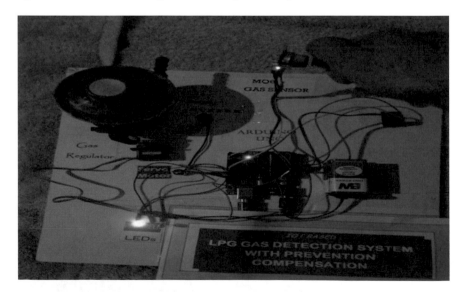

Fig. 7 Test at normal gas connection

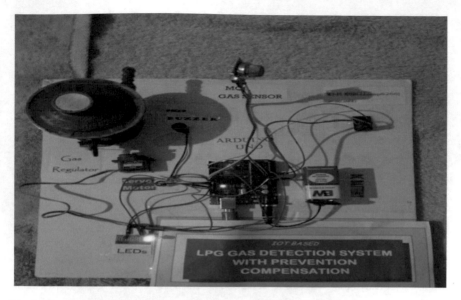

Fig. 8 Test to detect LPG leakage

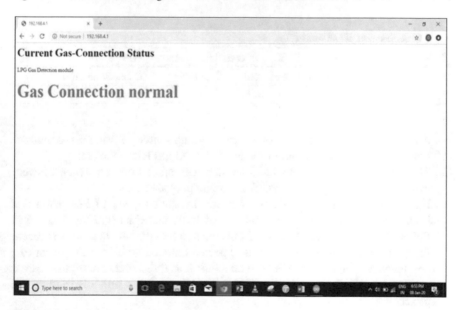

Fig. 9 Display showing normal gas connection

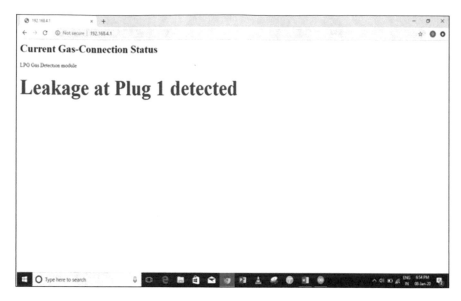

Fig. 10 Display showing leakage status

Table 1 Test condition and results

S. No.	Test condition	LED	Buzzer	Servo motor	Wi-Fi status
1	No leakage detected	OFF	OFF	OFF	Connections normal
2	Leakage detected	ON	ON	90–0	Leakage at Plug 1 detected

6. Automatic and abrupt closure of the gas from its source by using servo motors.
7. Can also be updated to monitor the level of LPG gas left in the tank.
8. The easy availability of this handy system can spread out and reach in every household who seek use of LPG for cooking purposes etc.
9. Figure 11 shows the Ujjwala scheme, run by the Ministry of Petroleum and Natural Gas of the central government of India launched on May 1, 2016 in Ballia, Uttar Pradesh [8]. In India, LPG consumption has grown rapidly in recent years as shown in Fig. 12, and it is expected demand would further reach to a new level. Mishaps due to LPG can conclude it as threat and in order to secure it and make it reliable, here we offer the solution through this simplified and candid project.

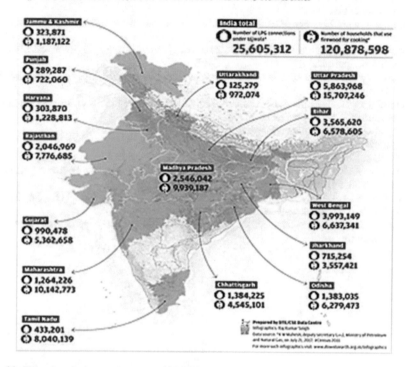

Fig. 11 Ujjwala scheme as per census 2011 [9]

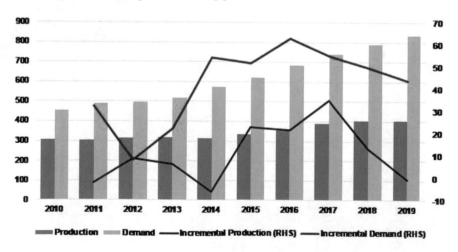

Fig. 12 Demand and production of LPG across India [10]

References

1. https://www.deccanchronicle.com/nation/in-other-news/270317/hyderabad-family-escapes-gas-cylinder-blast.html
2. https://kashmirobserver.net/2019/11/30/4-killed_3_injured-in-gas-cylinder-explosion-in-ramban/
3. https://m.tribuneindia.com/news/archive/29-people_injured-in_lpg-cylinder-blast-in_ludhiana-s_giaspura-580017
4. https://www.the-scientist.com/news-opinion/gas-cylinder-explosion-kills-researcher-at-indian-laboratory-65190
5. https://www.hindustantimes.com/india-news/5-killed-in-fire-lpg-cylinder-blast-in-assam-s-dibrugarh/storyN8XUIWk2eemFz37pb2gJIM.html
6. https://www.indiastat.com/crime-and-law-data/6/accidents/35/cooking-gas-cylinder-stove-burst/475549/stats.aspx
7. WLPGA: Guide to Good Industry Practices for LP Gas Cylinder Management, pp. 30
8. https://www.livemint.com/news/india/pmuy-how-to-avail-full-benefits-of-ujjwala-yojana-1568387408556.html
9. Mahesh, K.M.: Deputy Secretary (LPG), Ministry of Petroleum and Natural Gas, July 21 2012 #Census 2011. www.downtoearth.org.in/infographics
10. https://stratasadvisors.com/insights/2020/02182020-indias-run-away-lpg-demand-growth-spurs-imports

Short-Term Scheduling of Hydrothermal Based on Teaching–Learning Optimization

Rajanish Kumar Kaushal and Tilak Thakur

Abstract This chapter proposed an optimization technique based on teaching–learning (TLBO) for short-period scheduling of thermal and hydropower generation systems known as short-term hydrothermal scheduling (STHTS). The proposed problem with multiple objectives is conceived in two parts: (i) cost and (ii) emissions. The hydroelectric multireservoir hydropower system is considered with a nonlinear connection between hydrorelease, effective head, reservoirs volume, and generated power. The delay in the transfer of water is taken into account between the connected reservoirs. The actual fuel cost and pollution features of thermal power units are also considered for STHTS. The outcomes were verified by particle swarm optimization (PSO) for STHTS and for the standard three-generator framework with combined issues of emission and economic dispatch (CEED) taking into transmission losses on hourly demand for 24 h. The findings are provided from the implementation of the proposed technique and comparison is also done with the particle swarm optimization.

Keywords Economic · Emission · CEED · TLBO · STHTS

1 Introduction

One of the major challenges today in electrical systems is the efficient planning of hydrothermal systems. STHTS is a day-to-day power planning activity and aims primarily to reduce the overall running costs for the various hydraulic power network restrictions. The running charge of hydroelectric plants is negligible as the resource of hydropower is natural water supplies. The aim of reducing hydrothermal system operating costs thus reduces the cost of fuel for thermal systems significantly over

---

R. K. Kaushal (✉) · T. Thakur
EED, Punjab Engineering College, Chandigarh, India
e-mail: rajnish.nitham@gmail.com

T. Thakur
e-mail: tilak20042005@yahoo.co.in

© The Author(s), under exclusive license to Springer Nature Singapore Pte Ltd. 2021   317
H. Malik et al. (eds.), *AI and Machine Learning Paradigms for Health Monitoring System*, Studies in Big Data 86,
https://doi.org/10.1007/978-981-33-4412-9_18

a planning period, thus meeting different constraints. Increasing concern regarding air pollution requires the simultaneous minimization of harmful thermal emissions. A revised economic power dispatch system is therefore necessary, which takes into account fuel cost and emissions. Nonetheless, reducing pollution can lead to higher production costs and vice versa.

Energy generation from coal, natural gas, and oil releases various toxin into the atmosphere, such as CO_2, SO_2, water vapor (H_2O), NO_x, N_2O, ozone (O_3), and CO. Pollution of the environment affects humans as well as other forms of life such as cattle, animals, and vegetation. It also causes material dent, decreases visibility and global warming. While environmental issues continue to be concerned, society requires sufficient and healthy energy not only at the lowest charge available but also at low contamination levels. The operational power system tasks mentioned above are nonlinear multidimensional constrained optimization issues with single- or multiobjective functions. In order to resolve these problems, different optimization methods are recommended and applied. The bulk of these optimization methods has historically been deterministic techniques and derivative methods, while the majority of the recent approaches are heuristic in nature. Heuristic approaches, mostly focused on the various natural and biological phenomena, have gained that awareness due to numerous reasons such as straight forwardness, versatility, and generality. The digital computer is the only practical resource for solving these big nonlinear optimization problems in power system operations, whether for deterministic or heuristic methods.

Electric power systems need to be planned, established, and operated in such a manner that the major chunk of energy demand for loads is met reliably, cost-effectively, and environment-friendly through intelligent use of conventional energy sources. Practitioners aim to achieve these objectives by using various optimization methods for efficient planning and operations. The objectives to be met are often conflicting. Minimization of energy, fuel costs, environmental costs and gas emissions, in particular, is contradictory and inconsistent. Multiobjective optimization approaches are therefore used to create trade-offs between these conflicting objective features, to help decision-makers take appropriate decisions to capitalize benefits due to efficient use of energy resources.

A theoretical analysis was presented in [1, 2] on the relaxed classical hydrothermal scheduling algorithm. Yan et al. [3] presented a method based on Lagrangian relaxation in [3], which divided the STHTS issue into two subproblems. In [4], the STHTS issue was resolved by a diploid genotype GA. The superiorities of the first were demonstrated using the results obtained from several simulated experiments to compare the diploid genotype and haploid genotype GA approaches. Dhillon et al. [5] suggested a fuzzy method of deciding on the long period hydrothermal scheduling with pollution reduction in mind. With STHTS problem, a concomitant solution was proposed in [6] of the economic emission dispatch and unit commitment. In [7], considering the issue of pollution, another wording was put forward for a STHTS as a multiobjective issue. The issue of scheduling in [8] is divided into different sub-issues such as unit commitment, economic dispatch, and STHTS. A test model consisting of hydro and thermal units was used to test the process; however, there were no pumped-storage units used. In [9], an evolutionary method was developed to answer the hydrothermal systems predicament of the daily schedule. The STHTS problem was solving and the computational efficacy was compared in [10] using an actual GA and a binary coded GA system.

In [11], various versions of PSO were introduced, applied, and compared for the resolution of the STHTS problem. In [12], the cost characteristics of each thermal unit are taken into account. A PSO was used to answer the problem taking into account the consequence of the valve-point load both on the price function and various but not all realistic hydro and thermal restrictions. In [13], an evolutionary PSO-based solution for the solution of STHTS was offered to work out the problem of planning the pumped-storage devices. In [14], a dynamic search-space strategy has been applied for PSO algorithm to fix the STHTS problem. An additional application for the resolution of short-period hydrothermal generation scheduling by differential development-based techniques was introduced in [15]. The STHTS problem was introduced and extended in [16] for a stronger worth command and an improved Lagrange Hopfield neural network in light of various restrictions. The frequency tariff system in India is defined in great detail to charge a customer for electricity, considering the correct case for each situation in [17]. Some other optimization examples have been given in [18–20] for better understanding of the reader regarding optimization.

2 Optimization Technique

An effective population-based TLBO algorithm was developed by Rao et al. in [21]. This represents the teaching ability of the teacher and the learning ability of students in a classroom. A population is treated to be a group of students in a class during this process. The best solution up to now is like TLBO's teacher because he is regarded as the best learner in society. The TLBO cycle consists of two parts. One section concerns the phase of the teacher and the other is the phase of the student. Training from the instructor is the teacher process. Learning through interaction is also the student phase.

The mean of a class with the L student is as follows:

$$L_{\text{mean}} = 1/L \left(\sum_{i=1}^{L} L_i \right) \tag{1}$$

An equation to update the position of students:

$$L_{i,\text{new}} = L_{i,\text{old}} + \text{rand}.(L_{\text{instructor}} - T_F.L_{\text{mean}}) \tag{2}$$

A student communicates directly and improves performance with other students. Student L_i chooses another student L_j on a random basis and can express the following equation:

$$L_{i,\text{new}} = \begin{cases} L_i^{\text{old}} + \text{rand}.(L_i - L_j), & f(L_i) \le f(L_j) \\ L_i^{\text{old}} - \text{rand}.(L_j - L_i), & f(L_i) > f(L_j) \end{cases} \tag{3}$$

3 Problem Description

A multiobjective optimization issue is developed as a hydrothermal planning issue with a combination of economic emission scheduling. The aim is to reduce the cost of fuel and the release of green house gases from thermal units with maximum use of hydroresources. The subsequent objectives and constraints need to be in use into account in formulating the hydrothermal planning problem, while simultaneously satisfying linear and nonlinear constraints. Fuel price curves are without and with valve point effect are shown in (4) and (5).

3.1 Economic Dispatch

(i)   Without valve-point effect

$$f = \sum_{t=1}^{T} \sum_{i=1}^{N} a_i + b_i P_{git} + c_i P_{git}^2 \tag{4}$$

(ii) With valve-point effect

$$f = \sum_{t=1}^{T} \sum_{i=1}^{N} a_i + b_i P_{git} + c_i P_{git}^2 + \left| e_i * \sin\left(f_i * \left(P_{gi}^1 - P_{git}\right)\right)\right| \tag{5}$$

where

a_i, b_i, c_i, e_i, f_i ith generating unit fuel cost coefficients.
P_{gi}^1 Minimum generated power by the unit ith.
P_{git} Generated power from ith unit in scheduled period t.
N Number of total units in thermal plant.
T Total scheduled time.

3.2 Emission Dispatch

$$E = \sum_{t=1}^{T} \sum_{i=1}^{N} \left(\alpha_i + \beta_i P_{git} + \gamma_i^2 P_{git} + \eta_i \exp(\delta_i P_{git})\right) \tag{6}$$

α_i, β_i, γ_i, η_i, δ_i are ith generator unit's emission coefficients.
Linear and Nonlinear Constraints

(i)   Power balance limit

$$\sum_{i-1}^{N} P_{git} + \sum_{\varphi=1}^{N_h} P_{h\phi t} - P_{Dt} - P_{Lt} = 0 \tag{7}$$

P_{Lt} Transmission losses in scheduled period t.
P_{Dt} Demand in schedule period t.

(ii)   Generation limits

$$P_{gi}^l \leq P_{git} \leq P_{gi}^u \tag{8}$$

P_{gi}^l Lower power loading limit of ith unit.
P_{gi}^u Upper power loading limit by ith unit.

(iii) Discharge rates

$$Q_{h\phi,t}^l \leq Q_{h\phi,t} \leq Q_{h\phi,t}^u \tag{9}$$

(iv)   Reservoir storage volumes

$$(\text{VoR})_{h\phi,t}^l \leq (\text{VoR})_{h\phi,t} \leq (\text{VoR})_{h\phi,t}^u \tag{10}$$

(v)   The required water volume to be released throughout the planning period by
       each reservoir

$$(\text{VoR})_{h\phi,t}\big|^{t=0} = (\text{VoR})_{h,\phi}^{start}$$
$$(\text{VoR})_{h\phi,t}\big|^{t=T} = (\text{VoR})_{h,\phi}^{end} \tag{11}$$

(vi)   Hydropower generation features.
       The electricity produced from a hydroplant is based on the properties of the
       reservoir and the rate of drainage of water. The output of the hydrogenerator
       depends on general on the hydraulic head, H, volume of the reservoir, VoR and
       hydrodischarge rate, Q.

$$P_h(\phi_h, t) = f(Q_h(\phi_h, t), (\text{VoR})_h(\phi_h, t)) \tag{12}$$

Only relatively large reservoirs may ignore net head variations in which the
generation of electricity depends solely on water release.

4   Execution of the Proposed Method for STHTS

The procedures for solving the STHTS power system problem with the use of TLBO are described in detail in this section. The process of the STHTS approach can be expressed as follows.

4.1   Formation of Individuals

The hydrothermal planning structure of an entity consists of a collection of variables representing the discharge of hydropower and thermal power with help of this variable. Initial population is generated and which will update in further iterations. Generation of variables depends upon the problem, in proposed case four hydro and three thermal are considered so for generation of variable in this case first four of hydrodischarge considering their limits are generated and then for thermal considering their upper and lower power generation limits of thermal units. Total variable depends upon the total number of units taken in account for scheduling. More population size gives the more accuracy and in the results but it can take more time to optimize.

$$P_k = \begin{bmatrix} Q_{h11} & Q_{h21} & \cdots & Q_{hN_{h1}} & P_{g11} & P_{g21} & \cdots & P_{gN_1} \\ Q_{h12} & Q_{h22} & \cdots & Q_{hN_{h2}} & P_{g12} & P_{g22} & \cdots & PgN_2 \\ \vdots & \vdots & \cdots & \vdots & \vdots & \vdots & \cdots & \vdots \\ Q_{h1T} & Q_{h2T} & \cdots & Q_{hN_{hT}} & P_{g1T} & P_{g2T} & \cdots & P_{gN_T} \end{bmatrix} \tag{13}$$

4.2   Initialization Individuals

A number of individuals are generated at random during the initialization. In the feasible range, the solution for every individual is randomly initialized:

$$Q_{h\phi t} = Q_{hj}^l + r_h * \left(Q_{h\phi}^u - Q_{h\phi}^l\right)$$
$$P_{git} = P_{gi}^l + r_a * \left(P_{gi}^u - P_{gi}^l\right) \tag{14}$$

where r_h and r_a are the numbers between 0 and 1.

Combined emission and economic dispatch. The short-time, combined cost-effectiveness of hydrothermal scheduling with cascade reservoirs is a multiobjective challenge in attempting to simultaneously reduce fuel cost and thermal power plant emissions. This multiobjective problem needs to convert because of easy to optimize and for more optimal solution into a single objective with the use of the cost penalty factor (h_t).

$$\text{obj} = F(P_{git}) + h_t * E(P_{git}) \tag{15}$$

$F(P_{git})$ and $E(P_{git})$ represent the total fuel cost and total emission in a scheduled period t.

5 Thermal and Hydrocharacteristics

Reservoir inflows represent the flow of water at each interval in hydropower plant and hydroelectric power production coefficients depend upon the characteristics of hydropower plants.

6 Results and Discussion

For the proposed technique, population size is 50 and total number of iteration is 5000. The programming was written in MATLAB, using the Intel (R) Core(TM) i7-8565U, MATLAB R2015a, and the 1.99 GHz, 8 GB RAM. Load demand is taken from Table 1 [12] and the thermal characteristics are taken from Table 2 [12] and the hydrocharacteristics are taken from Tables 3 and 4 [7].

Table 5 represents the outcomes from hydrothermal scheduling as total fuel cost, total emission, total loss, and total cost; here, total cost is total of fuel cost and emission cost. Emission cost is obtained by multiplying penalty factor and emission at each scheduling interval. Table 6 represents the optimal water discharges of four hydropower plants and the optimal water volume of four hydropower plants for 24 h load demands.

Table 1 Hourly 24 h load [12]

Hour	Demand	Hour	Demand	Hour	Demand
1	750	9	1090	17	1050
2	780	10	1080	18	1120
3	700	11	1100	19	1070
4	650	12	1150	20	1050
5	670	13	1110	21	910
6	800	14	1030	22	860
7	950	15	1010	23	850
8	1010	16	1060	24	800

Table 2 Fuel cost coefficients, emission coefficients and operating limits [12]

Parameters	Unit 1	Unit 2	Unit 3
a_i	100	120	150
b_i	2.45	2.32	2.10
c_i	0.0012	0.0010	0.0015
e_i	160	180	200
f_i	0.038	0.037	0.035
P_{imin}	20	40	50
P_{imax}	175	300	500
γ_i	0.0105	0.0080	0.0120
β_i	−1.355	−0.600	−0.555
α_i	60	45	30
η_i	0.4968	0.4860	0.5035
δ_i	0.01925	0.01694	0.01478

Table 3 Hydroreservoir inflows ($\times 10^4$ m^3) [7]

Hour	Reservoir				Hour	Reservoir			
	1	2	3	4		1	2	3	4
1	10	8	8.1	2.8	13	11	8	4	0
2	9	8	8.2	2.4	14	12	9	3	0
3	8	9	4	1.6	15	11	9	3	0
4	7	9	2	0	16	10	8	2	0
5	6	8	3	0	17	9	7	2	0
6	7	7	4	0	18	8	6	2	0
7	8	6	3	0	19	7	7	1	0
8	9	7	2	0	20	6	8	1	0
9	10	8	1	0	21	7	9	2	0
10	11	9	1	0	22	8	9	2	0
11	12	9	1	0	23	9	8	1	0
12	10	8	2	0	24	10	8	0	0

Table 4 Hydrolimits [7]

Plant	V^l	V^{ini}	Q^l	P^l	V^u	V^{end}	Q^u	P^u
1	80	100	5	0	150	120	15	500
2	100	80	6	0	120	70	15	500
3	60	170	10	0	240	170	30	500
4	70	120	6	0	160	140	20	500

Table 5 Outcomes of hydrothermal scheduling

Outputs	PSO	TLBO (proposed)
Total fuel cost ($/h)	49879	50967
Total emission (lb/h)	35343	33336
Total loss (MW)	409.9	411.95
Total cost ($/h)	77266	69323

Table 6 Water discharge and water volume ($\times 10^4$ m^3) by TLBO

Hour	Q_1	Q_2	Q_3	Q_4	V_1	V_2	V_3	V_4
$h1$	13.90	11.01	20.07	13.57	96.1	77.0	158.0	109.2
$h2$	9.23	9.46	30.00	20.67	95.9	75.5	136.2	91.0
$h3$	11.79	12.79	27.59	25.00	92.1	71.7	126.5	70.0
$h4$	9.40	6.23	24.42	20.65	89.7	74.5	124.4	70.0
$h5$	12.24	10.46	17.82	21.26	83.4	72.0	130.8	70.0
$h6$	12.10	8.38	24.00	14.71	80.0	70.7	133.0	85.3
$h7$	9.04	10.31	21.98	16.95	80.0	66.4	132.5	95.9
$h8$	9.51	14.21	26.20	19.62	80.0	60.0	130.8	100.7
$h9$	11.14	11.02	18.55	17.16	80.0	60.0	130.7	101.4
$h10$	7.57	8.45	27.33	18.72	83.4	60.6	124.2	106.7
$h11$	12.23	11.84	13.92	18.07	83.2	60.0	136.6	110.6
$h12$	10.27	12.69	16.05	18.50	82.9	60.0	141.2	118.3
$h13$	6.81	11.13	18.49	23.00	87.1	60.0	147.4	113.8
$h14$	11.65	13.32	21.69	20.18	87.5	60.0	150.8	121.0
$h15$	11.47	8.25	14.13	20.01	87.0	60.7	159.2	114.9
$h16$	14.46	8.75	25.36	22.41	82.5	60.0	158.6	108.5
$h17$	13.32	14.54	17.59	18.14	80.0	60.0	167.8	108.9
$h18$	13.16	9.58	21.05	22.48	80.0	60.0	171.4	108.1
$h19$	10.45	13.51	21.34	19.52	80.0	60.0	173.2	102.7
$h20$	8.41	12.73	13.83	21.74	80.0	60.0	188.0	106.3
$h21$	8.33	11.15	27.08	16.75	80.0	60.0	183.0	107.2
$h22$	9.90	9.15	24.71	21.98	80.0	60.0	182.2	106.2
$h23$	10.90	7.73	20.08	22.30	80.0	60.3	184.2	105.3
$h24$	11.99	11.37	19.87	18.70	80.0	60.0	185.3	100.4

In Table 6, the optimal hydrodischarge is shown for four hydroplants considered in STHTS. Minimum and maximum discharge of first hydropower plant during 24 h is 6.81 and 13.90 and for second hydropower plant 6.23 and 14.54 and for third hydroplant 17.82 and 30 and for the forth plant 13.57 and 25.0 which are shown in Table 6 obtained by proposed technique. In Table 6, the optimal hydrovolumes are shown for four hydroplants considered in STHTS. Minimum and maximum volume of first hydrounit during 24 h is 80 and 96 which are shown in Table 6 results. In Table 7, the optimal hydrogenerations are shown for four hydroplants considered in STHTS. Minimum and maximum generation of first hydropower plant during 24 h is 62.9 and 95.6 MW which are shown in Table 7 results. In Table 7, the optimal thermal generations are shown for three thermal plants considered in STHTS. Minimum and maximum generation of first thermal unit during 24 h is 86 and 166.1 MW and for the second thermal unit 61.8 and 300 MW and for third thermal unit 103.5 and 472.8 which are shown in Table 7 results.

Table 7 Thermal and hydrogenerations in MW by TLBO

Hour	Hydrogenerations (MW)				Thermal generations (MW)		
	Plant 1	Plant 2	Plant 3	Plant 4	Unit 1	Unit 2	Unit 3
$h1$	95.6	75.0	40.9	204.4	86.0	97.9	156.1
$h2$	80.7	67.0	0.0	223.9	139.7	65.6	213.8
$h3$	89.4	77.4	0.0	199.6	128.7	107.5	103.5
$h4$	79.1	47.3	1.6	192.0	83.7	132.7	119.0
$h5$	86.0	69.2	39.9	193.8	118.5	61.8	106.0
$h6$	83.7	58.0	8.7	183.7	118.8	135.6	222.5
$h7$	72.9	64.3	21.5	212.7	128.1	147.5	321.8
$h8$	75.0	71.2	0.0	233.3	134.3	133.0	388.4
$h9$	81.1	62.2	37.3	221.1	112.1	195.4	408.8
$h10$	66.4	50.9	0.0	236.9	102.5	185.3	472.8
$h11$	85.8	65.1	50.3	238.3	146.7	168.7	370.0
$h12$	79.7	67.7	48.5	250.3	166.1	226.5	335.4
$h13$	62.9	62.6	43.6	263.7	99.2	192.5	412.7
$h14$	86.7	69.3	30.5	262.5	95.8	265.0	233.9
$h15$	85.9	50.0	56.3	253.9	82.7	222.9	272.4
$h16$	88.3	52.0	9.8	254.7	156.7	137.0	388.3
$h17$	85.8	71.8	52.5	236.5	49.5	214.6	360.0
$h18$	85.6	56.1	40.6	254.3	97.4	300.0	306.0
$h19$	78.8	69.7	39.8	235.5	153.5	300.0	209.5
$h20$	69.7	67.8	61.9	249.4	124.4	129.4	371.4
$h21$	69.3	62.7	5.4	225.9	94.1	235.1	229.5
$h22$	76.7	54.0	22.8	250.1	93.0	163.5	209.3
$h23$	80.4	46.7	48.3	249.8	88.7	113.2	233.0
$h24$	83.4	63.5	49.4	228.4	102.5	82.2	199.0

7 Conclusion

This chapter succeeded in implementing a teacher–learning-based optimization combined with new equity restricting strategies for solving the STHTS with non-convex fuel and environmental pollution costs of thermal units. Outcomes show that the presented technique can find improved quality results with much more accuracy than particle swarm optimization techniques discussed this research. The presented approach can, therefore, be generalized well to address the hydrothermal scheduling on large scales.

References

1. Ferreira, L.A.F.M.: A theoretical analysis of the classic hydro-thermal optimization algorithm in power system scheduling. In: IEEE International Symposium on Circuits and System (ISCAS 92), vol. 6, pp. 2757–2760 (1992)
2. Ferreira, L.A.F.M.: On the convergence of the classic hydro-thermal coordination algorithm. IEEE Trans. Power Syst. 9(2), 1002–1008 (1994)
3. Yan, H., Luh, P.B., Guan, X., Rogan, P.M.: Scheduling of hydrothermal power systems. IEEE Trans. Power Syst. 8(3), 1358–1365 (1993)
4. Yong-Gang, W., Chun-Ying, H., Ding Wang, H.: A diploid genetic approach to short-term scheduling of hydro-thermal system. IEEE Trans. Power Syst. 15(4), 1268–1274 (2000)
5. Dhillon, J.S., Parti, S.C., Kothari, D.P.: Fuzzy decision making in multiobjective long-term scheduling of hydrothermal system. Int. J. Electr. Power Energy Syst. 23(1), 19–29 (2001)
6. Gil, E., Bustos, J., Rudnick, H.: Short-term hydrothermal generation scheduling model using a genetic algorithm. IEEE Trans. Power Syst. 18(1), 1256–1264 (2003)
7. Basu, M.: An interactive fuzzy satisfying method based on evolutionary programming technique for multiobjective short-term hydrothermal scheduling. Electr. Power Syst. Res. 69(5), 277–285 (2004)
8. Onate, P.E., Ramirez, J.M.: Optimal operation of hydrothermal systems in the short term. In: 37th Annual Power Symposium Proceedings, pp. 113–119 (2005)
9. Yuan, X., Yuan, Y.: Application of cultural algorithm to generation scheduling of hydrothermal systems. Energy Convers. Manage. 47(9), 2192–2201 (2006)
10. Kumar, S., Naresh, R.: Efficient real coded genetic algorithm to solve the non-convex hydrothermal scheduling problem. Int. J. Electr. Power Energy Syst. 29(12), 738–747 (2007)
11. Yu, B., Yuan, X., Wang, J.: Short-term hydro-thermal scheduling using particle swarm optimization method. Energy Convers. Manage. 48(7), 1902–1908 (2007)
12. Mandal, K.K., Basu, M., Chakraborty, N.: Particle swarm optimization technique based short-term hydrothermal scheduling. Appl. Soft Comput. 8(4), 1392–1399 (2008)
13. Chen, P.H.: Pumped-storage scheduling using evolutionary particle swarm optimization. IEEE Trans. Energy Convers. 23(1), 294–301 (2008)
14. Hota, P.K., Barisal, A.K., Chakrabarti, R.: An improved PSO technique for short-term optimal hydrothermal scheduling. Electr. Power Syst. Res. 79(7), 1047–1053 (2009)
15. Mandal, K.K., Chakraborty, N.: Differential evolution technique-based short-term economic generation scheduling of hydrothermal systems. Electr. Power Syst. Res. 78(11), 1972–1979 (2008)
16. Dieu, V.N., Ongsakul, W.: Enhanced merit order and augmented Lagrange Hopfield network for hydrothermal scheduling. Int. J. Electr. Power Energy Syst. 30(2), 93–101 (2008)
17. Mughal, S.: The impact of frequency linked tariff system in India. In: Proceedings National Conference and Exhibition on Emerging and Innovative Trends in Engineering Technology (NCEEITET-2014), GCET Jammu (J&K), pp. 241–245, 9–10 Jan 2015

18. Iqbal, A., et al.: Metaheuristic algorithm based hybrid model for identification of building sale prices. In: Springer Nature Book: Metaheuristic and Evolutionary Computation: Algorithms and Applications. Studies in Computational Intelligence (2020). https://doi.org/10.1007/978-981-15-7571-6_32

19. Shahabuddin, M., Asim, M., Sarwar, A.: Parameter Extraction of a Solar PV Cell Using Projectile Search Algorithm. In: 2020 International Conference on Advances in Computing Communication & Materials (ICACCM), Dehradun, India, pp. 357–361 (2020). https://doi.org/10.1109/ICACCM50413.2020.9213005

20. Abu, S. et al.: Bacterial behaviour based swarm optimized PID controller tuning for high order system. Parameters 4.4 (2016)

21. Rao, R.V., Savsani, V.J., Vakharia, D.P.: Teaching–bearning-based optimization: a novel method for constrained mechanical design optimization problems. Comput. Aided Des. **43**, 303–315 (2011)

Simulation and Analysis of Rectifier-Based Four-Level Grid-Connected Inverter Using Genetic Algorithm

Anzar Ahmad, Mu Anas, Mohammad Zaid, Adil Sarwar, and Mohd Tariq

Abstract Renewable energy resources, especially solar PV, have become quite popular in recent decade especially because of the advancement in solar PV technology and power electronics. Solar PV can be used as a DC source in grid-connected converter for power transfer from load side to grid side. The waveform of line current in conventional line commutated AC to DC converter is not sinusoidal because of presence of higher-order harmonics. At power frequency, thyristors-based line commutated converter is used as they have better power handling capability and reliability. In the present work, four-level single-phase grid-connected converter is proposed and mathematically analyzed. Grid power, power factor, and line current THD are controlled by controlling the firing angle of switches. Results show that the average grid power increases, as well as line current THD reduces as compared to conventional line commutated converter. The input power factor, as well as smoothness in line current, is achieved to acceptable value. The genetic algorithm is implemented for optimizing the line current THD in terms of switching angles. The proposed model is simulated using MATLAB®/Simulink.

Keywords Grid-connected converter · THD · Multilevel inverter · Grid power · Input power factor

1 Introduction

Energy resources play a significant role in the development of any country. Electricity is one of them as its demand is increasing day by day throughout the world. At present, most of the energy requirement is fulfilled by fossil fuels (coal, petroleum, natural gases, etc.) [1]. Due to low energy cost, environmental issues shifted some of the energy demands from conventional energy resources to renewable energy resources. In case of solar PV, light energy (coming from the sun) is converted to electrical energy in DC form. Therefore, it is used as a DC source for power flow

A. Ahmad · M. Anas · M. Zaid · A. Sarwar (✉) · M. Tariq
Department of Electrical Engineering, AMU, Aligarh, UP 202002, India
e-mail: adil.sarwar@zhcet.ac.in

© The Author(s), under exclusive license to Springer Nature Singapore Pte Ltd. 2021
H. Malik et al. (eds.), *AI and Machine Learning Paradigms for Health Monitoring System*, Studies in Big Data 86,
https://doi.org/10.1007/978-981-33-4412-9_19

to grid [2, 3]. Several methods are available for conversion of DC to AC. At power frequency, PWM-based inverters (IGBT, GTO, MOSFET) are not used due to high switching losses, poor power handling capability, and reliability [2]. To overcome these difficulties, especially in terms of THD, multilevel inverter is used because as the number of level increases, a series of staircase waveforms of line current is obtained that exhibits sinusoidal waveform. The lower rating of switches is required as compared to the two-level converter. Switching and conduction losses are also less for the same value of current rating of switches [4]. Application of multilevel inverter with PV array for power transfer to the grid side (off-grid or interconnect to AC grid) is also beneficial because there is no voltage balancing problem with grid [5]. Moreover, in [6, 7], several recent examples are given for better understanding of optimization.

In present work, line commutated controlled bridge rectifier acts as an inverter. This is possible only when the firing angle of thyristors varies between 90° and 180° [6]. PV array is connected in series with small resistance and inductance, and the system behaves like a DC motor working in regenerative braking mode. Just like a DC motor (whose back emf depends upon flux per pole, speed, and number of poles), PV array voltage depends upon solar insolation and temperature of the surroundings. For obtaining less THD in line current, the number of levels increases. A significant amount of power flow to the grid side and input power factor has been achieved by choosing the proper values of switching angle of thyristors by these proposed circuits.

2   Photovoltaic Cell and Its Mathematical Modeling

The solar cell is the fundamental constituent of PV panel. The working principle of the PV cells is based on photovoltaic effect. It is commonly known as solar cells when light coming from the sun is taken as a source. Formation of PN junction in PV cell is same as PN junction diode. The connection of large number of PV modules in series is treated as PV panel. PV array is formed by series–parallel combination of PV panel [7]. Solar insolation, temperature, and choice of material affect the efficiency of PV panel. Figure 1 shows the basic model of PV cell which consists of a current

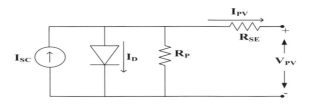

Fig. 1 Basic model of PV cell

source (I_{SC}), diode, parallel resistor (R_P), and series resistor (R_{SE}). V_{PV} and I_{PV} are the output voltage and output current of PV cell, respectively.

From the above model, using KCL

$$I_{SC} - I_D - \frac{V_D}{R_P} - I_{PV} = 0 \tag{1}$$

$$I_D = I_0\left(e^{V_D/V_T} - 1\right) \tag{2}$$

Using KVL,

$$V_{PV} = V_D - R_S I_{PV} \tag{3}$$

where,

V_D Diode voltage
I_0 Diode saturation current
I_D Diode current
V_T Thermal voltage.

3 Proposed Scheme

3.1 Inverted Mode of Operation of the Single-Phase Bridge Rectifier

Figure 3 shows the circuit of single-phase bridge rectifier, where T_1 T_4 and T_2 T_3 (switch pairs) are complementary to each other. For an inverter mode, it is not only to operate the converter in between 90° and 180° switching angle but also required to connect an active load in such a way that its internal voltage acts as a source that maintains the output current Io to flow in the positive direction as shown in Fig. 2.

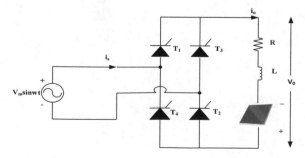

Fig. 2 Polarity of load emf E reversed with $\alpha_{inv} > 90$

Therefore, the converter operates in such a position to receive power from active load and output voltage is given by

$$V_O = \frac{2V_m}{\pi} \cos \alpha_{inv} < 0 \qquad (4)$$

In converter operation, the average value of output voltage V_O must be greater than active load circuit emf. But for an inverter mode of operation, load side emf must be more than inverter voltage V_O, and only then power would flow from DC source to grid. Here, the load is considered to be highly inductive and E is the PV voltage or maybe a back emf of a DC motor. Thyristors pair (T_1, T_2) is simultaneously triggered say at α Radian as well as (T_3, T_4) triggered together at $\pi + \alpha$ Radian. Figure 3 shows the waveform of output voltage, output current input voltage, and input current for the value of firing angle at α equal to $120°$.

For a nonlinear load, the active power in the AC side is given by the following formula

$$P = V_S I_{S1} \cos \varphi_1 \qquad (5)$$

where I_{S1} is the fundamental value of source current and φ_1 is the phase displacement between the fundamental value of source current and the supply AC voltage (V_S) at the rectifier input is considered sinusoidal.

3.2 Proposed Model

Figure 3 shows the circuit diagram of the proposed model. In proposed model, three bridge rectifier units are connected in parallel to a common voltage supply. All the rectifier units are operated in inverter mode. The working principle of this model is

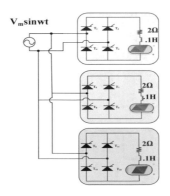

Fig. 3 Circuit diagram of four-level grid-connected inverter

same as we have discussed in Sect. 3.1. The proposed model has the capability to generate four levels of line current.

Power quality is an important issue nowadays, since the devices are designed for a particular frequency with narrow band of tolerances. Power quality in proposed topology is measured in terms of THD in line current. Two-level converters are not suitable because it injects a huge amount of harmonics into grid. High harmonic content in line current heats the core of distribution and power transformers above its rated temperature. Hence, line current should have low harmonic content and this is the most desirable feature of a grid inverter. Multilevel converters are usually preferred because it reduces the line current THD significantly. At low frequency, power handling capability and reliability of IGBT and MOSFET are quite low in comparison with thyristors. Therefore, in this model, grid operation thyristors are used. In each stage, two switches are operated in complementary fashion. Pulse generators are used for firing of switches. In the load side, a low resistance of (2Ω) is connected with inductor which is taken into account. Due to highly inductive load, the waveform of line current is continuous and ripple-free. But when switch to higher-level cost of hardware increases significantly, controlling of switches is also difficult. Due to these limitations, a suitable compromise has to be made between THD of line current and cost of hardware.

3.3 Control Strategy and Mathematical Analysis of Four-Level Inverter

Controlling of firing angle has been done in the same way as we have done in case of single-phase controlled rectifier. But firing angle should be between 90° and 180°. Let us suppose one pair of diagonal thyristors triggered at an angle a, then second pair of diagonal thyristors triggered at an angle (180° + a). The above firing scheme keeps remaining same for each stage. Figure 4 shows the waveform of each leg (stage) of line current and resultant of line current. The resultant line current is the algebraic sum of three leg currents. Fourier analysis has been done for obtaining the expression of input line current in terms of switching angle

According to the Fourier series, any non-sinusoidal periodic waveform can be represented in terms of cosine and sine wave. Mathematically,

$$I_{\text{line}} = a_o + \sum_{n=1}^{I_{\text{line}}n=\infty} a_n \cos n\omega t + b_n \sin n\omega t \tag{6}$$

where ω and T are angular frequency in (rad/s) and time period in (s), respectively.

$$a_n = \frac{-4I}{n\pi}[\sin na + \sin nb + \sin nc] \tag{7}$$

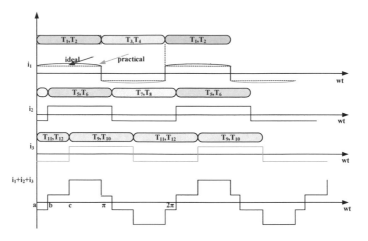

Fig. 4 Waveform of line current

$$b_n = \frac{4I}{n\pi}[\cos na + \cos nb + \cos nc] \tag{8}$$

Putting the value of a_n and b_n from Eqs. (7) and (8) in Eq. (6), we get the expression of line current.

For obtaining the fundamental value of line current (I_1), putting the value of $n = 1$ in Eq. (2) and Eq. (3), we get

$$a_1 = \frac{4I}{\pi}[\sin a + \sin b + \sin c] \tag{9}$$

$$b_1 = \frac{4I}{\pi}[\cos a + \cos b + \cos c] \tag{10}$$

$$c_1 = \sqrt{a_1^2 + b_1^2} \tag{11}$$

$$I_1 = \frac{C_1}{\sqrt{2}} \tag{12}$$

$$\phi_1 = \left\{\tan^{-1}\left(\frac{b_1}{a_1}\right)\right\} \tag{13}$$

Now obtaining the expression of RMS value of input line current

$$I_{\text{rms}} = \sqrt{\left[\frac{1}{\pi}\left\{\int_a^c I^2 d\omega t + \int_c^{\pi+a} 9I^2 d\omega t\right\}\right]} \tag{14}$$

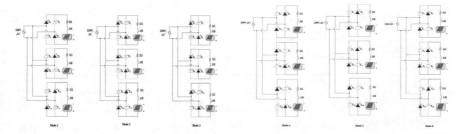

Fig. 5 Operating modes of proposed scheme

$$I_{rms} = I/\sqrt{\pi}\left(\sqrt{(c-a)} + 9(\pi + a - c)\right) \qquad (15)$$

$$THD = \sqrt{\frac{I_{rms}^2 - I_1^2}{I_1^2}} \qquad (16)$$

From Eq. (12), it is to be noted that the THD in line current is dependent on switching angles.

3.4 Modes of Operation

Figure 5 shows the operating modes of proposed topology. It is to be noted that at each instant of time six switches are in ON states.

4 Simulation Result

The model is tested with the parameters which are shown in Table 1. THD, input power factor, and grid power are calculated for different value of switching angle.

From Table 1, it is to be noted that for lower value of switching angle power factor as well as grid power is low as compared to higher value of switching angle. Line current THD is also improved for higher value of switching angle. THD level in line current becomes very large when one of the thyristors pair is fired beyond 170°. THD level remains same for the equal interval of firing angle. When one of the thyristors pair is fired at an angle of 180°, the inverter will become three-level and line current THD increases significantly. Figure 6 shows the waveform of line current and grid voltage at minimum THD in line current. Figure 7 shows the FFT analysis at minimum THD level. From Fig. 8, it is noted that negative area of instantaneous power is larger than the positive area. Therefore, average grid power flows from load to grid side. The output current is always positive. In other words, direction of current flow is from

Table 1 Circuit parameters

Grid voltage	230 V
Grid frequency	50 IIz
Inductance	0.1 H
Resistance	2Ω
Solar insolation	1000 W/m²
PV array temperature	25 °C
PV module	1soltech 1STH-215-P
Series connected module per string	25
Parallel string	5

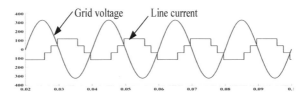

Fig. 6 Grid voltage and line current at switching angles ($a = 90.07°$, $b = 124.76°$, $c = 159.45°$)

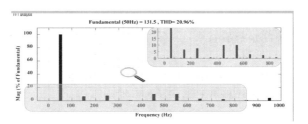

Fig. 7 FFT analysis at minimum THD in line current

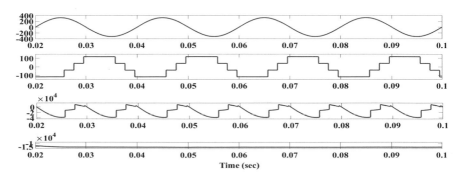

Fig. 8 Grid voltage, line current, instantaneous power, average power at switching angles ($a = 90.07°$, $b = 124.76°$, $c = 159.45°$)

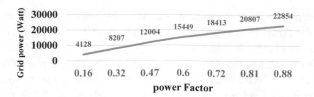

Fig. 9 Grid power versus power factor at switching angle interval of 10°

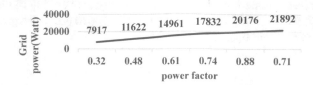

Fig. 10 Grid power vs power factor at switching angle interval of 20°

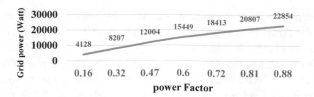

Fig. 11 Grid power versus power factor at switching angle interval of 30°

grid to load side. The minimum THD is 20.91% and is obtained in the four-level grid-connected inverter at an angle of $a = 90.07°, b = 124.76°$ and $c = 159.45°$ using genetic algorithm.

Line current THD remains approximately same at equal switching interval. But this is not to be true for grid power as well as input power factor. Figures 9, 10, and 11 show the effect of switching interval on grid power and input power factor. Grid power increases for higher switching interval of thyristors. The input power factor is also increased but decreases up to a certain point in case of 20° and 30° switching interval.

5 Conclusion

This paper reviewed the importance of solar PV in the present era and its application as a source of electricity production with a grid network. Due to better compatibility of cascaded H bridge with solar PV, grid power, as well as power factor, has been increased and improved by selecting proper value of firing angles of thyristors. The pulse generator has been used for the firing of thyristors pairs. At each instant, six out of twelve switches have worked. The mathematical expression of line current in terms of switching angle has been achieved. With the help of line current, power flow can be controlled from load side to grid side. Minimum THD achieved in line current is 20.96% and has been achieved at firing angles of ($a = 90.07°$, $b = 124.76°$, $c = 159.45°$). This result has been validated using genetic algorithm. At same interval of firing line current, THD has been observed approximately same value. Also, grid power has been obtained a large amount at a higher value of firing as compared to lower value. As the firing of one pair of thyristors is increased beyond $170°$, the THD level and the power factor decrease significantly. Also, the proposed four-level inverter has become three levels. Therefore, better operation of the multilevel converter with PV array will be provided a future scope to use it as a grid-connected converter up to a certain operating condition.

References

1. Ahmad, S., Johari, S.H., Halim, M.F.M.A., Ahmad, A.: Grid connected multilevel inverters for PV application. In: 2015 IEEE Conference on Energy Conversion, CENCON 2015, pp. 181–186 (2015)
2. Zahra, F., Moulay, A., Lamchich, T., Outzourhit, A.: Design control of DC/AC converter for a grid connected PV systems with maximum Power tracking using Matlab/Simulink (2010)
3. Sarwar, A., Asghar, M.S.J.: Multilevel converter topology for solar PV based grid-tie inverters. In: 2010 IEEE International Energy Conference, pp. 501–506 (2010)
4. Zhang, X., Ni, H., Yao, D., Cao, R.X., Shen, W.X.: Design of single phase grid-connected photovoltaic power plant based on string inverters, pp. 2–6 (2006)
5. Heldwein, M.L., Mussa, S.A., Barbi, I.: Three-phase multilevel PWM rectifiers based on conventional bidirectional converters. IEEE Trans Power Electron **25**(3), 545–549 (2010)
6. Iqbal, A., et al.: Metaheurestic algorithm based hybrid model for identification of building sale prices. In: Springer Nature Book: Metaheuristic and Evolutionary Computation: Algorithms and Applications. Studies in Computational Intelligence (2020). https://doi.org/10.1007/978-981-15-7571-6_32
7. FaizMinai, A., et al.: Metaheuristics paradigms for renewable energy systems: advances in optimization algorithms. In: Springer Nature Book: Metaheuristic and Evolutionary Computation: Algorithms and Applications. Studies in Computational Intelligence (2020). https://doi.org/10.1007/978-981-15-7571-6_2

Vector Control of Dual 3-ϕ Induction Machine-Based Flywheel Energy Storage System Using Fuzzy Logic Controllers

Mohamed Daoud and Atif Iqbal

Abstract In the renewable, islanded microgrid and transportation applications, the flywheel energy storage systems (FESS) will play a significant role due to its potential benefits, like long life span, fast dynamics and high charging/discharging range. The reliability of flywheel energy storage systems is an essential characteristic when it is applied to support critical loads or fault ride-through purposes. Therefore, this work proposes the exploitation of multiphase machines' reliability features in FESS applications. In this chapter, the vector control along with the fuzzy logic control (FLC) algorithms is proposed for a dual 3-ϕ induction machine (IM)-based FESS. The FLC ensures fast and smart vector control that suits the nature of critical applications. The validation of a proposed dual 3-ϕ IM-based FESS system is done in MATLAB/Simulink, where the case study under normal condition on FESS and machine mathematical model is presented in detail.

Abbreviations

FESS	Flywheel energy storage systems.
FLC	Fuzzy logic control.
IM	Induction motor.
L_m	Magnetizing inductance.
L_s	Self-inductance of stator.
L_r	Self-inductance of rotor.
λ_{ds}	Stator flux-linkages along d-axis.
λ_{qs}	Stator flux-linkages along q-axis.
r_s	Resistance of stator.
ω_e	Angular frequency of stator.
λ_{dr}	Rotor flux-linkages along d-axis.
λ_{qr}	Rotor flux-linkages along q-axis.

M. Daoud · A. Iqbal (✉)
Department of Electrical Engineering, Qatar University, Doha, Qatar
e-mail: atif.iqbal@qu.edu.qa

© The Author(s), under exclusive license to Springer Nature Singapore Pte Ltd. 2021   339
H. Malik et al. (eds.), *AI and Machine Learning Paradigms for Health
Monitoring System*, Studies in Big Data 86,
https://doi.org/10.1007/978-981-33-4412-9_20

r_r Resistance of rotor.
ω_r Angular frequency of rotor.
p Derivative.
T_e Electromagnetic torque.
θ Angular position.
P Pole pairs of a machine.
VSD   Variable speed drives.

1 Introduction

Nowadays, in all types industrial, commercial and residential applications, variable speed drives (VSD) are gaining momentous interest due to the requirement of adjustable speed as well as torque of the machineries. Among all types of electrical machines, IMs are horse-powering the industry due to the low cost, good self-starting, simple design, high reliability and high robustness. Because of these reasons, in the FESS applications, IMs are best promising candidate. The FESS is a combination of electrical machines, flywheel, power electronic circuitry and the bearings, which is emerged as a dynamic energy storage system assigned to several grid-connected applications [1, 2]. In the FESS, IM is driving the flywheel and works as a motor while storing energy than as a generator during releasing energy.

The FESS is dedicated in this work to support critical loads, where the reliability is crucial constraint [3]. Multiphase induction machines (MIM) exhibit high reliability levels compared to three-phase counterparts because of the fault tolerance (high reliability) w.r.t faults, minimized ratings of the power semiconductor devices, higher efficiency due to the reduced magnitude of space harmonics as well as losses in the system. In addition, the MIMs will give the torque ripple with higher frequencies, on-board charging for electric vehicles, minimized toque/power per phase, etc. With these reasons, in this work, an MIM (i.e. dual 3-ϕ or asymmetrical six-phase IM)-based FESS is considered.

One of the IM's richest topics is its control strategies. The simplest control schemes for IMs are scalar control as volt/hertz control [4], which does not require complicated measurements as all the required data are available on machine's name plate [5–7]. Yet, such a control strategy is not suitable if fast dynamic operation is required, so other techniques of IM control are developed such as direct and indirect vector control, as well as direct torque control. However, the conventional proportional integral (PI) controllers are sensitive to parameters change, temperature variation and magnetic flux saturation. Therefore, several nonlinear controllers have been developed lately to avoid undesirable features of conventional controllers, such as fuzzy logic controllers (FLC) and artificial neural networks (ANN) [8, 9]. This chapter proposes FLCs along with indirect vector control to generate the voltage references supplied to the machine converter. FL is a sort of artificial intelligence (AI) approach. FLCs can easily manage nonlinearity regardless the system model, which makes them feasible for any system model. They link the input–output pattern based on human logic. Therefore, the need of exact mathematical models can be omitted. In case of drive systems, FLCs are tolerant to parameter variation [10–12].

With the advantages of the MIM drives, in the present chapter, a dual 3-φ IM is employed for FESS. The FESS is devoted to support a critical load connected to the grid so that the FESS stores energy during low demand periods then release energy during peak demand periods. A vector control technique is performed using FLCs. The control algorithm's aim is to ensure proper charging/discharging of the flywheel system during off-peak/peak intervals. With the MATLAB/Simulink, the modelling of the MIM as well as case study on FESS w.r.t different control algorithms for charging and discharging has presented.

2 Proposed System Description

The dynamic model of the proposed IM as well as the control strategy is presented in this section.

2.1 Dual 3-φ IM or Asymmetrical 6-φ IM

The dual 3-φ IM is nothing but an asymmetrical 6-φ IM, where the windings are grouped as 2 set of 3-φ windings which are phase displaced shifted by an angle of 30^0 with the two isolated neutral points [13–17]. In each three-phase winding, the three windings are symmetrically distributed by angle of 120°. The stator as well as rotor winding distributions of the dual 3-φ IM are presented in Fig. 1.

Fig. 1 A dual 3-φ phase IM representation

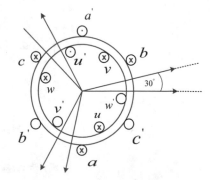

2.2 Mathematical Modelling of Dual 3-φ IM

In general, for a 3-φ phase machine mathematical model equations consist of one orthogonal α-β plane components and one zero-sequence component for symmetrical transformation of Park's matrix. The dual 3-φ IM mathematical equations consist of two orthogonal α-β frame, x-y frame, planes and a zero-sequence components $(0^+, 0^-)$. In the multiphase machine, two orthogonal α-β frame components are useful for required torque producing. The x-y frame and zero-sequence components will not be useful for the torque production; these components will cause the losses in the system. Moreover, the x-y plane components are helpful for torque enhancement by injecting the harmonics into the stator phase currents. In the present work, because of the isolated dual 3-φ winding sets, the zero-sequence components are neglected.

The phase variable *(abcuvw)*-based modelling of the machine involves in the time-dependent inductance matrices as well as modelling equations, which has limitations w.r.t the computational times, complexity to solve differential equations, inverse calculation matrices, etc. For avoiding these issues, the phase variable equations of the machine *(abcuvw)* can be transferred into $\alpha\beta o$ domain (i.e. stationary reference frame) by using the Park's transformation presented in Eq. (1) [15]. The machine modelling equations in $\alpha\beta o$ domain are further transformed into dqo domain (i.e. rotating reference frame) by using the rotational matrix shown in Eq. (2). The final stator and rotor voltage equations of dual 3-φ IM are given in Eqs. (3) to (10)

$$
\begin{bmatrix} \alpha \\ \beta \\ x \\ y \end{bmatrix} = \frac{1}{\sqrt{3}} \cdot \begin{bmatrix} 1 & -0.5 & -0.5 & 0.866 & -0.866 & 0 \\ 0 & 0.866 & -0.866 & 0.5 & 0.5 & -1 \\ 1 & -0.5 & -0.5 & -0.866 & 0.866 & 0 \\ 0 & -0.866 & 0.866 & 0.5 & 0.5 & -1 \end{bmatrix} \begin{bmatrix} a \\ b \\ c \\ u \\ v \\ w \end{bmatrix} \tag{1}
$$

$$
\begin{bmatrix} d \\ q \\ x' \\ y' \end{bmatrix} = \begin{bmatrix} \cos\theta & \sin\theta & 0 & 0 \\ -\sin\theta & \cos\theta & 0 & 0 \\ 0 & 0 & \cos\theta & -\sin\theta \\ 0 & 0 & \sin\theta & \cos\theta \end{bmatrix} \begin{bmatrix} \alpha \\ \beta \\ x \\ y \end{bmatrix} \tag{2}
$$

$$
v_{ds} = r_s i_{ds} + p\lambda_{ds} - \omega_s \lambda_{qs} \tag{3}
$$

$$
v_{qs} = r_s i_{qs} + p\lambda_{qs} + \omega_s \lambda_{ds} \tag{4}
$$

$$
0 = r_r i_{dr} + p\lambda_{dr} - (\omega_s - \omega_r)\lambda_{qr} \tag{5}
$$

$$0 = r_r i_{qr} + p\lambda_{qr} + (\omega_s - \omega_r)\lambda_{dr} \tag{6}$$

$$\lambda_{ds} = L_s i_{ds} + L_m i_{dr} \tag{7}$$

$$\lambda_{qs} = L_s i_{qs} + L_m i_{qr} \tag{8}$$

$$\lambda_{dr} = L_r i_{dr} + L_m i_{ds} \tag{9}$$

$$\lambda_{qr} = L_r i_{qr} + L_m i_{qs} \tag{10}$$

The xy orthogonal subplane and zero-sequence component equations in rotating reference frame are given in Eqs. (11)–(14).

$$v_{xs'} = r_s i_{xs'} + p\lambda_{xs} \tag{11}$$

$$v_{ys'} = r_s i_{ys'} + p\lambda_{ys} \tag{12}$$

$$\lambda_{xs} = L_s i_{xs'} \tag{13}$$

$$\lambda_{ys} = L_s i_{ys'} \tag{14}$$

The electromagnetic torque equation of the dual 3-φ IM is presented in Eq. (15),

$$T_e = P L_m (i_{qs} i_{dr} - i_{ds} i_{qr}) \tag{15}$$

The slip frequency of machine is given in Eq. (16)

$$\omega_{\text{slip}} = \frac{r_r i_{qs}}{L_r i_{ds}} \tag{16}$$

2.3 Fuzzy Logic-Based Vector Control Algorithm for IMs

In this work, an indirect field-oriented vector control for dual 3-φ IM drives has been implemented [13, 14], as shown in Fig. 2. Firstly, the machine phase currents are sensed and transformed into the rotating reference frame by using Eqs. (1) and (2). From these sensed currents, slip speed as well as frequency are calculated according to the Eq. (16). The rotor flux angle is calculated from the sensed mechanical speed of the machine as well slip frequency. With this vector control, the d-q components

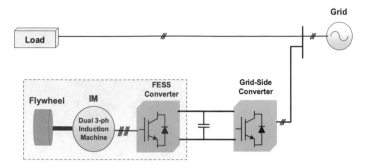

Fig. 2 Vector control of dual 3-φ IM-based FESS

are useful for modulating the active as well as reactive power flows of FESS, and the
x-y components are used for minimizing the losses.

The current components of rotating reference frame i_{ds}, i_{qs}, i_{xs}' and i_{ys}' are
compared to their reference values and the errors are applied to FLCs. FLCs are
useful for applications based on power electronics such as machine drives as no
exact mathematical model or closed-loop parameters are required. FLCs consist of
a group of logic rules set by a human being. In a common platform domain, the
input as well as output variables of the membership function (MF) are predefined.
MFs can be described as curves with different shape; however, triangle is the most
common shape. For proper design of FLCs, the tuning of input/output scaling gains
is an essential task. The basic rules for any FLC are based on If-conditions about the
MFs using logic functions of OR, AND and NOT. The reference of the d-axis current
is defined with respect to the rated magnetization current as well rated flux of the
machine. This i_{ds}^* is compared with the transformed components (i_{ds}) of actual phase
currents. FLCs observe the pattern of the error signals and correspondingly update
their output signals to match the reference values. In general, the FLC requires two
inputs, i.e., error (e) and the change in error or error derivative (ce). In this work,
the fuzzy sets are defined as in Table 1. Using the fuzzy sets, then the MFs can be
formed. Seven MFs are selected for input signals, while nine MFs are selected for
the output signal. Therefore, 49 rules can be created as shown in the table in Fig. 3.
The torque component of the machine is nothing but the q-axis current reference
component of the machine. This q-axis reference current is generated based on the
control parameters on grid side, like grid voltage, frequency and power. This i_{qs}^* is
compared with the actual i_{qs} current, and the error is fed to the FLC-based controllers.

Table 1 Fuzzy sets

Z = Zero	PS = Positive Small
PM = Positive Medium	PB = Positive Big
PVS = Positive Very Small	NS = Negative Small
NM = Negative Medium	NB = Negative Big
NVS = Negative Very Small	

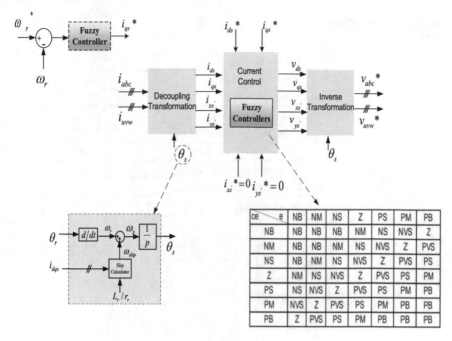

Fig. 3 FLC diagram for dual 3-φ IM-based FESS system

The FLC generates the reference d-q voltages, which are transformed into original phase variables (*abcuvw*) by using the inverse transformation of Park's transformation given in Eqs. (1) and (2). The control logic and fuzzy sets of FLC used in vector control of IM are presented in Fig. 3 and Table 1, respectively.

3 Simulation Case Study

The vector control of dual 3-φ IM for FESS using the FLC is implemented in MATLAB/Simulink. FESS delivers the power for critical loads through the machine (dual 3-φ IM) and a six-phase conventional two-level inverter. The mathematical model is implemented according to the modelling equations presented in Sect. 2 from Eqs. (1) to (16). The machine design details are power 1 kW, voltage 100 V, frequency 50 Hz, rotor is squirrel cage type and others are presented in Table 2. The proposed system is validated at two various cases. The healthy condition is considered as first case, which gives the performance of overall system during charging and discharging cycles, the associated results are presented in Fig. 4a–e. The system behaviour under fault condition is considered as a second case, shown in Fig. 4f–i.

The current reference d-q components are derived according to the grid-side control parameters, like voltage, power and frequency. With the fuzzy logic-based

Table 2 Design parameters
of dual 3-ϕ IM

Rated phase voltage (V)	100
Rated power (kW)	1
Rated frequency (Hz)	50
Full-load current (A)	2.35
Rated speed (rpm)	960
Stator resistance (Ω)	6.1
Stator leakage resistance (Ω)	7.75
Rotor referred resistance (Ω)	5.155
Rotor referred reactance (Ω)	7.75
Magnetizing reactance (Ω)	75
No. of pole pairs	6

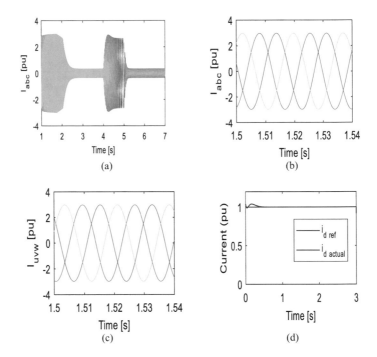

Fig. 4 Simulation results per unit values: **a** abc currents during charging/discharging, **b** abc currents
(2 cycles), **c** uvw currents (2 cycles), **d** direct current, **e** quadrature current, **f** i_x, **g** i_y, **h** flywheel
speed and **i** machine torque

vector control, the reference voltage vectors are generated and that are used to modu-
late the six phase inverter through current regulators, which helps in control of
charging and discharging cycles. The machine actual currents in healthy condition
are given in Fig. 4a–c, where the *abc* winding currents are given in Fig. 4a, b and
uvw winding currents are given in Fig. 4c. The charging and discharging can be

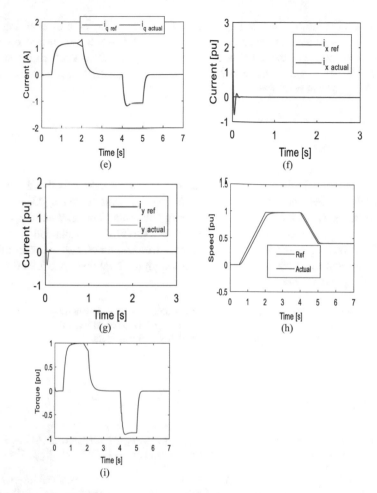

Fig. 4 (continued)

observed in Fig. 4a. During the constant speed operation, the machine consumes the power in terms of losses only. Form these figures, it is observed that the currents are symmetrical and balanced in both charging and discharging modes.

The d-axis current component which is helpful for regulating the flux inside the machine is given in Fig. 4d. The torque component is regulated by the q-axis current component which is given in Fig. 4e. From this figure, it can be observed that the positive q-axis current represents the charging mode of system and acceleration state of the machine. And negative q-axis current represents the discharging mode of system and deceleration state of the machine. The x-axis and y-axis current components (i_x and i_y) representing the losses of the system are presented in Fig. 4f, g, respectively, where the controller commands are tracking the zero value to minimize the losses. The speed of a IM for charging as well as discharging states is shown in Fig. 4h, where from 0 to 2 s machine is in charging state and 4–5 s machine is in discharging state. The FLC helps in accurate speed control with respect to the d-q current response. The torque response of the machine during charging as well as discharging states is shown in Fig. 4i, where positive and negative torques are representing the charging and discharging states of system.

4 Conclusion

A dual 3-ϕ IM-based FESS with FLC-based vector control is described in this chapter. The simulation results have shown that the control system managed to operate machine properly under charging/discharging intervals. The measured quantities exhibited good response compared to references. The FLC reveals good decoupling of machine frames. Moreover, FLC is simpler to implement, faster for simulation and independent on machine parameters. Employing a dual three phase in this work reduced the power converter rating as well.

Acknowledgements This publication was made possible by Qatar University-Marubeni Concept to Prototype Development Research grant # [**M-CTP-CENG-2020-2**] from the Qatar University. The statements made herein are solely the responsibility of the authors.

References

1. Zhang, J.: Research on flywheel energy storage system using in power network. In:International Conference on Power Electronics and Drives Systems, PEDS 2005, vol. 2, pp. 1344–1347, 28–01 Nov 2005
2. Sough, M.L., Depernet, D., Dubas, F., Boualem, B., Espanet, C.: PMSM and inverter sizing compromise applied to flywheel for railway application. In:Vehicle Power and Propulsion Conference (VPPC), pp. 1–5, 1–3 Sept 2010. IEEE (2010)
3. Cimuca, G., Breban, S., Radulescu, M.M., Saudemont, C., Robyns, B.: Design and control strategies of an induction-machine-based flywheel energy storage system associated to a variable-speed wind generator. IEEE Trans. Energy Convers. 25(2), 526–534 (2010)
4. Morsy, A.S., Abdelkhalik, A.S., Abbas, A., Ahmed, S., Massoud, A.:Open loop V/f control of multiphase induction machine under open-circuit phase faults. In: IEEE Applied Power Electronics Conference and Exposition (APEC), 2013, pp. 1170, 1176, 17–21 March 2013
5. Park, J.-D.:Simple flywheel energy storage using squirrel-cage induction machine for DC bus microgrid systems. In:IECON 2010—36th Annual Conference on IEEE Industrial Electronics Society, pp. 3040–3045, 7–10 Nov 2010
6. Cardenas, R., Pena, R., Asher, G., Clare, J.: Power smoothing in wind generation systems using a sensorless vector controlled induction Machine driving a flywheel. IEEE Trans. Energy Convers. 19(1), 206–216 (2004)
7. Cardenas, R., Pena, R., Asher, G.,Clare, J.: Control strategies for energy recovery from a flywheel using a vector controlled induction machine. In: 2000 IEEE 31st AnnualPower Electronics Specialists Conference, 2000. PESC 00, vol. 1, pp. 454–459 (2000)
8. Kukker, A., et al.: Reinforcement learning based genetic fuzzy classifier for transformer faults. IETE J. Res.https://doi.org/10.1080/03772063.2020.1732844

9. Sharma, R., et al.: Fuzzy reinforcement learning based intelligent classifier for power transformer faults. ISA Trans. (2020). https://doi.org/10.1016/j.isatra.2020.01.016https://doi.org/10.1016/j.isatra.2020.01.016
10. Beierke, S., von Altrock, C.: Fuzzy logic enhanced control of an induction motor with DSP. In: 5th IEEE International Conference on Fuzzy Systems, New Orleans, LA, September 1996
11. Spiegel, R.J., Turner, M.W., McCormick, V.E.: Fuzzy-logic-based controllers for science optimization of inverter-fed induction motor drives. ELSEVIER J. (2003)
12. Zilouchian, A., Jamshidi, M.: Intelligent Control Systems Using Soft Computing Methodologies. CRC Press LLC (2001)
13. Zhao, Y., Lipo, T.A.: Space vector PWM control of dual three-phase induction machine using vector space decomposition. In:IEEE Trans. Ind. Appl. **31**(5), 1100, 1109 (1995)
14. Kianinezhad, R., Nahid, B., Betin, F., Capolino, G.A.: A new field orientation control of dual three phase induction machines. In:IEEE International Conference on Industrial Technology, vol. 1, pp. 187, 192, 8–10 Dec 2004
15. Che, H.S., Levi, E., Jones, M., Duran, M.J., Hew, W.-P., Abd Rahim, N.: Operation of a six-phase induction machine using series-connected machine-side converters. IEEE Trans. Ind. Electron. **61**(1), 164, 176 (2014)
16. Xiang-Jun, Z., Yongbing, Y., Hongtao, Z., Ying, L., Luguang, F., Xu, Y.:Modelling and control of a multi-phase permanent magnet synchronous generator and efficient hybrid 3L-converters for large direct-drive wind turbines. IETElectr. Power Appl. **6**(6), 322, 331 (2012)
17. Levi, E., Bojoi, R., Profumo, F., Toliyat, H.A., Williamson, S.: Multiphase induction motor drives - a technology status review. IETElectr. Power Appl. **1**(4), 489, 516 (2007)
18. Ashoush, A., Gadoue, S.M., Abdel-Khalik, A.S., Mohamadein, A.L.:Current optimization for an eleven-phase induction machine under fault conditions using Genetic Algorithm. In:IEEE International Symposium on Diagnostics for Electric Machines, Power Electronics & Drives (SDEMPED), pp. 529, 534, 5–8 Sept 2011
19. Abdelkhalik, A., Masoud, M., Barry, W.: Eleven-phase induction machine: steady-state analysis and performance evaluation with harmonic injection. IET Electr. Power Appl. **4**(8), 670–685 (2010)

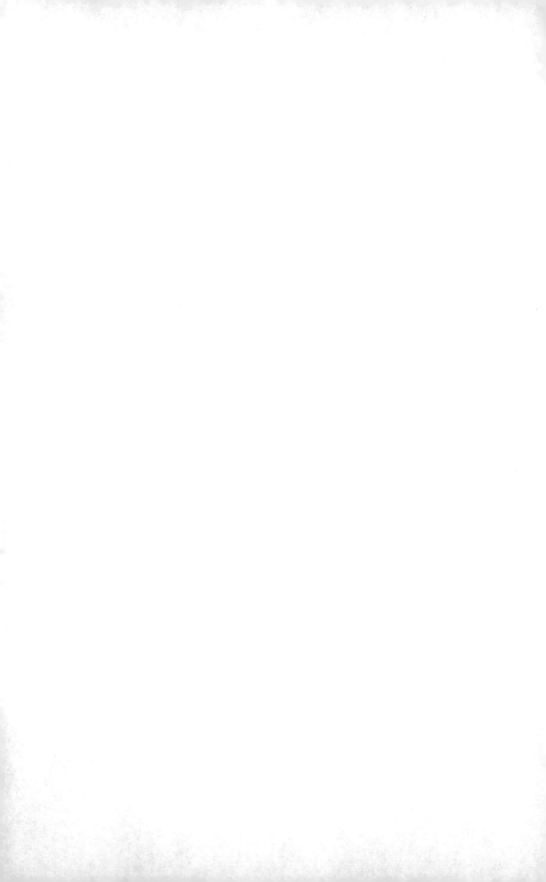

Hotspot Detection in Distribution Transformers Using Thermal Imaging and MATLAB

Monika Sahu, Saurabh Ranjan Sharma, Rajesh Kumar, and Yog Raj Sood

Abstract Condition monitoring of transformer and failure is of great concern in power industries. Temperature is one of the most well-known pointers of the basic well-being of hardware and its segments. Infrared thermal imaging (IRT) or thermography is a highly engrossing method in electric preventive maintenance credit to it being precise and sensitive to simulation of heat signatures. As of present-day scenario, ITI is a mature and hugely appreciated condition-monitoring tool wherein temperature measurements can be done at real time in pseudo-contact manner. Infrared thermography is utilized as a tool to identify the variations from the norm within the transformer. Slight variations in temperature are acceptable, but any unnatural rise must be taken note of, which may be an indicator to a probable fault and must be dealt with in a timely manner. Unusual high temperatures can harm or devastate transformer insulation and, in this way, diminish the life span. In this paper, an approach for transformer abnormality diagnosis based on thermography using thermal imaging camera 'HOTSHOT-HD' and image processing using MATLAB is proposed.

Keywords Infrared thermography (IRT) · Condition monitoring (CM) ·
Transformer preventive maintenance

1 Introduction

It is an important and challenging task nowadays to monitor the condition of electrical machines and to identify the factors which may affect the quality, cost and productivity of any industry. The application of condition monitoring (CM) is to avoid a sudden break-down, reduce downtime, minimize maintenance cost and increase the life of machine before any fault occurs. Thermal imaging as a CM technique has been utilized in numerous applications such as observing of civil structures, deformation monitoring, assessment of machinery, weld monitoring, atomic industries,

M. Sahu (✉) · S. R. Sharma · R. Kumar · Y. R. Sood
Department of Electrical Engineering, NIT Hamirpur, Hamirpur, HP, India
e-mail: monikasahu264@gmail.com

© The Author(s), under exclusive license to Springer Nature Singapore Pte Ltd. 2021
H. Malik et al. (eds.), *AI and Machine Learning Paradigms for Health Monitoring System*, Studies in Big Data 86,
https://doi.org/10.1007/978-981-33-4412-9_21

monitoring of electrical/electronic components, IRT-based condition monitoring in aerospace industries, corrosion monitoring, etc. [1].

The transformer is a crucial equipment in the power grid; any problem in the transformer will influence electrical power-system composure. The failure in a transformer may occur due to different causes or conditions. The types of failure in transformer described in [2–4] can be divided into two parts: external and internal. Internal faults include corrosion of the insulation, overheating, moisture, solid contamination in the insulating oil (furan content), partial discharge (PD), design flaw and manufacturing defects, and external faults such as overvoltage strikes, system overload, system failures (short circuit). To sum up, these can be categorized as electrical, mechanical and thermal faults and can in some way cause transformers to overheat or temperature variations. Therefore, early awareness of transformer abnormality and the ability to evaluate the problems will prevent the transformer from getting damaged.

The basic theory is that every object with a temperature more than 0 K (i.e., 273 °C) emits EM radiation in the IR region of the electromagnetic spectrum. Meola [5] explains thermal radiation theory, where he defines a blackbody as an imaginary object which absorbs all incident energies and emits a constant spectrum whose power is in accordance to Planck's law. Upon integrating Planck's law over the frequency range, the Stefan–Boltzmann's law is derived which can be shown as Eq. 1.

$$\frac{W}{A} = \varepsilon \sigma T^4 \tag{1}$$

where

W rate of energy emission (W),
T absolute temp (K),
A emitting surface area (m^2),
σ Stefan–Boltzmann's constant ($\sigma = 5.676 \, \text{W} \times 10^{-8} \, \text{m}^{-2}\text{K}^{-4}$), and
ε emissivity at constant wavelength.

Over the past decade, the image recognition approach was commonly employed that applied to many applications such as agricultural engineering, facial recognition, electrical inspection, biomedical and assist-aided vehicle driving [6–9]. The fault occurs in induction motor due to various reasons, and its inspection and feature extraction is described in [10, 11]. Transformer condition monitoring by thermal images and error diagnostic methods dependent on image processing and AI tools were suggested in [12, 13]. An image processing technique was used to examine the analysis and outputs of this thermal sequence. MATLAB programming is implemented in the present study to describe the transformer's abnormal condition and detect the highest known temperature point as HOTSPOT.

Infrared thermal imaging tool for condition monitoring eliminates the idea of predictive maintenance team to be harmed during an inspection. In this paper, image processing toolbox in MATLAB is used to process the images of the transformer to describe the temperature variations. An expert system can be used for fault diagnosis of any electrical system, for instance, an alarm system for fault isolation in distributed networks. Taking inputs from sensors, an AI based online diagnostic tool was made that evaluates condition of equipment and performs appropriate action. This coupled with thermography can have higher degrees of accuracy while monitoring thus providing a much-needed improvement over present monitoring system that simply sounds an alarm based on sensed parameter [14]. AI-based technique for detection of incipient fault and condition-based assessment of transformer is well explained in [15]. Then, a step-by-step process on thermal images is carried out to detect any abnormal temperature. The abnormal temperature in the image above the threshold value is obtained. The results obtained through MATLAB programming analyze and recommend the best suitable diagnostic method [14–20]. Some other recent applications in domain are represented in [21–26].

The proposed approach for detecting hotspot in a transformer is discussed in Sect. 2 of this paper; in Sect. 3, algorithm for implementation for the suggested scheme is discussed. In Sect. 4, the obtained results are analyzed, which is then followed by conclusion in the last section.

2 Methodology

Experimental setup consists of thermal camera style Hotshot HD, which was used as hardware tool. It has a resolution of 640 * 480 pixels to capture pattern of thermal radiation. The observed sections are transformer tank, tap changer, radiator and bushing to determine anomaly location. Abnormally high-temperature erratic transformer tank thermal patterns point to problems within. The testing process involves dividing the transformer into three parts, namely top, middle and bottom, which include bushing, radiator and transformer tank, respectively. Under normal conditions, thermal heat pattern of the tank and radiators looks relatively 'cooler at the bottom' and 'gradually warmer' toward the higher side.

3 Algorithm and Implementation

The algorithm for image recognition in pictorial form is given in Fig. 1 for a better understanding.

- *Image Acquisition.* The first step, i.e., collecting the image samples, called the 'method of image acquisition', i.e., the setup of experiments with a thermographic camera and image of a 630-kVA distribution transformer. Collect the thermal images of transformer and store it in personal computer [PC]. Then, recognize the parts of the transformer, i.e., bushings, winding, main tank, conservator from top to bottom (Fig. 2)
- *Conversion of RGB to Grayscale image.* (Images involving only intensity are called grayscale images) for further processing the image.

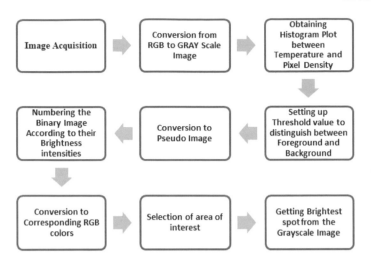

Fig. 1 Algorithm for image recognition

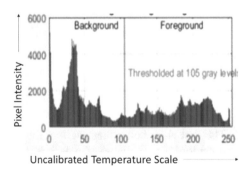

Fig. 2 Original RGB image

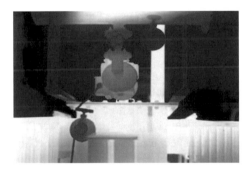

Fig. 3 Histogram of thermal image

- Obtaining the *histogram* of image plotted between temperature and pixel intensity and find the characteristics of the image (Fig. 3). This contains following two processes

  - Setting up a threshold value based on the standard value of the transformer temperature operating region
  - Distinguishing the foreground and background on the basis of the threshold value.

- *Thresholding*: Conversion from grayscale image to binary image. A threshold value of 105 Gy level is chosen based on which pixels in foreground (white or 1) and background (black or 0) are classified (Fig. 4)
- *Labeling*: Conversion of binary to pseudo-color image using matrix maps, where each label is identified and associated with a color map matrix (Fig 5)
- Based on the temperature level, binary image is numbered to distinguish the area of the highest temperature and conversion to RGB image corresponding to grayscale levels matching RGB colors filled in the image (Fig. 6)
- Finding the region of interest is that outlining the areas with higher than threshold temperature (Fig. 7)

Fig. 4 Binary image

Fig. 5 Labeled image

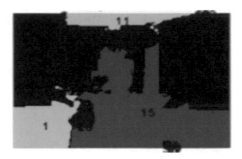

Fig. 6 Pseudo-colored image

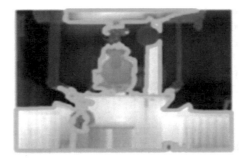

Fig. 7 Outlines from boundaries

- Hotspot detection is that the highest temperature point in the region of interest (Fig. 8)
- Getting the brightest spot in the grayscale image (Fig. 9)

Fig. 8 Brighter spots

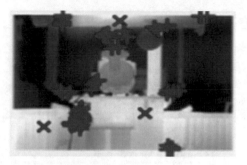

Fig. 9 Resultant grayscale image

4 Analysis and Result

Histogram obtained by the image processing is one of the best methods to represent the image characteristics and analyze the data. By this histogram, we can represent the image in various forms like binary image, labeled image, pseudo-colored image and image with boundaries. This programming includes the finding the hottest temperature zone as well as the hottest points in the thermal image.

Various sensors, including acoustic sensors, sound emission sensors, current transducers and rotating encoders, have been developed in the field of fault diagnostics. Yet in real applications, these devices have their own limits. The IRT-based fault diagnostic approach provides several significant advantages compared to conventional vibration-based approaches. First, the IRT method is fast, non-contact and non-invasive; hence, there is no surface damage. Second, it has ability to track multiple objects simultaneously and high scalability. The third and perhaps most critical thing is that IRT is resilient to running conditions.

Most major faults get linked to thermal issues that may occur due to erratic loading or abnormality. Table 1 lists the recommended actions one must take when hotspot is detected in the various parts.

The real-time application of thermal image processing of fault detection is to locate the hotspot and finding the hottest temperature region. By this, we can measure the temperature of the winding and top oil temperature by various methods and can estimate the per unit insulation life and aging acceleration factor of the transformer. The future scope of this approach is to find hotspot in the various parts like bushing, winding, radiator, etc.

5 Conclusion

In this paper, thermographic imaging method is suggested to locate the hottest temperature region to differentiate the transformer's normal and abnormal states. We may suggest the possible diagnosis and maintenance techniques of different parts of the

Table 1 Recommended action(s)

Parts of transformer	Recommended actions
Winding	• Eliminate excessive vibration • Increase clamping pressure • Increase frequency of monitoring • Periodical checking • Solidly bolting earthing connection
Main tank	• Replacement of worn-out gaskets • Monitoring gas pressure • Checking for corrosion
Bushing	• Proper tightening of terminals and joints • Through examination of cracks and crevice
Radiator	• Replacement of faulty subsystem • Clearing blockages
Others	• Rectification of mechanical failure • Clearing or replacement of oil

transformer, based on the hottest temperature region. In terms of economy, thermal imaging for defect detection, because of the maintenance of thermal imaging detectors, is the cheapest compared to current sensors. It is commonly used because of its non-invasive high-temperature measurement technique. Sensors cannot conduct high-temperature measurements if subjected to a higher limit than recommended, sensors may be affected. The diagnostic method recommends the introduction of thermograms that boosts the working conditions of machines and additionally reduces fault clearing time. Continual productivity and optimal schedule for maintenance are also discussed. The use of thermal imaging together with the presence of AI technologies would reduce the risks involved when tracking the electrical equipment for human safety.

References

1. Bagavathiappan, S., Lahiri, B.B., Saravanan, T., Philip, J., Jayakumar, T.: Infrared thermography for condition monitoring—a review. Infrared Phys Technol **60**, 35–55 (2013)
2. Wang, M., Van der Maar, A.J., Srivastava, K.D.: Review of condition assessment of power transformers in service. IEEE Elect. Insulation. Mag. **18**(6), 12–25 (2002)
3. CIGRÉ Working Group 05: An international survey on failures in large power transformers in service. Electra, no. 88 (1983)
4. Kogan, V.I., Fleeman, J.A., Provanzana, J.H., Shih, C.H.: Failure analysis of EHV transformers. IEEE Trans. Power Delivery **3**(2), 672–683 (1988). https://doi.org/10.1109/61.4306https://doi.org/10.1109/61.4306
5. Meola, C.: Origin and theory of infrared thermography. In: Meola, C. (ed.), Infrared Thermography Recent Advances and Future Trends, pp. 3–28 (2012)
6. Asiegbu, G., Haidar, A.M., Hawari, K.: Non-destructive defect detection on electrical equipment using thermographic technology. Int. Rev. Comput. Softw. **7**(3), 919–927 (2012)

7. Jadin, M.S., Taib, S.: Recent progress in diagnosing the reliability of electrical equipment by using infrared thermography. Infrared Phys. Technol. **55**(4), 236–245 (2012)
8. Bortoni, E.C., Siniscalchi, R.T., Jardini, J.A.: Hydro generator efficiency assessment using infrared thermal imaging techniques. In: Power and Energy Society General Meeting, IEEE (2010)
9. Bin Ghazali, K.H., Ma, J., Xiao, R.: Multi-angle face detection using back propagation neural network. J. Appl. Mech. Mater. **121–126**, 2411 (2011)
10. Lopez-Perez, D., Antonino-Daviu, J.: Application of infrared thermography to failure detection in industrial induction motors: case stories. IEEE Trans. Ind. Appl. **53**(3) (2017)
11. Khamisan, N., Ghazali, K.H., Zin, A.H.M.: A thermograph image extraction based on color features for induction motor bearing fault diagnosis monitoring. APRN J. Eng. Appl. Sci. **10**(22), (2015)
12. Utami, N.Y., Tamsir, Y., Pharmatrisanti, A., Gumilang, H., Cahyono, B., Siregar, R.: Evaluation condition of transformer based on infrared thermography results. In: IEEE 9th International Conference on the Properties and Applications of Dielectric Materials, pp. 1055–1058 (2009)
13. Abu-Siada, A., Islam, S.: Image processing-based on-line technique to detect power transformer winding faults. In: Proceedings of the 39th Annual Conference of the IEEE Industrial Electronics Society, pp. 5549–5554 (2013)
14. Malik, H., Mughal, S.N., Jarial, R.K., Sood, Y.R.: Application and implementation of artificial intelligence in electrical system. In:International Conference on Advances in Computing & Communication (ICACC-2011), pp. 499–505. ISBN 978-81-920874-0-5, Sponsored by IEEE-MTTS
15. Malik, H., Mughal, S.N., Azeem, A.:Artificial intelligence techniques for incipient faults diagnosis and condition assessment in transformer. In: International Conference on Emerging Trends in Engineering (ICETE-2011), pp. 5–8. ISBN 978-93-81195-07-9
16. Khan, Q, Khan, A.A., Ahmad, F.: Condition monitoring tool for electrical equipment–thermography. In: International Conference on Electrical, Electronics, and Optimization Techniques (ICEEOT) (2016)
17. Qidwai, U., Chen, C.H.: Digital Image processing an Algorithm approach with MATLAB. Champman& Hall/CRC
18. Vollmer, M., Mollman, K.-P.: Infrared Thermal Imaging: Fundamentals, Research and Application, 2nd edn
19. Patil, A.J., Singh, A., Jarial, R.K.: A novel fuzzy based technique for transformer health index computation. In: International Conference on Advances in Computing, Communication and Control (ICAC3), pp. 1–6 (2019)
20. Malik, H., Iqbal, A., Yadav, A.K.: Introduction to condition monitoring of electrical systems. In: Soft Computing in Condition Monitoring and Diagnostics of Electrical and Mechanical Systems. Advances in Intelligent Systems and Computing (AISC), vol. 1096, pp. 91–120 (2020)
21. Mishra, S.: Application of gene expression programming (GEP) in Power transformers fault diagnosis Using DGA. IEEE Trans. Ind. Appl. **52**(6), 4556–4565 (2016). https://doi.org/10.1109/TIA.2016.2598677https://doi.org/10.1109/TIA.2016.2598677
22. Yadav, A.K., et al.: Application of neuro-fuzzy scheme to investigate the winding insulation paper deterioration in oil-immersed power transformer. Electr. Power Energy Syst. **53**, 256–271 (2013). https://doi.org/10.1016/j.ijepes.2013.04.023https://doi.org/10.1016/j.ijepes.2013.04.023
23. Mishra, S., et al.: Selection of most relevant input parameters using waikato environment for knowledge analysis for gene expression programming based power transformer fault diagnosis. Int. J. Electr. Power Compon. Syst. **42**(16), 1849–1862 (2014). https://doi.org/10.1080/15325008.2014.956952https://doi.org/10.1080/15325008.2014.956952
24. Mishra, S., et al.: Selection of most relevant input parameters using principle component analysis for extreme learning machine based power transformer fault diagnosis model. Int. J. Electr. Power Components Syst. **45**(12), 1339–1352 (2017). https://doi.org/10.1080/15325008.2017.1338794https://doi.org/10.1080/15325008.2017.1338794

25. Kukker, A., et al.: Reinforcement learning based genetic fuzzy classifier for transformer faults. IETE J. Res. (in Press). https://doi.org/10.1080/03772063.2020.1732844
26. Mishra, S., et al.: Fuzzy reinforcement learning based intelligent classifier for power transformer faults, in Press. ISA Trans. (2020). https://doi.org/10.1016/j.isatra.2020.01.016https://doi.org/10.1016/j.isatra.2020.01.016

An Innovative Fuzzy Modelling Technique for Photovoltaic Power Generation Farm's Failure Modes and Effects Analysis

Vivek Kumar Tripathi, Arush Singh, Atul Jaysing Patil, and Yog Raj Sood

Abstract The yield of a photovoltaic system is highly influenced by its consistent operation without any unexpected shutdown. The availability of this system is vastly dependent on the unhindered and trouble-free operation of the various components incorporated in the photovoltaic system. These components have interdependence among each other, and their coordinated operation provides the most optimum result promised to the grid and consumers. An investigation is conducted in this research for the identification of the most prominent causes of failures in the components of a photovoltaic system. Subsequently, using crisp data associated with various failure modes, a fuzzy-logic-based FMEA model is also developed for risk assessment and maintenance prioritization. Particular attention is given to address the drawbacks of the conventional FMEA approach and a comparative analysis between the conventional and fuzzy-based FMEA approach improving the reliability and performance of the system. This research will be assist researchers, practising engineers from utilities and agencies dealing with risk assessment and maintenance prioritization of photovoltaic power generation farm.

Keywords Photovoltaic · Failure Mode (FM) · Detection (D) · Severity (S) · Occurrence (O) · Fuzzy inference system (FIS)

V. K. Tripathi · A. Singh (✉) · A. J. Patil · Y. R. Sood
Department of Electrical Engineering, NIT Hamirpur, Hamirpur, HP 177005, India
e-mail: arushsingh.contact@gmail.com

V. K. Tripathi
e-mail: vivek.vt95@gmail.com

A. J. Patil
e-mail: atul2322nith@gmail.com

Y. R. Sood
e-mail: yrsood@gmail.com

© The Author(s), under exclusive license to Springer Nature Singapore Pte Ltd. 2021   361
H. Malik et al. (eds.), *AI and Machine Learning Paradigms for Health Monitoring System*, Studies in Big Data 86,
https://doi.org/10.1007/978-981-33-4412-9_22

1 Introduction

Integration of renewables to an electric power system has its own associated challenges. Solar power generation farms are renewable energy generation units whose capacity depends upon the availability of solar irradiance. These farms span over a large landmass and require frequent maintenance for their reliable operation. Failure in a solar farm due to mal-operation of various components deteriorates the availability of the grid. Quantization of the frequency of occurrence, their associated severity and the ease with which they can be detected is used as a collaborative indicator for risk assessment of various failure modes (FMs) in a solar farm while using failure mode and effects analysis (FMEA). Initially, FMEA originated as a tool for failure analysis in the aerospace industry, but soon it became a critical element of defence, chemical, nuclear, electrical and electronics industries. FMEA is a flexible risk assessment tool for proactive FM identification and maintenance prioritization. The conventional FMEA approach involves a product of three crisp values consisting of occurrence (O), severity (S) and detection (D) and terms it as risk priority number (RPN). This multiplicative risk assessment strategy has several inherent limitations, for instance, possibility of assignment of same RPN values for different O, S and D values and significant variation in RPN values with small deviation in O, S and D.

In [1], it is observed that FMEA has its satisfactory performance in finding solutions for proper working of a rooftop PV system, while it is observed that conventional FMEA models having discrete values for rate of failures are basically dependent on the geographical region of installation the method used. In [2], it is evident that using FMEA a stage-dependent system developed to prioritize various compensation solution and their effectiveness for the matching risks discussed by them. Also, it can be concluded that FMEA approach can be applied simultaneously on individual as well as sets of measures under the resource constraints. The theoretical background related to a typical photovoltaic farm is discussed in [3–6], and methods for performing FMEA are discussed in [7]. Thus, going by existing literature so far, a dedicated fuzzy methodology for FMEA of photovoltaic power generation farm does not exist and have the potential to augment the risk assessment methodology for a typical photovoltaic power generation farm.

In this research, a fuzzy-modelling-based FMEA strategy is developed for risk assessment and removing causes for such by setting priority. For this purpose, the solar farm is firstly segregated into various components and subsequently FMs for each component are identified. Thereafter based on expert assigned values for O, S and D, a fuzzy model for risk assessment and maintenance prioritisation is developed. In order to create a fuzzy model, membership functions are assigned to O, S and D values, and a fuzzy rule base of 125 rules is made for the calculation of the RPN. The Mamdani inference technique is used for fuzzy linguistic inference if–then rules, and the centroid methods are used for defuzzification.

The proposed method to the creation of a fuzzy model is enlightened upon in Sect. 2 of this paper. The description of the various FMs, along with their respective effects and control mechanisms, is discussed in Sect. 3. The main design of the fuzzy model, which includes the development of a rule base, expert evaluation and maintenance prioritisation, is discussed in Sect. 4. Finally, in Sect. 5, the model is applied by collecting data on failure of the solar power generation farm supplying electricity.

2 Proposed Approach for PV Generation Farm's FMEA

For performing FMEA, the PV generation farm is initially segregated into its various subcomponents, and their respective FMs are identified along with their effects and control measures. Subsequently, O, S and D values are given to each FM. Formulation of membership function for O, S, D and RPN is based on crisp values in [8–11]. Thereafter, fuzzy RPN is computed for each FM, and maintenance work is prioritized accordingly. The flowchart highlighting the proposed FMEA approach is shown in Fig. 1.

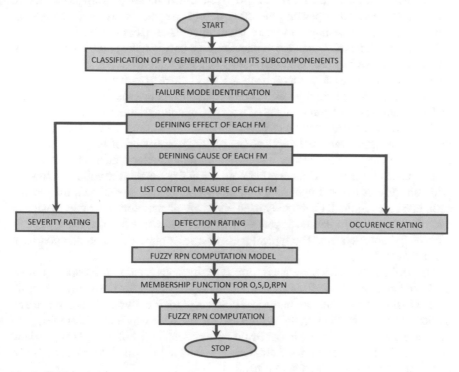

Fig. 1 FMEA model developing algorithm

3   FMs in a Typical Solar Power Generation Farm

A solar PV system uses the principle of photovoltaics for generation of usable power. The system is an assembly of different components and subcomponents with the sole purpose of absorption of solar power and its conversion to usable electrical energy in the most optimized manner. The system uses an inverter for conversion of output DC power to AC by means of several accessories like mounting cabling and monitoring equipment for the formation of an overall working system. The core part of a solar PV system is the solar panel as it converts photons energy directly into usable electrical form by means of crystalline silicon cells, thin film cells and organic multijunction cells. The individual cell has a very low voltage generation, so cells are arranged in series/parallel forming a solar array. A charge controller controls the flow of charges in the solar cell, i.e. it basically manages overcharging and undercharging of solar cells by directing the voltage and current through the cells. Maximum Power Point Tracking (MPPT) is a technique through which maximum utilizable energy is collected through the solar array and stored in the batteries.

The MPPT system uses resistors to track down the maximum power point throughout the variable power generation output. As per the generation systems, location cables are designed to be resistant towards temperature fluctuations and UV radiations. The cables are the connecting link between the components of a PV system, thus collecting the generated energy and storing it in batteries; they are unaffected by temperature and climate changes. PV system uses rechargeable batteries for storage during low-demand periods and later usage of the generated energy during high-demand periods. Commonly used battery technologies are valve-regulated lead acid, lithium ion, nickel cadmium batteries, etc. Applications where AC current is must such as grid-connected applications require conversion of the DC-generated energy to AC requires an inverter, and the PV system inverter synchronizes the alternating current frequency with the grid frequency and maintains the voltage below the grid voltage. For optimal operation and protection against breakdown, monitoring equipment are required. Commonly used photovoltaic monitoring strategies depend upon the output and its nature. Separate smart meters measure the total energy generation of PV array system. The typical parts of a solar photovoltaic generation farm are shown in Fig. 2.

For performing FMEA, the solar farm is firstly segregated into separate components, and their respective FMs are identified. Subsequently, for assessment of the O, S and D values, an exhaustive analysis is conducted for the causes of occurrence of a particular FM, their effect on the system and the methods which can be employed to minimize the impact of a particular FM on the system. A list of 29 FMs is provided in Table 1 for FMEA of a typical solar power generation farm. Additional FMs can be seamlessly added to the model if needed.

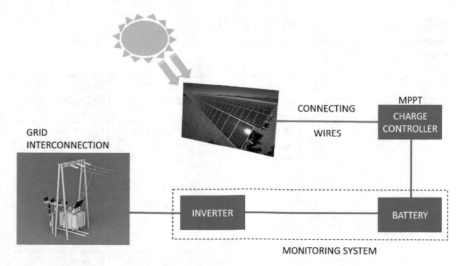

Fig. 2 Typical parts of a solar photovoltaic generation farm

4 Fuzzy FMEA Model Formulation

Any fuzzy model has five functional blocks (fuzzy inference unit, rule base, database, decision making unit and a defuzzification unit) which are helpful in developing a fuzzy inference system (FIS). Triangular and trapezoidal membership functions are used for formulation of various membership functions using crisp values shown in [11, 20–23]. The membership functions for O, S, D and RPN are shown in Figs. 3, 4, 5 and 6, respectively.

Mamdani FIS, proposed by Ebhasim Mamdani in 1975, is chosen as the inference engine for this model due to its ability to train with limited number of rules when compared to Sugeno FIS. A set of 150 if–then rules constitutes the rule base for the fuzzy model. These rules are shown in Table 3 (Appendix). Centroid method is used for defuzzification in this model. Figure 7 shows the fuzzy model.

The output surface plots are shown in Fig. 8, 9 and 10, respectively.

For maintenance and assessment by experts prioritization, traditional and fuzzy RPN values are calculated for each FM, and a comparative analysis of maintenance prioritization is performed in Table 3.

5 Fuzzy Model Implementation

For implementing the fuzzy FMEA model and performing a comparable analysis on traditional and fuzzy FMEA, based upon exhaustive analysis and data collected from [12–16, 18–23], a hypothesis is performed on identification of typical FMs of PV. Figure 11 shows an illustrative distribution of the malicious components.

Table 1 Determination of failure modes [6, 12–18]

Component name and ID	Failure mode (FM) name and ID	Description	Effect	Controls
PV panel (CMP1)	Orientation failure of panels (FM1)	Improper geographical site due to lack of data	Decrement in output energy	Use sun trajectories and solar tracker data
	Short circuiting of bypass diode (FM2)	Material defects/lightning and surges	Decrement in open-circuit voltage produced	Proper material selection/lightning and surge protectors
	Improper connection of bypass diode (FM3)	Due to lack of maintenance and improper connection of batteries	PV panel mal-operation	Proper maintenance and battery operation
	Terminal failure (FM4)	Slack connections and corrosion	Arcing, electric shocks and prone to hazards	Regular maintenance and proper material selection
	Connection failure (FM5)	Forced/pressurized connections	Arcing, electric shocks and prone to hazards	Proper maintenance and installation practices
	Cracking of panels (FM6)	Vandalism, improper material and site selection	Electric shocks and prone to hazards	Proper care and fragile handling with hail storm prevention
	Failure in proper panel mounting (FM7)	Improper geographical site selection and mounting practices	Damage to panels and mounting hazards	Proper maintenance practices and material selection
	Heat fading of panels (FM8)	MPPT failure and PV module failure	Decrement in open-circuit voltage produced	Proper MPPT testing and shading tests
Inverter and charge controller (CMP2)	IC control failure (FM9)	Low quality and design deficiency	Battery damaging	Proper design and quality selection
	Short circuiting (FM10)	Connection problems	Protection equipment failure	Proper maintenance guide and procedures
	Electrical connection failure (FM11)	Inoperable material/connector failure	Incomplete circuit and no current flow	Proper protection equipment usage and load calculation study
	Overloading (FM12)	Inoperable or defective heat sink	PCB failure and fire hazards	Operational inspections and proper material selection

(continued)

Table 1 (continued)

Component name and ID	Failure mode (FM) name and ID	Description	Effect	Controls
	MPPT failure (FM13)	Controller operational failure	Low energy generation	Effective controller selection
	Decreased voltage output (FM14)	Leads to overloading and battery failure	Low output voltage	Load flow and study of power flow calculations with proper material selection
	Overheating (FM15)	Inoperable or defective heat sink	PCB failure and fire hazards	Operational inspections and proper material selection
	Terminal failure due to burning or corrosion (FM16)	Inoperable connections corrosion and overheating	Arcing, electric shocks and prone to hazards	Proper and regular maintenance and trained operators
Battery (CMP3)	Casing failure due to swelling and breaking (FM17)	Excessive charging	High injury probability	Inspectional control
	Dusty or corroded battery connectors (FM18)	Corrosion and improper maintenance and cleaning	High battery discharge	Proper and regular maintenance and trained operators
	Sulfation of battery (FM19)	Low charging and stagnant operation	Deterioration in battery performance	Battery charging and field test
	Improper or reverse connection of battery (FM20)	Polarization and indexing problem	Incomplete circuit	Inspectional control and testing
	Failure due to reduced capacity (FM21)	Ageing and lifespan problem	Low output voltage production	No available control
	Failure due to low-voltage battery operation (FM22)	Ageing and lifespan problem	Low energy output production	No available control

(continued)

Table 1 (continued)

Component name and ID	Failure mode (FM) name and ID	Description	Effect	Controls
	Drained or discharged battery (FM23)	Complete lifespan and aged battery	No output	No available control
Protection and monitoring system (CMP4)	Fuse wire faulty operation (FM24)	Overloaded usage and improper maintenance	No response on overloading and overheating	Proper maintenance and protection equipment testing
	Resolution problem of measuring instruments (FM25)	Underrated and improper calibrated instrument usage	Improper testing results	Calibrated and proper rated instrument usage
	String module problem (FM26)	Connection failure between adjacent panels and improper arrangement of PV array	Low voltage and energy generation	Proper mounting and array arrangements
Connecting wire (CMP5)	Overloading of wires (FM27)	Due to system fault and conductor high conductivity	Fire hazards and overheating	Protection equipment usage, testing and maintenance
	Failure of insulation (FM28)	Mechanical damage	No power output due to short circuiting and shock/ fire hazards	Proper packaging and handling
	Failure of conductors (FM29)	Twisting and flexing of wires	No output power developed as open circuited	Control through continuous testing

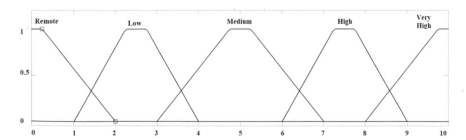

Fig. 3 Occurrence rated membership function

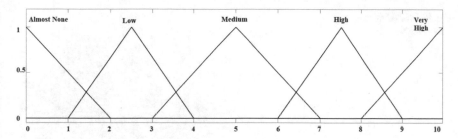

Fig. 4 Severity rated membership function

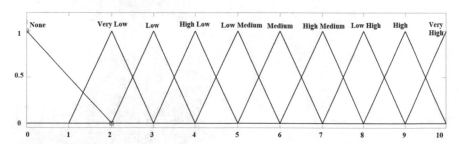

Fig. 5 Detection rated membership function

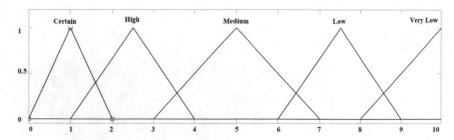

Fig. 6 RPN rated membership function

Fig. 7 RPN computating fuzzy model

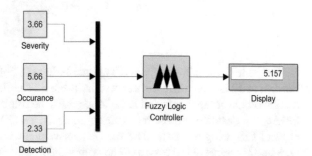

Fig. 8 Plot (O versus D versus RPN)

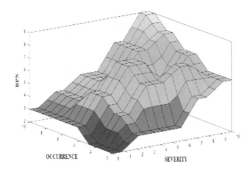

Fig. 9 Plot (O versus S versus RPN)

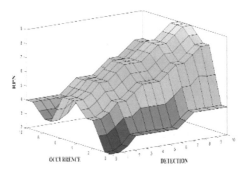

Fig. 10 Plot (D versus S versus RPN)

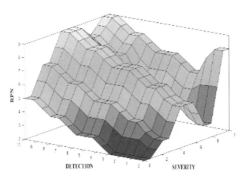

The FMEA sheet is established by considering the failure data set and the identification of FMs from different surveys in Table 3. The FMEA sheet provides information on the components that are likely to fail, the role of the FM type, the cause of failure, the obstacle and the recognition controls. The FM is defined by the knowledge of FIS using this data. The fuzzy RPN values are determined by the average O, S and D values of the experts. The comparative analysis of one-tenth of the standard RPN and fuzzy RPN is shown in the table. The FMEA sheet is established by considering the failure data set and the identification of FMs from different surveys in Table 3. The FMEA sheet provides information on the components that are likely to fail, the role of the FM type, the cause of failure, the obstacle and the recognition

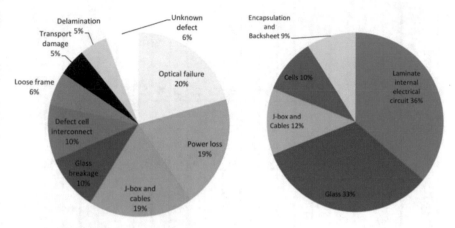

Fig. 11 PV generation farm components' failure percentages [13]

controls. The FM is defined using this data by the information of the fuzzy inference method. The fuzzy RPN values are determined by the average O, S and D values of the experts. The comparative analysis of values obtained by both is visualized in Table 2 (Fig. 12).

Later, the accepted procedures and acts are carried out, and the ambiguous RPN values are updated and re-calculated. The revision of the fuzzy RPN values is based on the quantification of the results of the prescribed behaviour using the method set out in Table 18. The comparative comparison of the original and updated values by the proposed method can be visualized in Fig. 13.

6 Conclusion

Solar farm productivity can be greatly enhanced by recognizing failure modes and proactively prioritizing maintenance action. Solar farms employ a wide range of components whose reliable operation is necessary to improve overall availability. A fuzzy-based FMEA model is built using modified and more practical data that not only eliminates the limitations of conventional RPN computational logic, but also offers predictive repairs and steps based on comprehensive and thorough condition monitoring. A stable and productive system is built where faults and defects are dramatically reduced depending on the importance of maintenance work. In case of the usual insufficiency modes occurring at a solar farm using this fluid-flow model, the insufficiency and effect analysis (FMEA) sheet is developed and the approach to prioritize maintenance is also explained. This logic of FMEA will be helpful for designers to test practises for appropriate maintenance of photovoltaic power generation plants.

Table 2 Assessment by experts for O, S and D ratings

FM CODE	EXPERT 1			EXPERT 2			EXPERT 3			RPN	Prioritization by RPN	Fuzzy RPN	Prioritization by fuzzy RPN
	O	S	D	O	S	D	O	S	D				
FM5	4	8	9	4	6	7	3	7	8	205.3333	3	7.419	1
FM13	4	5	6	3	6	7	4	7	7	146.6667	9	7.259	2
FM7	4	8	8	4	7	7	5	7	8	243.6296	1	7	3
FM4	4	8	9	4	7	7	5	6	7	232.5556	2	7	4
FM25	5	4	6	4	5	6	4	4	6	112.6667	11	7	5
FM24	4	4	5	5	5	5	5	6	4	108.8889	12	7	6
FM11	2	9	5	2	8	6	3	5	6	96.96296	13	7	7
FM10	2	9	5	2	7	5	3	5	7	92.55556	14	7	8
FM3	2	9	4	3	8	5	3	7	4	92.44444	15	7	9
FM27	3	8	3	2	8	4	3	7	5	81.77778	18	7	10
FM26	6	4	3	5	4	4	6	4	4	83.11111	17	6.596	11
FM19	3	8	3	2	7	4	3	7	4	71.7037	20	6.596	12
FM29	2	8	4	1	7	6	2	7	5	61.11111	21	6.378	13
FM16	4	9	4	3	9	5	4	8	5	148.2963	8	6.131	14
FM8	4	9	4	3	8	5	4	8	5	142.5926	10	5.872	15
FM22	4	9	6	3	7	5	4	7	5	149.9259	6	5.868	16
FM28	1	9	5	1	8	5	2	7	6	56.88889	22	5.849	17
FM20	1	9	4	1	8	5	2	7	4	46.22222	25	5.849	18
FM9	3	9	2	3	8	3	4	7	5	88.88889	16	5.61	19
FM1	3	6	2	4	6	3	4	5	2	48.48148	24	5.581	20

(continued)

Table 2 (continued)

FM CODE	EXPERT 1			EXPERT 2			EXPERT 3			RPN	Prioritization by RPN	Fuzzy RPN	Prioritization by fuzzy RPN
	O	S	D	O	S	D	O	S	D				
FM15	1	8	3	1	6	4	2	7	4	34.22222	28	5.507	21
FM14	1	8	3	2	6	4	2	5	7	49.25926	23	5.22	22
FM21	5	9	7	4	8	5	4	7	5	196.4444	4	5	23
FM23	5	9	4	5	7	5	6	8	4	184.8889	5	5	24
FM18	4	9	4	4	8	5	4	7	5	149.3333	7	5	25
FM12	3	8	3	4	7	2	4	8	3	74.96296	19	4.868	26
FM6	1	8	5	1	7	6	2	4	5	45.03704	26	4.852	27
FM2	1	7	5	2	6	4	1	6	6	42.22222	27	4.852	28
FM17	1	9	2	2	7	2	1	7	4	27.25926	29	4.849	29

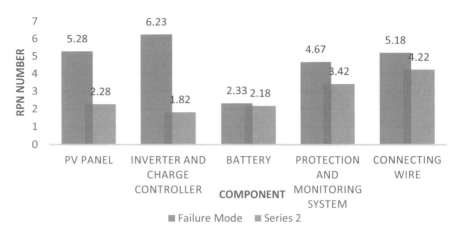

Fig. 12 Fuzzy versus one-tenth of conventional RPN values

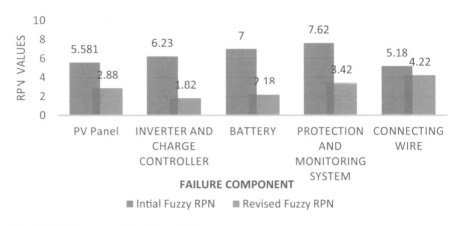

Fig. 13 Initial versus updated fuzzy RPN values

Appendix

See Table 3.

Table 3 FMEA worksheet

S. No.	Component	Functions	Failure Mode	Failure Effect	Controls	Risk ratings (fuzzy-model)				Revised risk (fuzzy-model)			
						O	S	D	RPN	O	S	D	RPN
1	PV panel	To convert light energy into electrical energy	Orientation failure of panels	Decrement in output energy	Use sun trajectories and solar tracker data	3.67	5.67	2.33	5.581	1	3	4	2.88
2	Inverter and charge controller	Conversion of output dc power to ac	Short circuiting	Protection equipment failure	Proper maintenance guide and procedures	3.33	7.33	4.33	6.23	1	4	2	1.82
3	Battery	To store electric power	Casing failure due to swelling and breaking	Excessive charging	High injury probability	2.33	7	5.67	7.00	1	4	3	2.18
4	Protection and monitoring system	To ensure reliable operation	Resolution problem of measuring instruments	Underrated and improper calibrated instrument usage	Improper testing results	4.67	6.67	8.33	7.62	1	5	6	3.42
5	Connecting wire	To establish electric connection	Failure of insulation	Mechanical damage	No power output due to short circuiting and shock/fire hazards	5.33	6.33	2.67	5.18	1	5	6	4.22

References

1. Basu, J.B.: Failure modes and effects analysis (FMEA) of a rooftop PV system. Int. J. Sci. Eng. Res. (IJSER) **3**(9) (2015)
2. Valdes, M.E.: Adapting failure mode and effects analysis (FMEA) to select hazard mitigation measures. In: IEEE Conference on Petroleum and Chemical Industry Conference (PCIC), pp. 1–10 (2014)
3. Czanderna, A.W., Jorgensen, G.J.: Service lifetime prediction for encapsulated photovoltaic cells/minimodules. In: AIP Conference Proceedings, pp. 295–311 (1997)
4. Feldman, D., Barbose, G., Margolis, R., Bolinger, M., Chung, D., Fu, R., Seel, J., Davidson, C., Wiser, R.: Photovoltaic system pricing trends: historical, recent, and near-term projections. In: 2015, NREL/PR-6A20–64898. March 2015
5. Renewable Energy Policy Network for the 21st century (REN21), Renewables 2010 Global Status Report, Paris, 2010, pp. 1–80, Document Available at: https://www.ren21.net/Portals/0/documents/activities/gsr/REN21_GSR_2010_full_revised%20Sept2010.pdf
6. Woofenden, I.: Photovoltaic... cell, module, string, array (PDF). Word Power Publication, pp. 106–107 (2006)
7. Bian, J., Sun, X., Yang, X.: Failure mode and effect analysis of power transformer based on cloud model of weight. TELKOMNIKA Telecommun. Comput. Electron. Control **13**(3), 776–782 (2015)
8. Franzen, A., Karlsson, S.: Failure modes and effects analysis of transformers. KTH Electrical Engineering. Stockholm, Sweden. Document Available At: Available: eeweb01.ee.kth.se/upload/publications/reports/2007/TRITA-EE-2007–040.pdf
9. Filo, G., Fabiś-Domagała, J., Domagała, M., Lisowski, E., Momeni, H.: The idea of fuzzy logic usage in a sheet-based FMEA analysis of mechanical systems. MATEC Web Conf. 183 (2018). https://doi.org/10.1051/matecconf/201818303009
10. TaufiqImmawan, W.S., Rachman, A.K.: Operational risk analysis with Fuzzy FMEA (Failure Mode and Effect Analysis) approach (Case study: Optimus Creative Bandung). In: The 2nd International Conference on Engineering and Technology for Sustainable Development (ICET4SD 2017), vol. 154 (2017)
11. MIL-STD-1629A, Military standard: procedures for performing a failure mode, effects, and criticality analysis. Every Spece, NOV 1980, Document Available At: https://everyspec.com/MIL-STD/MIL-STD-1600-1699/MIL_STD_1629A_1556/
12. Marc, K., Sarah, K., Corinne, P., Karl, A.B., Kazuhiko, K., Thomas, F., Haitao, L., Iseghem, M.V.: Review of failures of photovoltaic modules. International Energy Agency Photovoltaic POWER Systems Programme, Document Available At: https://iea-pvps.org/fileadmin/dam/intranet/ExCo/IEA-PVPS_T13-01_2014_Review_of_Failures_of_Photovoltaic_Modules_Final.pdf.
13. DeGraaff, D., Lacerda, R., Campeau, Z.: Degradation mechanisms in si module technologies observed in the field; their analysis and statistics. Presentation at PV Module Reliability Workshop, NREL, Denver, Golden, USA (2011). Document Available At: https://www1.eere.energy.gov/solar/pdfs/pvmrw2011_01_plen_degraaff.pdf
14. IEC Standard International Electro technical Commission (IEC) 61215: 2nd edn, 2005: Crystalline Silicon Terrestrial Photovoltaic (PV) Modules—Design Qualification and Type Approval, 2nd edn, 2005-04
15. IEC Standard International Electrotechnical Commission (IEC) 61646: 2nd edn, 2008: Thin-Film Terrestrial Photovoltaic (PV) Modules—Design Qualification and Type Approval, 2 edn, 2008-05
16. IEC Standard International Electro technical Commission (IEC) 61730-2: "Photovoltaic (PV) module safety qualification—Part 2: Requirements for testing, 1st edn, 2004-10
17. Schulze, K., Groh, M., Nieß, M., Vodermayer, C., Wotruba, G., Becker, G.: Untersuchung von Alterungseffektenbeimonokristallinen PV-Modulenmitmehrals 15 BetriebsjahrendurchElektrolumineszenz- und Leistungsmessung, Proceedings of 28. Symposium PhotovoltaischeSolarenergie, (OTTI, Staffelstein, Germany, 2012)

18. Honecker, S.L., Yenal, U.: Quantifying the effect of a potential corrective action on product life. In: IEEE Conference 2017 Annual Reliability and Maintainability Symposium (RAMS), pp. 1–5 (2017)
19. Mughal, S.N., Sood, Y.R., Jarial, R.K.: A review on Solar Photovoltaic technology and future trends. Int. J. Sci. Res. Comput. Sci. Eng. Inf. Technol. (IJSRCSEIT-2018) **4**(1) (2018). ISSN: 2456-3307
20. Hassan, M.S., Mughal, M.S., Jarial, R.K., Sood, Y.R.: A comparative analysis of different maximum power point tracking algorithms of solar photovoltaic system. In: Applications of Computing, Automation and Wireless Systems in Electrical Engineering. Lecture Notes in Electrical Engineering, vol. 553, pp. 217–229. Springer, Singapore
21. Mughal, S., Sood, Y.R., Jarial, R.K.: Design and techno-financial analysis of solar photovoltaic plant. In: School of Engineering and Technology at BGSB University, Rajouri (J&K).Applications of Computing, Automation and Wireless Systems in Electrical Engineering. Lecture Notes in Electrical Engineering, vol. 553, pp. 231–243. Springer, Singapore
22. Patil, A.J., Singh, A., Jarial, R.K.: A novel fuzzy based technique for transformer health index computation. In: International Conference on Advances in Computing, Communication and Control (ICAC3), pp. 1–6 (2019)

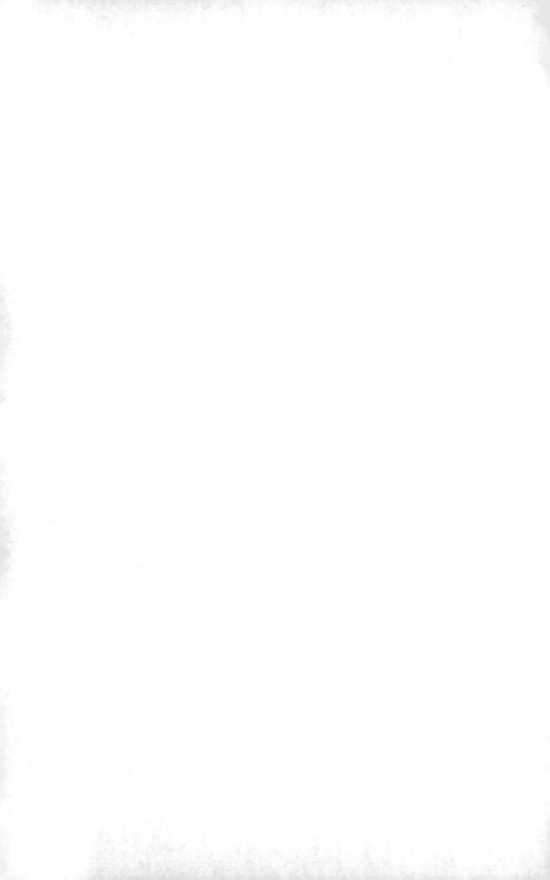

Analysis and Application of Nine-Level Boost Inverter for Distributed Solar PV System

Deepak Upadhyay, Shahbaz Ahmad Khan, Mohammad Ali, Mohd Tariq, and Adil Sarwar

Abstract In this chapter, a nine-level multilevel topology based on the switched capacitor technique which is capable of boosting the output voltage to twice the input voltage is presented for distributed solar PV system. There is no need for an external balancing circuit as the topology has the characteristic of inherently balance the capacitors. There is lower voltage stress at the switches incorporated and which makes it more cost-effective. Also, in this chapter, the integration of two PV modules with the grid is done and the simulation results validating the boosting capability and the low total harmonic distortion at the output side are presented.

Keywords Boost converter · PV distributed system · Multilevel inverter · High power applications · Solar energy

1 Introduction

MVSIs have come up as power inverter in different applications in UPS, renewable energy systems, machine drives, and active power filters. Recently, established topologies like neutral point converter (NPC), flying capacitor (FC), and cascaded inverter topologies (CHB) were the first generations of multilevel inverter topologies [1, 2]. Earlier attempts were made to increase the levels of output voltage levels.

D. Upadhyay · S. A. Khan · M. Ali · M. Tariq (✉) · A. Sarwar
Department of Electrical Engineering, Z.H.C.E.T, Aligarh Muslim University, Aligarh, India
e-mail: tariq.ee@zhcet.ac.in

D. Upadhyay
e-mail: deepak.dsta@gmail.com

S. A. Khan
e-mail: shahbazkhan8067@gmail.com

M. Ali
e-mail: mohad_ali92@yahoo.com

A. Sarwar
e-mail: adil.sarwar@zhcet.ac.in

© The Author(s), under exclusive license to Springer Nature Singapore Pte Ltd. 2021   379
H. Malik et al. (eds.), *AI and Machine Learning Paradigms for Health Monitoring System*, Studies in Big Data 86,
https://doi.org/10.1007/978-981-33-4412-9_23

Amid the modular MVIs, latest topology packed U cell (PUC) inverter is catching lots of interest because of its merits over the previous well-established topologies [3, 4]. Hybrid of flying capacitor and cascaded H-bridge in which U cell was placed compactly was modified further. PUC using six switches was initially designed, and then some modifications were done to improve its voltage level and THD percentage. It has 6 switches and 1 capacitor to generate seven-level voltage by using a capacitor voltage to one-third of the capacitor voltage to generate seven-level output voltage. The main issue with the packed U cell is voltage balancing capability which is deteriorated as the U cells are increased [5]. The second problem is designing of voltage controllers in a control strategy. Another single-phase multilevel inverter topology and many advances in its features are packed E cell which has only seven switches and two capacitors balanced at $V_{dc}/4$ and in turn the DC link of $V_{dc}/2$. This inverter generates nine-level output voltage, and capacitor voltages are charged and discharged instantaneously. In addition to that, reduction of the voltage stress across the switches which results in a reduction rating of the switch also remains concern of the researchers. These efforts result in the need of the filters, cut down of cost and space requirements. In spite of a myriad of multilevel topologies already been introduced but still comprehensive work is being carried out to propose promising topology. For instance, the present investigated multilevel inverter topology which has been presented in the chapter [6–8] uses a switched capacitor approach. Although a noticeable cut down in the number of devices is attained in this MLI as compared to traditional ones, there is a requirement of H-bridge for the generation of bipolar voltages. This results in the sudden increase in the standing voltage and hence the cost of switches.

In the presented nine-level inverter topology for a single-phase system, switches having the low peak inverse voltage (PIV) are being employed [6]. Also, there is a reduction in the number of devices and cost of implementation compared to conventional/leading edge. In addition to that, the presented topology faces no issue with capacitor balancing as the capacitor charging is inherently self-balancing in nature [7, 8]. Due to its ability to effectively boost the voltage, the topology finds various applications in UPS, electric drives, grid-tied non-conventional energy resources (such as solar and wind energy conversion systems), particularly in the systems where the low voltages at the input side are needed to boost up to attain the admissible voltage.

The chapter is divided into five sections. In Sect. 2, a description of the circuit topology and the modification carried out in the circuit are discussed. In Sect. 3, the control strategy used, and the pulse width modulation technique is being explained. In Sect. 4, various simulation results (output voltage and current and the associated total harmonic distortion) are explained through simulation results. In the end, conclusions are explained Sect. 5.

2 Nine-Level Boost Inverter Topology

In the following chapter, an inverter based on the switched capacitor technology has been presented, which has the ability to produce nine levels stepped waveform having the magnitude of output voltage levels equal to zero, twice, thrice, half and same as that of input voltage(Vs) in both positive and negative directions ($\pm 2V_s$, $\pm 1.5V_s \pm V_s \pm 0.5V_s$, and 0). The presented topology consists of 12 switches, 2 capacitors (C1 & C2), and a single DC source at the input side with the additional ability of regenerative ability. The voltage can be step up to twice the applied voltage at the input side (Fig. 1).

This can be achieved by the series connection of the already charged capacitors. The most striking feature of the configuration is that the voltage stress across all of all the switches is the same as that of V_{in} except S7, S8, and S12 switches which need to block only half of the applied voltage (V_{in}). The inverter generates a bipolar voltage at the output and does not use H-bridge at the end. This capability of the switch has been considered as a very useful feature as lower the voltage rating of the switch, lesser the cost.

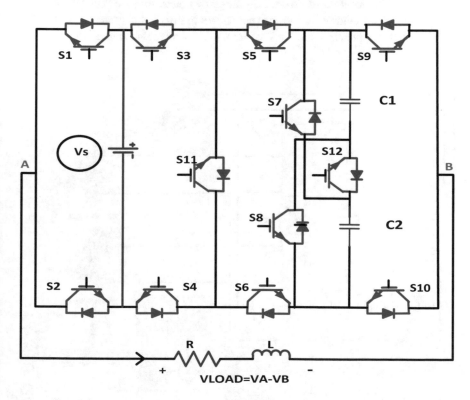

Fig. 1 Nine-level boost inverter topology for PV distribution application

As the electrical energy generation from renewable energy resources (sources like solar energy, wind energy, micro-hydro turbines, etc.) experience a boost in the recent decade and the penetration of these in the grid increase, because which the necessity of technology required for their integration is soon realized. In this chapter, three PV modules having the voltage equal to V_{in}, 0.5 V_{in}, and 0.5 V_{in} are employed to obtain the output voltage boosted two times as that of the PV module having voltage V_{in}.

3 Integrated Photovoltaic Distributed System

3.1 System Description

Renewable energy has a great demand in this modern era of the energy crisis, and solar energy demand is accelerating with its unbeatable advantages. One of the major advantages is distributed PV system can be easily incorporated in the micro- and mini gird. PV sources of different power and voltage rating can be easily connected to this investigated nine-level boost inverter topology by connecting PV panel of different voltage ratings. Its controls and circuit are shown in Fig. 2. Solar panel 1 is of 200 V and the other two panels 2 and 3 are of 100 V. They are connected across the place

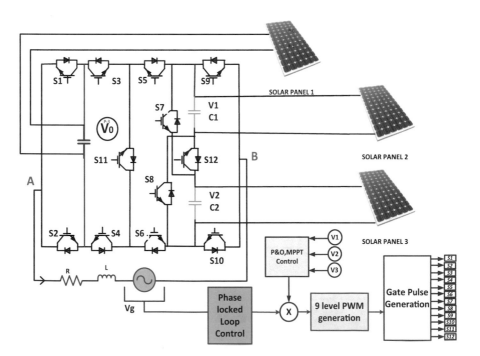

Fig. 2 Grid-connected PV distributed system with its control blocks

of three sources that are to be connected in the investigated topology. P&O and Maximum Power Point Tracking (MPPT) control are used to maintain constant and maximum output from solar panels. Phase-locked loop control is used to control the power factor of the grid voltage and current fed by inverter. Voltages V1, V2, and V3 are controlled by closed-loop control strategy and maintained at terminals of topology. When all other parameters are incorporated the reference, a signal is generated which is used to generate the Nine PWM signals, and finally, gate pulse is generated for all switches and gate pulse generation is shown in Fig. 3. Nine-level PWM is generated by using half parabola carrier wave so that the pulse generated to follow the capacitor charge and discharge waveforms.

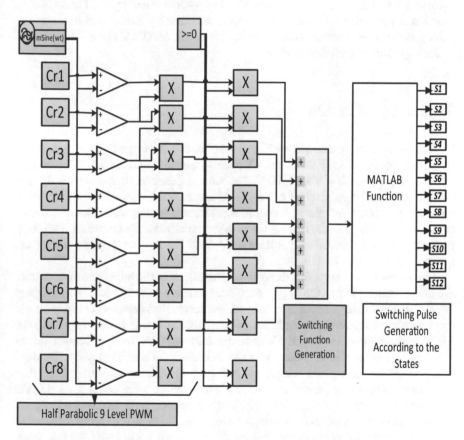

Fig. 3 Nine-level PWM generation and switching gate pulse generation

3.2   Control Strategy and PWM Generation

The control strategy for controlling the topology is depicted in the block diagram. Eight vertically shifted half parabolic carriers are generated for generating nine states, and this wave is them compared with sinusoidal signal of the fundamental frequency of 50 Hz and unit magnitude and frequency of carrier wave are 4000 Hz. After comparing, the new pulse output is achieved for every level within the range from 0 to 1. For changing the levels to desired states, these pulse signals are now used to oscillate between different states by using the way switches and proper gate logic. In the next stage, we get nine-level output pulses from 0–1, 1–2, 2–3, 3–4 upper half cycle and 0 to −1, −1 to −2, −2 to −3, −3 to −4 lower half cycle. The switching function is generated by adding these values and making them input to switching pulse generation according to the switching table. The MATLAB function is used to create logic for the different switches.

4   Simulation Results

Simulation is done to show the effectiveness of the investigated topology in the integration of distributed PV sources, PV panels are used in multiples, 24 V connected in series to generate 200 V and 100 V. The voltage generated in nine levels of peak voltage 400 V and current of 3.9 A. Multilevel inverters are known for their harmonic reduction capability and directly controlling current harmonics, and also, the size of components required in the passive filters is very small as we increase the switching frequency. In our simulation, we have used 2000 Hz frequency, and still, we are getting under the standard limit.

Simulation results show that the voltage waveforms of the integrated system have not much changed in fact the ripples have been reduced as was in the actual chapter. We are getting a voltage boost of two times, and current has become very smooth and came within the required standard. The calculated current was 4 A, and it came to be 3.95 A voltage approximately 396 V and expected was 400 V. It can be seen clearly in Fig. 4. that the power factor of the grid is approximately 0.9 which is a great advantage of applying this topology for integration. In Figs. 5 and 6, harmonic analysis is given for both synchronizing current and voltage and readings were taken for a specific load. Voltage THD percentage is 9.62%, and the current THD percentage is 1.53% which is the biggest advantage of using this topology. Also, we can see that the value THD percentage has a significant peak on 2000 Hz, as it is the switching frequency which is as per the desired parameters.

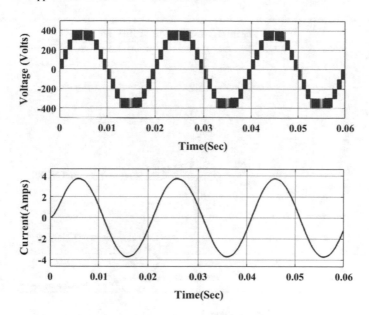

Fig. 4 Load voltage and current waveforms for specified load

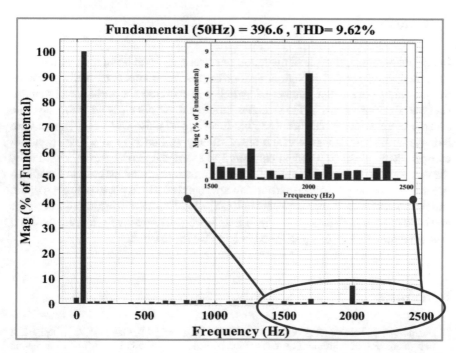

Fig. 5 Harmonic spectrum for load voltage

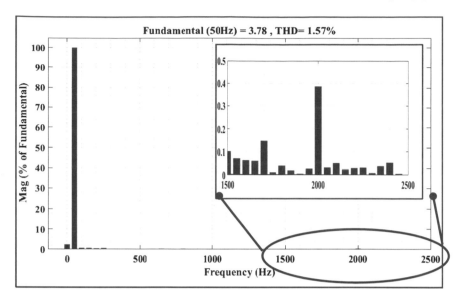

Fig. 6 A Harmonic spectrum for load current

5 Conclusions

In this chapter, the principle of operation of novel nine-level boost inverter has been presented and confirmed through simulation results. The comparative analysis reveals that not only the smaller number of switches is required for a nine-level genera-tion but also the ratings of the switches employed are also less which makes this inverter comparatively cheaper. The nine-level hybrid pulse width modulation with half parabolic carrier waves which are vertically shifted is used which results in comparatively lower THD when compared to triangular carrier waves. Ultimately, the very low total harmonic distortion in the output voltage and the current waveform is verified. The output voltage and current are found nearly in phase with each other, and the power factor is approximately unity. The total harmonic distortions in voltage and current are 9.62% and 1.57% (% of fundamental), respectively, and are depicted through simulation results performed in MATLAB/Simulink.

References

1. Bharatiraja, C., Selvaraj, R., Chelliah, T.R., Munda, J.L., Tariq, M., Maswood, A.I.: Design and implementation of fourth arm for elimination of bearing current in NPC-MLI-Fed induction motor drive. IEEE Tran. Ind. Appl. **54**(1), 745–754 (2018). https://doi.org/10.1109/TIA.2017. 2759204
2. Bharatiraja, C., Munda, J.L., Bayindir, R., Tariq, M.: A common-mode leakage current mitiga-tion for PV-grid connected three-phase three-level transformerless T-type-NPC-MLI. In: 2016

IEEE International Conference on Renewable Energy Research and Applications (ICRERA), Birmingham, pp. 578–583 (2016). https://doi.org/10.1109/ICRERA.2016.7884401

3. Sharifzadeh, M., et al.: Hybrid SHM-SHE pulse-amplitude modulation for high-power four-leg inverter. IEEE Trans. Ind. Electron. **63**(11), 7234–7242 (2016). https://doi.org/10.1109/TIE.2016.2538204

4. Tariq, M., Meraj, M., Azeem, A., Maswood, A.I., Iqbal, A., Chokkalingam, B.: Evaluation of level-shifted and phase-shifted PWM schemes for seven level single-phase packed U cell inverter. CPSS Trans. Power Electron. Appl. **3**(3), 232–242 (2018). https://doi.org/10.24295/CPSSTPEA.2018.00023

5. Upadhyay, D., Khan, S.A., Tariq, M.: Design and simulation of front end converter based power conditioning unit. In: International Conference on Emerging Trends in Electro-Mechanical Technologies and Management, New Delhi, India (2019)

6. Saeedian, M., Pouresmaeil, E., Samadaei, E., Manuel Godinho Rodrigues, E., Godina, R., Marzband, M.: An innovative dual-boost nine-level inverter with low-voltage rating switches. Energies **2**, 207 (2019)

7. Sebaali, F., Vahedi, H., Kanaan, H.Y., Moubayed, N., Al-Haddad, K.: Sliding mode fixed frequency current controller designed for grid-connected NPC inverter. IEEE J. Emerg. Select. Topics Power Electron. **4**(4), 1397–1405 (2016)

8. Sharifzadeh, M., Vahedi, H., Sheikholeslami, A., Labbé, P., Al-Haddad, K.: Hybrid SHM–SHE modulation technique for a four-leg NPC inverter with DC capacitor self-voltage balancing. IEEE Trans. Industr. Electron. **62**(8), 4890–4899 (2015)

Performance Evaluation of a 500 kWp Rooftop Grid-Interactive SPV System at Integral University, Lucknow: A Feasible Study Under Adverse Weather Condition

Ahmad Faiz Minai, T. Usmani, and Atif Iqbal

Abstract Currently, power generation using solar PV source is in advance stage in India. Government policies and subsidies attract citizens of India to install solar PV system at their commercial and domestic places. Some of the design models and tariffs are also very favorable for them, such as RESCO and CAPEX. To cope with the world in the field of power generation using renewable sources, Integral University opt a RESCO model to install 1 MW rooftop grid-interactive solar PV system. In this paper, a feasibility study of 500kWp is done under adverse weather condition, i.e., in every month of January for last 3 years because maximum variation of temperature and insolation takes place in this month and that is why the system generates minimum amount of energy. Comparison of real data through SCADA with solar PVGIS and PVSYST is also presented in this paper with the complete description of installed system and detailed results at different temperature and insolation at the end.

Keywords Rooftop · SPV system · Grid-interactive · SCADA · Solar PVGIS · PVSYST · Performance ratio

1 Introduction

High demand of power and limitation of non-renewable energy sources has triggered the researcher to develop new means of power generation using solar energy, which comes under the non-conventional source of energy [2]. The scope of power generation using sun in India is incredible. The geographical location is the main cause behind it because most of the places in India receive solar insolation throughout the year, which is about 3000 h of daylight form sun. This is equivalent to 5000 trillion kWh or more. In fact 3–7 kWh/m^2-day of solar radiation is received by India

A. F. Minai (✉) · T. Usmani
Integral University, Lucknow, India
e-mail: fzminai@gmail.com

A. Iqbal
Qatar University, Doha, Qatar

© The Author(s), under exclusive license to Springer Nature Singapore Pte Ltd. 2021   389
H. Malik et al. (eds.), *AI and Machine Learning Paradigms for Health Monitoring System*, Studies in Big Data 86,
https://doi.org/10.1007/978-981-33-4412-9_24

[7]. According to the National Solar Mission, India has tremendous goal to achieve giant grid-interactive sun-based power generation systems, with a total assembled capacity of 20,000 MW by 2020 [5]. At Integral University, apart from 30 to 40% revenue saving the plant abates around 700 tons of carbon dioxide annually and reduces emissions from grid power and backup diesel generators. For power generation, solar photovoltaic (PV) panels are used which are made of semiconductor material that can convert radiant energy of sun into electricity [3, 4].

These solar photovoltaic (PV) panels can give a safe, less maintenance, eco-friendly, and reliable option of energy for a large duration throughout the year [1, 6, 8]. Some other examples are I [9, 10]. The performance of 500 kWp rooftop grid-interactive solar PV plant at Integral University for the month of January is carried out in this work because at this site, January has the maximum temperature and insolation variation, which results as adverse weather condition for solar PV system. The following objectives are fulfilled in this paper.

1. To investigate the occasional variations in the response of solar PV system using solar PVGIS planner.
2. To assess the technical response through assessment of daily yield of energy, using the installed SCADA system and study for adverse weather condition.
3. To analyze the real daily data response of the monitored SCADA data system with PVSYST and solar GIS planner.

2   Overview of the Rooftop Grid-Interactive SPV Plant

2.1   Geographical Description of the Site

Integral University is located in Lucknow, Uttar Pradesh, India. From the last two years, a 500 kWp rooftop grid-interactive system is in working condition. This plant was installed under RESCO model. The latitude of the site is 26.95°, and longitude is 80.99°. Tilt angle and orientation of the modules for the given plant are 15⁰ facing the South.

2.2   Overall Plant Description

A 500 kWp grid-interactive rooftop SPV system is installed through RESCO model at phase-1 Integral University. Total number of 1877 panels are used of 320 Wp each. Different ratings of inverters, i.e., 20 kVA, 25 kVA, and 66 kVA, are used according to the requirement. Earth pits and lightening arresters are provided as per the need for protection. Specification of the modules which are installed in all four buildings is same but there are different number of modules present on the rooftop of the building, i.e., 400 in Medical Block Phase-1, 340 in Academic Block-4, 417

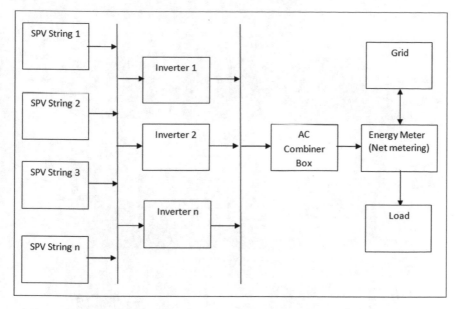

Fig. 1 Rooftop SPV Grid-Interactive General Plant Layout at Integral University

in Academic Block-2, and 720 in Academic Block-1. Figure 1 shows general layout of the SPV system installed at each four buildings.

3 Methodology and Data Monitoring

Whole year study of 500 kW rooftop grid-interactive solar PV plant at Integral University reveals that the variation of temperature and insolation is very high in the month of January. So this month is selected for the analysis for the adverse weather condition. Also in the study of complete year, lowest solar insolation and energy generation are recorded through data monitoring system as well as through the software PVSYST and PVGIS which is also presented in results and discussion section. At the site, data monitoring has been done through supervisory control and data acquisition (SCADA) system installed with the SPV system. This system has recorded the daily energy generation for the year 2018, 2019, and 2020 and is shown in Fig. 2 specifically for the month of January including performance ratio (PR), whereas the PR of the system is the ratio of final yield (Y_f) to the reference yield (Y_r).

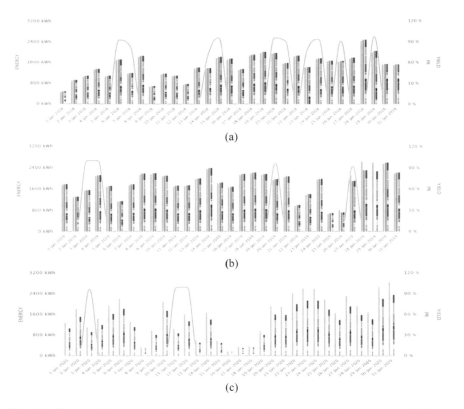

Fig. 2 Daily recorded energy and PR using SCADA for the year **a** 2018, **b** 2019, and **c** 2020

4 Results and Discussions

4.1 Energy Generation at Different Temperature and Insolation

For the month of January, following data of energy generation is recorded which matches the energy generation data from solar GIS planner and PVSYST. This shows that the different plant factors like its functioning, installation, maintenance, and site selection has been done very carefully. The energy generation is near about 50000kWh for the year 2018, 2019, and 2020 in January which is a month of adverse weather condition (for Lucknow region) for solar plant clearly shows that in other months generation is much higher than this and installer gets payback in very less time. Figure 3a shows total energy generation in the month of January for the year 2018, 2019, and 2020. Variation in energy takes place due to variation in temperature and insolation which is comparatively shown in Fig. 3b–d.

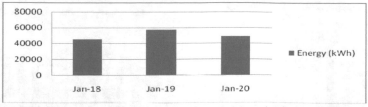

(a) Total Encrgy Generation for January, recorded through SCADA (Yearly)

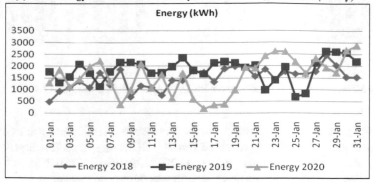

(b) Total Energy Generation for January, recorded through SCADA (Daily)

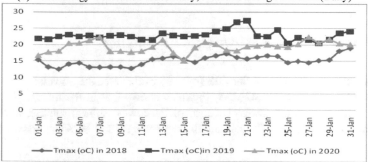

(c) Temperature (T_{max}) for January, recorded through SCADA (Daily)

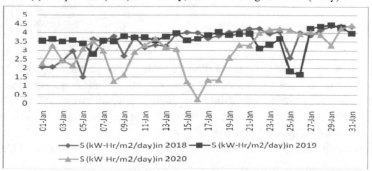

(d) Insolation (S) for January, recorded through SCADA (Daily)

Fig. 3 Data recorded through SCADA

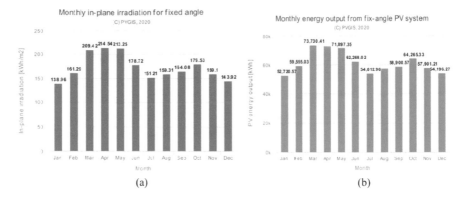

Fig. 4 a Monthly in-plane irradiation and **b** Energy output at the site using PVGIS

Energy generation is increasing with the increase in solar insolation and decrease in tempearature. Real data is recorded through SCADA system for the month of January over the period of three years (i.e., 2018, 2019, and 2020). Figure 4 shows the recorded energy generation at different temperature and insolation.

4.2   Simulation Using Solar GIS-PV Planner

Simulation is done through solar GIS for the given site of the university to validate the recorded data through SCADA. Figure 4 shows that in the month of January, energy generation is the lowest because of the lowest solar insolation at the site. These results of solar PVGIS validate the recorded data of SCADA installed at the site.

4.3   Simulation Using PVSYST

For the given site, recorded data is also validated through very reputed software PVSYST which is used for the study and assessment of SPV systems. Using this software attempt is made to calculate the energy generation and PR of the plant. According to Fig. 5, the normalized energy generation in the month of January is lowest, when it is compared with the other months.

Performance ratio of the different months throughout the year is also shown in Fig. 5.

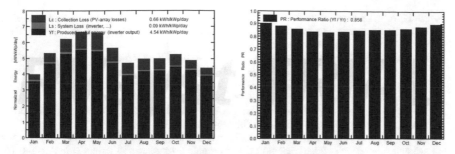

Fig. 5 Normalized Energy Generation and Performance Ratio (PR) using PVSYST

5 Performance Comparison

It is seen from the solar PVGIS planner and PVSYST that the plant generates minimum energy in the month of January. The response obtained from the installed SCADA system is analyzed with solar PVGIS planner and PVSYST Software. The responses are presented in Figs. 3, 4, and 5. The real performance of the system is identical with the performance of solar PVGIS and PVSYST simulation software throughout the study.

6 Conclusion

The analysis done in this paper is for only month of January, 2018, 2019, and 2020. January is taken because whole year study reveals that this month has the adverse weather condition for solar PV plant (for the given site). On the other hand, it is also proved that the generation is high at low temperature and high insolation. The average energy generation is near about 50,000 kWh (i.e., 45,761 kWh in Jan. 18, 57,278 kWh in Jan. 19, and 49,123 kWh in Jan. 20). Although for the whole year the recorded average PR of the plant is 86%, the system losses are about 14%. Actual recorded data through the SCADA is also validated through simulated performance of solar PVGIS planner and PVSYST. The authors are highly thankful to the authority of the Integral University, Lucknow, for accessing the data used in this study.

References

1. Dondariya, C., Porwal, D., Awasthi, A., Shukla, A, K., Sudhakar, K., Manohar, S.R.M., Bhimte, A.: Performance simulation of grid-connected rooftop solar PV system for small households: a case study of Ujjain, India. Energy Rep. **4**, 546–553 (2018)
2. Goura, R.: Analyzing the on-field performance of a 1–641 megawatt-grid –tied PV system in South India. Int. J. Sustain. Energy **34**, 1–9 (2015)

3. Hioki, A.T., da Silva, V.R.G.R., Vilela Junior, J.A., Loures, E.D.F.R.: Performance analysis of small grid connected photovoltaic systems. Braz. Arch. Biol. Technol. **62**(spe), e19190018 (2019). ISSN 1678-4324 Online Edition
4. Kumar, S.B., Sudhakar K.: Performance evaluation of 10 MW grid connected solar photovoltaic power plant in India. Energy Rep. **1**, 184–192 (2015)
5. Ministry of New and Renewable Energy, Solar energy in India. https://mnre.gov.in/schemes/decentralized-systems/solar-systems. 12 Feb 2014
6. NASA Homepage: https://power.larc.nasa.gov/downloads/POWER_SinglePoint_Daily_201 90101_20190131_026d88N_080d93E_30bd2446.txt
7. Sudhakar, K., Srivastava, T., Satpathy, G., Premalatha, M.: Modelling and estimation of photosynthetically active incident radiation based on global irradiance in Indian latitudes. Int. J. Energy Environ. Eng. **4**(21), 2–8 (2013)
8. Shuvho, M.B.A., Chowdhury, M.A., Ahmed, S., Kashem, M.A.: Prediction of solar irradiation and performance evaluation of grid connected solar 80KWp PV plant in Bangladesh. Energy Rep. **5**, 714–722 (2019)
9. Minai, A.F., et al.: Metaheuristics paradigms for renewable energy systems: advances in optimization algorithms. In: Springer Nature Book: Metaheuristic and Evolutionary Computation: Algorithms and Applications. Studies in Computational Intelligence (2020). https://doi.org/10.1007/978-981-15-7571-6_2
10. Mahto, T., et al.: Condition monitoring and fault detection & diagnostics of wind energy conversion system (WECS). In: Springer Nature Book: Soft Computing in Condition Monitoring and Diagnostics of Electrical and Mechanical Systems, pp. 121–154 (2019). https://doi.org/10.1007/978-981-15-1532-3_5

Fuzzy Logic-Based Cycloconverter for Cement Mill Drives

Iram Akhtar and Sheeraz Kirmani

Abstract In cement mill application, the different equipments are used to grind the solid clinker from the furnace into the fine powder. Further, in a cement mill drives, different motors are used with frequency and voltage converters. Besides, the frequency of produced electricity is 50 Hz in India, which is not useful in many applications. Many drives need the variable frequency than the constant frequency such as cement mills drives. Therefore, it is required to get the variable frequency and variable voltage for proper operation of the cement mills. The cycloconverters are widely used for this purpose, as it is not possible to change a number of poles during the operating condition. The cycloconverter output voltage and frequency can be changed uninterruptedly using a fuzzy logic based control circuit. In this chapter, the fuzzy logic controller is used to control the output of the converter. This work shows how to get variable voltage and frequency to control the cement mill drives with the help of a fuzzy-based controller. Hence, an idea of controlling the cement mill drives with the fuzzy controller has been given in the chapter so the complete system is made in such a manner that it is efficient and reliable. Further, results show the effectiveness of the proposed scheme.

Keywords Cement mills drives · Cycloconverter · Fuzzy logic controller

1 Introduction

In cement mill applications, different types of motors are used which require AC power for proper operation. The AC power at one frequency is changed into an AC power at a different frequency with the help of cycloconverter without having the converter–inverter combination. The converter–inverter combination makes the

I. Akhtar (✉) · S. Kirmani
Department of Electrical Engineering, Faculty of Engineering & Technology, Jamia Millia Islamia, New Delhi 110025, India
e-mail: akhtariram12@gmail.com; iram1208@gmail.com

S. Kirmani
e-mail: sheerazkirmani@gmail.com

system heavy and complicated; hence, the proper choice is cycloconverter which is used to run the AC motors in cement mill drives. There are two types of cycloconverter available in the market, step-up and step-down cycloconverter. These cycloconverters have a switch which can be controlled by different controllers like PI, PID, PD, fuzzy logic, model predictive controller to control the output of the cycloconverter. In this chapter, the fuzzy logic controller is used to controlling the output of cycloconverter or input of the different AC machines used in the cement mill drives. Whereas in industries, the speed control of induction motor is very important, because many industries use the induction motor, but it very important to take care of the efficiency of the machine while controlling the machine. There are so many ways to control the speed of induction motor, i.e., by changing the poles of induction motor or by using the inverter circuit. The changing of poles in the running condition of the motor is not worthy, and inverter circuit needs the DC supply for their operation. Hence, firstly AC power is converter into the DC power with the help of controlled rectifier, and then this DC power is given to the inverter circuit; this needs two-step conversions. Again this is not a good choice to control the output of induction motor [1]. Induction motors are very useful and hence used in many applications like domestic, industrial, and commercial purpose. The cycloconverter has a switch, and by controlling the on–off period of switches, the output voltage and frequency of cycloconverter are controlled. The pulse modulation technique can be used to control the switching sequence that is required to permit the current to off naturally without any distortion. The earlier used techniques need the large inductors to less the undesired current, thus cooperating efficiency [2]. The pulse width modulation method can control the output voltage of cycloconverter even in the case of the undesired input voltage. This method can be applied for any type of cycloconverter. Another important factor in cyclolconverter is switching losses, because there so many switches, hence are switching losses. To control the switching losses, different techniques are used. In fact, the change of switch type also affects the losses. Pulse width modulation technique also reduces the switching losses. The proper pattern of switching can reduce switching losses. In electric traction applications, cycloconvertes are used to control the input voltage and frequency of the AC motors, and earlier times, DC motors are used in traction drive. But due to the advancement of the power electronics devices, the speed of AC motors is controlled in the wide range. In fact, this is cost-effective solution for traction applications [3], whereas, sometime, the power electronics devices are also failed to work properly due to an undesired breakdown in the device. The failure also detects using different techniques nowadays [4]. Integration of different sources to the grid is also an important issue in power system [5–8]; hence, keeping above-mentioned points, cycloconverters are used to control the drives in the cement mill application. Further, in this chapter, cycloconverter is controlled by a fuzzy logic controller circuit; this reduces the harmonic distortion and increases the efficiency of the system. It is confirmed by the outcomes that the proposed technique gives the best results for cement mill applications.

In this chapter, the three-phase to three-phase cycloconverter in cement mill drives is presented in Sect. 2. In Sect. 3, the control strategy of three-phase to three-phase cycloconverter for cement mill drives is described. Results and discussion are defined in Sect. 4. Finally, concluding statements are offered in Sect. 5.

2 Three-Phase to Three-Phase Cycloconverter in Cement Mill Drives

Cycloconverter is basically used to converter input power at one frequency into output power at the desired frequency in one stage change. In step-up cycloconverter, the output frequency is more than the input frequency, whereas, in step down cyclocon-verter, the output frequency is lower than the input frequency. The AC motor when operates in lower frequency gives better results; hence, cycloconverter can be used to control the output of AC motors. The cycloconverter can be used in induction heating, VAR compensation, etc. In the three-phase to three-phase cycloconverter, three sets are connected which are displace 120° to each other. There are so many ways to get the three-phase to three-phase cycloconverter to take the best results in cement mill applications. As the number of switches increase, the magnitude of the output voltage is changed; hence, this circuit changes the frequency and voltage.

Figure 1 shows the three-phase to three-phase cycloconverter for cement mill drives with employing 18 switches. These switches are controlled with a fuzzy logic controller circuit. This circuit gives good changes in the output voltage; hence, the input of motor can be varied in a wide range. This circuit is basically a dual converter but runs as to get an AC voltage. Each switch in a circuit works as a controlled

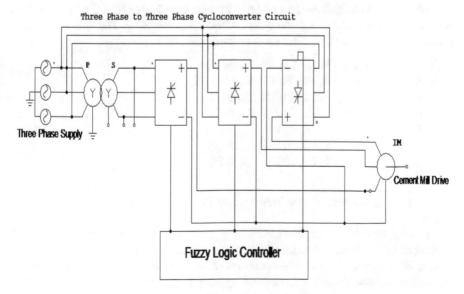

Fig. 1 Three-phase to three-phase cycloconverter for cement mill drives

rectifier with a variable firing angle range. Hence by controlling the switches of cycloconverter, the input of the AC motor in cement mill drives can be controlled.

3   Control Strategy of Three-Phase to Three-Phase Cycloconverter for Cement Mill Drives

The simple control method is employed for controlling the cement mill drives by the help of fuzzy logic controller based cycloconverter. The fuzzy logic technique is the best one that improves the general design with expertise [9–11]. The fuzzy logic use can provide help for hard mathematical modeling. It is dissimilar from classical logic, and the main goal of this technique is modeling based on inexact and vague information.

The fuzzy logic controller gives the reference signal which is used to produce the gate pulses after comparing with the carrier signal. In the suggested work, the controller system gets the reference signal V_{drf} from the error signal (i.e., AC output voltage and desired voltage) and the change of error signal. To get the suggested controller, error signal E_{rr} and change of error signal E_{ch} are taken as the inputs of the controller and reference signal V_{drf} are selected as the output of the controller which is the reference signal to produce the firing pulses for the cycloconverter switches. The triangular membership functions are taken for the input and output fuzzy sets, and the linguistic variables are defined as negative peak (NP), negative moderate (NM), negative low (NL), zero (ZX), positive low (PL), positive moderate (PM), and positive peak (PP).

The pulse width modulation can be achieved, which produces the firing pulses for the switches in the fuzzy logic-controlled cycloconverter. The fuzzy rules are presented by the IF–THEN rules as described below:

IF E_{rr} is NP and E_{ch} is NP THEN V_{drf} is NP
IF E_{rr} is NP and E_{ch} is NM THEN V_{drf} is NM
IF E_{rr} is NP and E_{ch} is NL THEN V_{drf} is NP
IF E_{rr} is NP and E_{ch} is ZX THEN V_{drf} is ZX
IF E_{rr} is NP and E_{ch} is PL THEN V_{drf} is NL
IF E_{rr} is NP and E_{ch} is PM THEN V_{drf} is PL
IF E_{rr} is NP and E_{ch} is PP THEN V_{drf} is PL
And so on.

The 49 rules are described in Table 1, and Fig. 2 is to get the preferred reference signal.

Many applications require the variable frequency than the constant frequency such as cement mills drives. Consequently, it is compulsory to acquire variable frequency and variable voltage for suitable operation of the cement mills. So, three-phase to three-phase cycloconverter is controlled by a fuzzy logic-based controller, and this

Table 1 Fuzzy rule table

V_{drf}		Error (E_{rr})						
		NP	NM	NL	ZX	PL	PM	PP
Change of error (E_{ch})	NP	NP	NM	NL	NL	PL	NL	PP
	NM	NM	NM	NL	ZX	PL	ZX	PM
	NL	NP	NP	NM	PL	ZX	PM	PL
	ZX	ZX	NL	ZX	PL	PM	PP	ZX
	PL	NL	ZX	PL	PM	PM	PM	PP
	PM	PL	PM	PL	PP	PP	PP	PM
	PP	PL	PM	PP	PP	PP	PP	PP

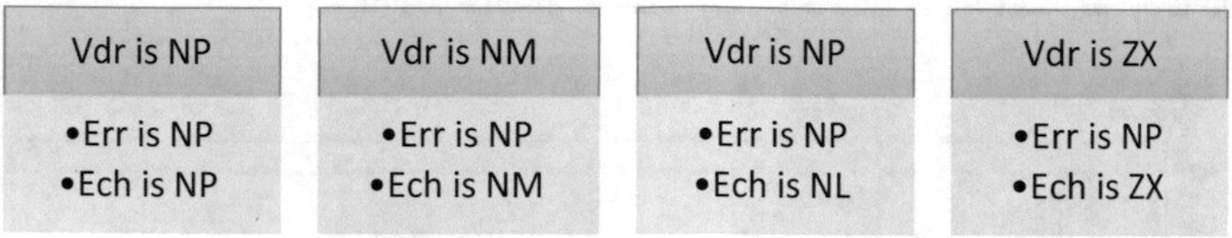

Vdr is NP
•Err is NP
•Ech is NP
Vdr is NM
•Err is NP
•Ech is NM
Vdr is NP
•Err is NP
•Ech is NL
Vdr is ZX
•Err is NP
•Ech is ZX

Fig. 2 Fuzzy rules to control the cycloconverter

V3
400
200
0
-200
-400
0
0.1
0.2
0.3
0.4
Time (s)

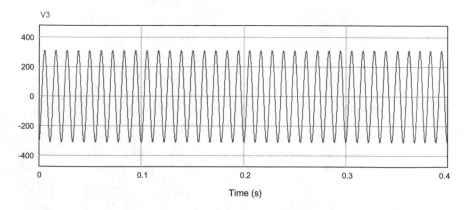

Fig. 3 Input voltage of cycloconverter with frequency 90 Hz (Phase a)

controller also reduces the harmonic distortion and hence rises the efficiency of the entire system.

4   Results and Discussions

Figures 2 and 3 show the waveform of input voltage at 90 Hz and output voltage
15 Hz, respectively. As these figures, it can be said that the output voltage frequency
is less than the input voltage frequency. Since the cycloconverter load is induction
motor, but the output voltage contains low harmonic distortion because of using a
fuzzy-based controller. Hence, cycloconverter acts as a harmonic mitigation device
which provides less number of harmonic distortion in comparison with no controller.
The THD of the output voltage is 3.45% which is under the suitable range.

Figures 4 and 5 show the waveform of input voltage at 150 Hz and output voltage
25 Hz, respectively. Therefore, it can be seen from these figures that the output
voltage frequency is less than the input voltage frequency. The THD of the output
voltage for this case is 2.62% which is under a suitable range.

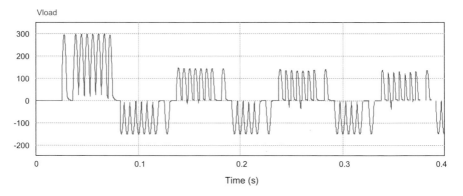

Fig. 4 Output voltage of cycloconverter with frequency 15 Hz (Phase a)

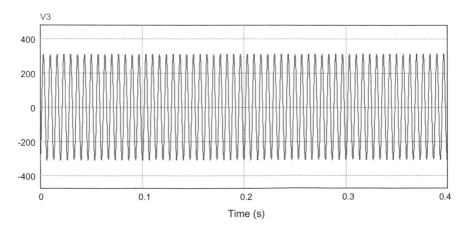

Fig. 5 Input voltage of cycloconverter with frequency 150 Hz (Phase a)

The outcomes show that the proposed fuzzy logic-based control method can provide the desired value of output voltage and frequency to control the cement mill drives. As it can be seen from Figs. 3, 4, 5 and 6 that output and input voltage frequencies are different. The output of cycoloconveter is applied to the input of induction motor, as voltage and frequency vary; the speed of induction motor also varies. Hence, this is the best solution to control the cement mill drives.

The input and output voltage waveforms are presented for phase an only because of the complexity of the circuit. Figures 7 and 8 show the harmonic spectrum analysis of the output voltage at frequency 15 Hz and 25 Hz, respectively. These figures show that by using the proposed techniques, harmonics also reduce. The pulse modulation technique can also be applied to control the sequence of the switches that are required

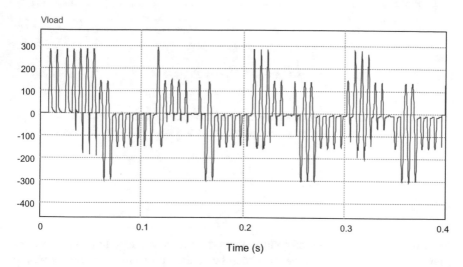

Fig. 6 Output voltage of cycloconverter with frequency 25 Hz (Phase a)

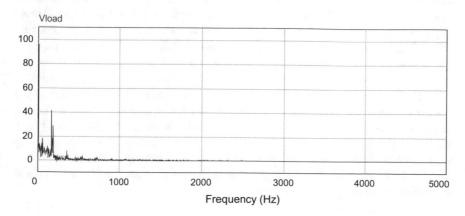

Fig. 7 Harmonic spectrum at output voltage frequency 15 Hz

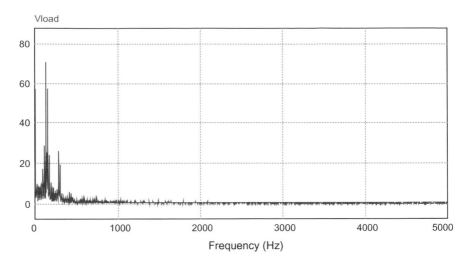

Fig. 8 Harmonic spectrum at output voltage frequency 25 Hz

to control the output voltage and frequency of the cycloconverter, but it needs a large circuit. Hence, fuzzy logic control approach is the best solution for cement mill drives.

5 Conclusion

An effective fuzzy logic-based control method for three-phase to three-phase cyclo-converter for cement mill drives has been presented in this chapter. The proposed technique can provide the desired output voltage and frequency even with unbalanced cycloconverter input voltages. Further, the harmonic can be reduced with this method and cycloconverter acts as a harmonic mitigation device. The proposed technique effectively controls the speed of AC motors which are used in cement mill drives. The proposed control technique promises that there is no circulation current and higher value of harmonic contains in the output of the cycloconverter. As, the cycloconverters are generally used in many drives, as it is not possible to change the operating condition of the drives. Hence, this circuit easily controls the output of drives in terms of speed. The cycloconverter output voltage and frequency can be changed uninterruptedly using a fuzzy logic-based control circuit. This work displays how to acquire flexible voltage and frequency to control the cement mill drives using the fuzzy-based controller. Therefore, an idea of adjusting the cement mill drives with the fuzzy controller has been given in the chapter; consequently, results show the usefulness of the proposed scheme.

References

1. Lole, P.R., Adhav, K.D., Gholap, S.D., Karkade, S.R., Medewar, P.G.: Speed control of induction motor by using cyclo-converter. IOSR J. Electr. Electron. Eng., 50–54 (2017)
2. Balog, R.S., Krein, P.T.: Commutation technique for high-frequency link cycloconverter based on state-machine control. IEEE Power Electron. Lett. **3**, 101–104 (2005)
3. Babaei, E., Heris, A.A.: PWM-based control strategy for forced commutated cycloconverters. In: 2009 IEEE Symposium on Industrial Electronics & Applications (ISIEA 2009)—Proceedings, vol. 2, pp. 669–674 (2009)
4. Kirmani, S., Jamil, M., Akhtar, I.: Effective low cost grid-connected solar photovoltaic system to electrify the small scale industry/commercial building. Int. J. Renew. Energy Res. **7**(2) (2017)
5. Akhtar, I., Kirmani, S., Jamil, M.: Analysis and design of a sustainable microgrid primarily powered by renewable energy sources with dynamic performance improvement. IET Renew. Power Gener. **13**(8), 1024–1036 (2019)
6. Kirmani, S., Jamil, M., Akhtar, I.: Economic feasibility of Hybrid Energy Generation with Reduced Carbon Emission. IET Renew. Power Gener. **12**(8), 934–994 (2018)
7. Asim, M., Tariq, A., Sarwar, A.: Simulation and analysis of a directly coupled solar PV based water pumping system. J. Electr. Eng. **2** (3) (2009)
8. Asim, M., Tariq, M., Mallick, M.A., Ashraf, I.: An improved constant voltage based MPPT technique for PMDC motor. Int, J. Power Electron. Drive Syst. (IJPEDS) **7**(4), 1330–1336 (2016)
9. Sharma, R., et al.: Reinforcement learning based Genetic fuzzy classifier for transformer faults. IETE J. Res. (in press). https://doi.org/10.1080/03772063.2020.1732844
10. Sharma, R., et al.: Fuzzy reinforcement learning based intelligent classifier for power transformer faults. ISA Trans. (2020). https://doi.org/10.1016/j.isatra.2020.01.016https://doi.org/10.1016/j.isatra.2020.01.016 in Press
11. Kushwaha, N., et al.: Paper insulation deterioration estimation of power transformer using fuzzy-logic: part-2. In: Proceedings of the IEEE International Conference on Engineering Sustainable Solutions, pp. 1–5, INDICON-2011. https://doi.org/10.1109/INDCON.2011.6139532

Comparative Control Study of CSTR Using Different Methodologies: MRAC, IMC-PID, PSO-PID, and Hybrid BBO-FF-PID

Neha Khanduja and Bharat Bhushan

Abstract This chapter presents different control methodologies for CSTR, i.e., continuously stirred tank reactor. More broadly two control methodologies, i.e., model-based controllers and optimization-based controllers are used. Model-based controllers, i.e., internal model controller (IMC) and model reference adaptive controller (MRAC) are used for time response analysis of CSTR and further two metaheuristic optimization-based methods, i.e., hybrid biogeography. Firefly optimization algorithm and particle swarm optimization (PSO) are applied on CSTR for a comparative study between model-based control and optimal control.

Keywords Model reference adaptive control · Particle swarm optimization (PSO) · Internal model control · Biogeography-based optimization (BBO) · Firefly optimization (FF)

1 Introduction

During the previous decades, there has been an incredible progression in the process control. Different control strategies, for example, fuzzy control, neural network control, model-based control, optimal control, etc., have been used for controlling purposes [1]. Practically all the modern procedure parameters change over time for different reasons like hardware change, change in working states of the units, change in showcase request. Subsequently, a regular control strategy may not give viable control of complex procedures where process parameter changes can happen essentially; however, it cannot be estimated or foreseen. The old-style control techniques are regularly a criticism technique which depends on checking the change in the process variable as for the set point and control intended for most pessimistic scenario conditions. Then again, versatile control systems are accessible where controller parameters or potential control structure are altered online as conditions change [2].

N. Khanduja (✉) · B. Bhushan
Delhi Technological University, New Delhi 110042, India
e-mail: nehakhanduja.dce@gmail.com

© The Author(s), under exclusive license to Springer Nature Singapore Pte Ltd. 2021   407
H. Malik et al. (eds.), *AI and Machine Learning Paradigms for Health
Monitoring System*, Studies in Big Data 86,
https://doi.org/10.1007/978-981-33-4412-9_26

Increasing complexity like a dead zone, saturation in process control is giving rise to the need for model-based controllers. An adaptive controller is a model-based controller that can alter its conduct in light of the changing elements of the process and the character of the unsettling influences. An adaptive framework has the most extreme application when the plant experiences advance or show nonlinearity and when the structure of the plant is unknown. Adaptivity is known as a control framework, which can change its parameter naturally to make up for varieties in the attributes of the procedure it control [3]. Another kind of model-based control is IMC having an open- and closed-loop frameworks. IMC tuning is alluded to as a tuning method dependent on the inside model rule [4].

The challenges related to utilizing scientific improvement for enormous large-scale process control issues have added to the advancement of alternative arrangements. Linear programming and dynamic programming procedures, for instance, frequently come up short (or arrive at nearby ideal) in taking care of NP-difficult issues with the enormous number of factors, what is more, nonlinear fitness or objective function. To defeat these issues, scientists have proposed developmental based calculations for looking at optimal solutions for issues [5].

The particle swarm optimization (PSO) which was first introduced by Kennedy and Eberhart [6] in 1995 is a parallel evolutionary computation method and based on the simulation of the social system of metaphors. It begins with the random population having random velocity and lead to an optimum solution with small computation time and stable convergence [7].

As of late, another idea of enhancement has been proposed by Simon in the year 2008. It is another populace-based transformative calculation. BBO has the element of sharing data between arrangements. The BBO calculation has a few favorable circumstances in contrast with different calculations [8].

The FF calculation which is created by Y. Xin-She in 2009 depends on the blazing qualities of fireflies. The FA is likewise ready to proficiently get local optima together with global optima [9]. Regarding optimization understanding [18, 19], can be referred by the reader.

Chapter is organized in following subsequent sections: Sect. 2 describes model reference adaptive controller, Sect. 3 explains IMC-PID controller; PSO, Hybrid BBO-FF is explained in Sects. 4, 5, and 6, respectively; CSTR is explained in Sect. 6; Simulink results and comparative analysis are done in Sect. 7.

2   Model Reference Adaptive Control (MRAC)

The MRAC framework is a significant controller. It might be viewed as a versatile servo framework in which the ideal execution is communicated as far as a source of the perspective model, which gives the desired output for the set point. This is an advantageous method to give detail for a servo issue. It consists of two feedback loops: one consists of process and controller and another one consists of adjustment mechanism [10].

2.1 MIT Rule

The MIT rule also termed as gradient strategy, changes the parameters dependent on the gradient of the error, concerning that parameter. The parameters are changed according to the negative error gradient. This implies on the off chance that the error concerning a predetermined parameter is expanding at that point by the MIT decide the estimation of that parameter will be decreased [1].

2.2 Lyapunov Rule

To design a controller using Lyapunov rule of MRAC, following steps are followed:

(1) Determine the controller structure; (2) Derive the error condition; (3) Find a Lyapunov condition; (4) Determine adaption law that fulfills the Lyapunov hypothesis [2, 10].

3   IMC-PID Controller

A progressively complete model-based plan technique, internal model control (IMC), was created by Garcia and Morari and Rivera et al. in 1982. The IMC strategy solves the issue of instability and vulnerability which is most common in an open-loop control framework. IMC controller is an invertible piece of plant. It has a solitary parameter for tuning, i.e., filter coefficient which makes IMC a simple and straightforward controller [11].

4   Particle Swarm Optimization (PSO)

PSO algorithm is motivated by the social conduct of living life forms in nature like a group of feathered creatures, the swarm of honeybees, the school of fish, and so on. Higher convertibility qualities inside a brief timeframe toward the optimality are the key point of PSO [12].

The execution of PSO starts with the generation of starting particles with arbitrary position and speed; fitness function calculation of every particle; calculate particle's personal best and populace global best; and finally, updated speed and position of the particle.

5   Biogeography-Based Optimization (BBO)

The BBO movement system is like the worldwide recombination approach of developmental systems in which numerous guardians can add to a solitary posterity. BBO relocation is utilized to change existing arrangements [13].

Following steps are followed for BBO.

1. Initialize the fitness function for the given optimization problem.
2. Introduce habitat variables randomly.
3. Perform BBO migration and mutation operation respectively and calculate HIS.
4. The emigration and immigration paces of every arrangement are helpful in probabilistically sharing the data between the habitats. Every arrangement can be changed with the territory change likelihood to yield great arrangement. Recompute HSI and change the habitats.
5. Check the halting criteria. If not accomplished, rehash from step 3.

BBO does not include the generation of arrangement as in GA. In every age, the recreation of each arrangement (environment) is used to discover the migration rates [14].

6   Firefly Optimization (FFO)

The firefly calculation (FA) is a metaheuristic advancement calculation that is organically motivated by their conduct. The firefly calculation as portrayed above uses themselves as the collaborating specialists of nature. The calculation is built up dependent on the accompanying guidelines:

1. The fireflies are pulled in to one another as they are unisex.
2. The appeal of the fireflies is corresponding to brilliance. Accordingly, the fireflies are pulled in and this movement depends on a more significant state of brilliance. The brilliance is conversely corresponding to separation.
3. The degree of brilliance speaks to the goal work esteem [9].

FA relies upon two significant components: the variety of the light force and the detailing of the attractiveness [15]. For effortlessness, we can expect that the allure of a firefly is controlled by its brilliance which thus is associated with the encoded target work.

7   Hybrid BBO-FF Algorithm

The essential inspiration driving hybridization of at least two calculations is to beat the limitations of individual calculation and to give indications of progress. It is in like manner required to find the nature of the half and half calculation so the investigation can be cultivated rapidly. Hybridization not just uses the upsides of both the computation yet keeps up a key good way from their inadequacy too. FA is used to find overall optima while BBO has an extraordinary blending trademark, and besides, it has an elitism method that holds the best plan. The accomplishment of any advancement calculation is in balancing among investigation and exploitation. The process begins with FFA and proceeds for a certain number of cycles to guarantee global optimality and afterward moved to BBO to assist speedy convergence and lead to the best arrangement [11].

8 Continuously Stirred Tank Reactor (CSTR)

CSTRs are significant gear in the substance and biochemical industry, having a differing scope of inquires for concoction and control building. The CSTR framework has the attributes of time fluctuating, nonlinear, and time delay [16].

Right now, control issue of a perfect CSTR framework (Fig. 1) is considered, where it is assumed that reaction is exothermic and irreversible first-order [17]:

$$f_1(C_A, T) = \frac{dC_A}{dt} = \frac{F}{V}(C_{Af} - C_A) - r \tag{1}$$

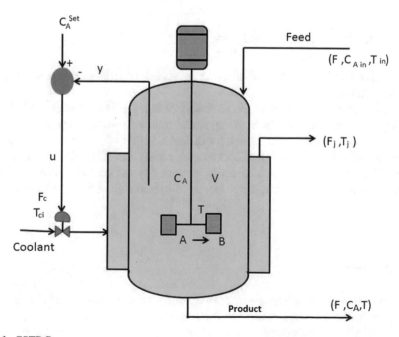

Fig. 1 CSTR Process

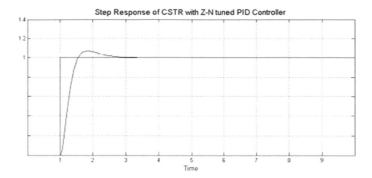

Fig. 2 ZN-PID Controller

$$f_2(C_A, T) = \frac{dT}{dt} = \frac{F}{V}(T_f - T) + \left(\frac{-\Delta H}{\rho c_p}\right)r - \frac{UA}{V\rho c_p}(T - T_j) \qquad (2)$$

The kinetic rate law is given by:

$$r = k_0 \exp\left(\frac{-\Delta E}{RT}\right)$$

9 Simulation Results and Discussion

The comparative investigation of different types of the controller is organized in the following manner:

Figure 2 gives the output of CSTR with ZN tuned PID controller, and Figs. 3 and 4 give the output of CSTR by using model reference adaptive control, i.e., MIT rule and Lyapunov rule, respectively, for different values of γ. Figures 5 and 6 give the output of CSTR with PSO-PID controller and hybrid BBO-FF-PID controller. Different time response specifications for various types of controllers are presented in Table 1. Figure 7 represent the response of hybrid BBO-FF-PID Controller for CSTR.

10 Conclusion

This chapter presents a comparative study for a model-based controller as well as the optimization-based controller for a nonlinear control process, i.e., CSTR. Among all metaheuristic strategies for advancement, the hybrid BBO-FF indicated the best outcomes, and through this, we acquired the PID controller parameters

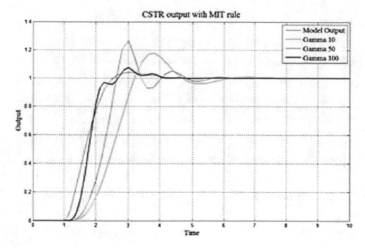

Fig. 3 MIT rule [1]

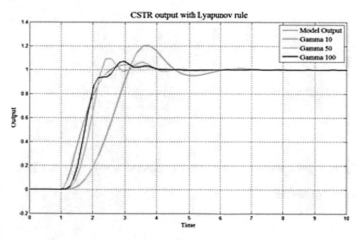

Fig. 4 Lyapunov rule [1]

which demonstrated the brilliant outcomes especially for rise time and settling time. Model-based controllers are easy to implement but give more overshot as compared to optimization-based controllers. PSO-PID gives the best result among all in terms of maximum overshoot and settling time. Further, this study can be extended by considering other recent metaheuristic algorithms and some more nonlinear control problems like surge tank and servo motor.

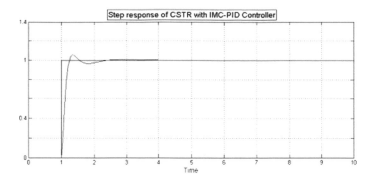

Fig. 5 IMC-PID Controller [11]

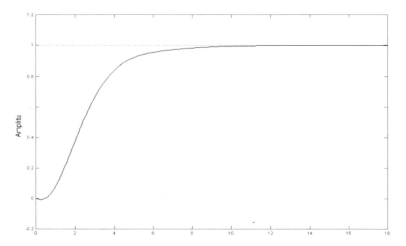

Fig. 6 PSO-PID Controller

Table 1 Performance specification for various types of controllers

Performance Specification	ZN-PID	MRAC MIT Rule			Lyapunov rule			IMC-PID	PSO-PID	FF-PID	BBO-FF-PID
		$\Gamma = 10$	$\Gamma = 50$	$\Gamma = 100$	$\Gamma = 10$	$\Gamma = 50$	$\Gamma = 100$				
Rise Time	1.5	3.27	2.65	2.78	3.1	2.3	2.6	1.20	4.51	0.0036	1.1123e−05
Maximum Overshoot	6.7	17.83	26.7	7.5	7.5	20.3	9.6	5.34	0	0.00325	0.00286
Settling Time	Very high	7	6.2	4.5	6.4	4.0	3.9	High	8.65	0.00315	5.1315e−06
ISE	0.1691	0.405	0.21	0.02	0.37	0.04	0.614	0.06748	0.03		1.93

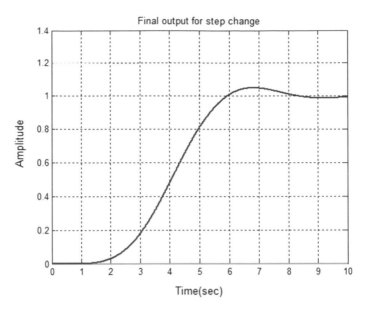

Fig. 7 Hybrid BBO-FF-PID Controller

References

1. Khanduja, N.: CSTR control by using model reference adaptive control and PSO. World Acad. Sci. Eng. Technol. Int. J. Mech. Aerospace, Ind. Mechatron. Manuf. Eng. **8**(12), 2144–2149 (2014)
2. Kumar, N.: Control of CSTR by using Lyapunov's rule of MRAC and PSO. In: Proceeding of 3rd International Conference on "Advance Trends in Engineering, Technology and Research" ICATETR-2014; 22–24th, Dec 2014, no. August 1991, pp. 686–693 (2014)
3. Anbu, S., Jaya, N.: Design of adaptive controller based on Lyapunov stability for a CSTR. Int. J. Electr. Comput. Energ. Electron. Commun. Eng. **8**(1), 183–186 (2014)
4. Zuhwar, Z.F.: The control of non Isothermal CSTR using different controller strategies. Iraqi J. Chem. Pet. Eng. **13**(3), 35–45 (2012)
5. Elbeltagi, E., Hegazy, T., Grierson, D.: Comparison among five evolutionary-based optimization algorithms. Adv. Eng. Informatics **19**(1), 43–53 (2005)
6. Kennedy, J., Eberhart, R.: Particle swarm optimization. In: Proceedings of ICNN'95—International Conference on Neural Networks, pp. 1942–1948 (1995)
7. Nekoui, M.A., Khameneh, M.A., Kazemi, M.H.: Optimal design of PID controller for a CSTR system using particle swarm optimization. In: Proceedings of the EPE-PEMC 2010—14th International Power Electronics Motion Control Conference, pp. 63–66 (2010)
8. Jain, J., Singh, R.: Biogeographic-based optimization algorithm for load dispatch in power system. Int. J. Emerg. Technol. Adv. Eng. **3**(7), 549–553 (2013)
9. Yang, X.S., He, X.: Firefly algorithm: recent advances and applications. Int. J. Swarm Intell. **1**(1), 36 (2013)
10. Aruna, R., Kumar, M.S.: Adaptive control for interactive thermal process. In: 2011 International Conference on Emerging Trends in Electrical and Computer Technology (ICETECT 2011), pp. 291–296 (2011)

11. Khanduja, N., Bhushan, B.: CSTR control using IMC-PID, PSO-PID, and hybrid BBO-FF-PID controller. In: Advances in Intelligent Systems and Computing, vol. 697, pp. 519–526. Springer, Singapore (2019)
12. Baruah, S., Dewan, L.: A comparative study of PID based temperature control of CSTR using Genetic Algorithm and Particle Swarm Optimization. In: 2017 International Conference on Emerging Trends in Computing and Communication Technologies (ICETCCT 2017), vol. 2018-Jan, pp. 1–6 (2018)
13. Malik, S., Dutta, P., Chakrabarti, S., Barman, A.: Survey on biogeography based optimization algorithm and application of biogeography based optimization to determine parameters of PID controller. Int. J. Adv. Res. Comput. Commun. Eng.3(2), 5625–5629 (2014)
14. Kalaivani, R., Lakshmi, P.: Biogeography-based optimization of PID tuning parameters for the vibration control of active suspension system. Control Eng. Appl. Informatics 16(1), 31–39 (2014)
15. Ali, E.S.: Firefly algorithm based speed control of DC series motor. WSEAS Trans. Syst. Control 10, 137–147 (2015)
16. Chaudhari, Y.: Design And implementation of intelligent controller for a continuous stirred tank. Int. J. Adv. Eng. Technol.6(1), 325–335 (2013)
17. Khanduja, N., Sharma, S.: Performance analysis of CSTR using adaptive control. Int. J. Soft Comput. Eng. 2(2), 80–84 (2014). ISSN 2231-2307
18. Iqbal, A., et al.: Metaheurestic algorithm based hybrid model for identification of building sale prices. In: Springer Nature Book: Metaheuristic and Evolutionary Computation: Algorithms and Applications. Studies in Computational Intelligence (2020). https://doi.org/10.1007/978-981-15-7571-6_32
19. FaizMinai, A., et al.: Metaheuristics paradigms for renewable energy systems: advances in optimization algorithms. In: Springer Nature Book: Metaheuristic and Evolutionary Computation: Algorithms and Applications. Studies in Computational Intelligence (2020). https://doi.org/10.1007/978-981-15-7571-6_2

Performance Analysis of Nine-Level Packed E Cell Inverter for Different Carrier Wave PWM Techniques

Shahbaz Ahmad Khan, Deepak Upadhyay, Mohammad Ali, Mohd Tariq, and Adil Sarwar

Abstract Multilevel inverter topology has been investigated in this chapter. The investigated inverter called as packed E-Cell has the capability of generating nine levels at reduced switch counts with low total harmonic distortion (THD). In addition to that, the comparative analysis of the THD levels in the output voltage and current obtained by applying different modulation techniques are also presented. Sine, triangular and half parabolic carriers have been used for analysis. The simulation is done in MATLAB and Simulink and the results obtained for THD in the output voltage and current are presented and discussed in the chapter.

Keywords Multilevel voltage source inverters · Packed E-Cell · Half parabolic carrier wave · Renewable energy conversion

1 Introduction

In the last few years, extensive work has been performed on the multilevel converter topologies due to several advantages like their potential in various industrial applications, interruptible power supplies, electric drives, active power filters, and integration of electricity generated from renewable energy resources to the grid [1, 2]. The

S. A. Khan · D. Upadhyay · M. Ali · M. Tariq (✉) · A. Sarwar
Department of Electrical Engineering, Z.H.C.E.T, Aligarh Muslim University, Aligarh, India
e-mail: tariq.ee@zhcet.ac.in

S. A. Khan
e-mail: shahbazkhan8067@gmail.com

D. Upadhyay
e-mail: deepak.dsta@gmail.com

M. Ali
e-mail: mohad_ali92@yahoo.com

A. Sarwar
e-mail: adil.sarwar@zhcet.ac.in

© The Author(s), under exclusive license to Springer Nature Singapore Pte Ltd. 2021
H. Malik et al. (eds.), *AI and Machine Learning Paradigms for Health Monitoring System*, Studies in Big Data 86,
https://doi.org/10.1007/978-981-33-4412-9_27

multilevel converters are not only able to produce an increased number of voltage levels but also withstanding voltage stress on the switches is comparatively less.

Some of the earliest multilevel inverter topologies are neutral point clamped (NPC), flying capacitor converter (FCC), and cascaded H-bridge converter (CHB) which are being treated as the conventional multilevel inverters [3–5]. These inverters proved superior as compared to the bipolar voltage source inverters due to the low electromagnetic interference, low voltage, and current changing stress and improved voltage and current harmonic profile.

A lot of attempts have been made to increase the number of voltage levels and inspired by the concept of CHB, hybrid of the traditional multilevel inverters, for instance, asymmetrical and symmetrical series configuration has been used because of its capability of getting the low THD values by increasing the number of levels in output voltage wave and improve energy efficiency [6]. Comparing the two, the asymmetrical ones have higher efficiency as it can produce more number of levels and utilize less number of cells.

Researchers started focusing on the establishment of MVSIs operate optimally by trading-off between the factors like components count, number of voltage level, and converter replacement of the DC sources by using capacitors [7]. That is why, multilevel inverter topologies employing the single DC source has been analyzed extensively as a competitive and cost-effective configuration as compared to other multilevel voltage source inverter and is being seen as one of the suitable to be used in asymmetrical and symmetrical asymmetrical cascaded connections [8], but the balancing of capacitors must be taken into account while designing stage by providing the proper charging and discharging paths [9].

The chapter is structured in the following manner as in the next to the introduction in Sect. 2, and the circuit diagram of the basic PEC topology has been described with a circuit diagram. In Sect. 3, various modulation techniques that are being used with PEC are discussed in brief. Next to this section, in Sect. 4, the simulation results of the comparative analysis of the voltage and current harmonics using different carrier waves are depicted and the conclusions derived are being outlined.

2   Packed E Cell Topology

The packed E cell (PEC-9) structure comprises six active bidirectional current devices T1, T2, T3, T4, T5, and T6; one DC source E, single four-quadrant switch T7 and to form a single-phase nine-level converter topology, and two capacitors also incorporated. The topology is structured on the basic concept of employing an E-Cell type of arrangement in order to develop the horizontal structuring of auxiliary capacitors arranged in a row as depicted in Fig. 1. The redundant switching states obtained in this topology can be effectively used to balance both the capacitors in charging as well as discharging mode, which is required to balance the secondary DC link to maintain the voltage level across the DC link formed by the two capacitors and have to maintain the voltage level to $V_{dc}/2$ as it is required for the attainment of nine

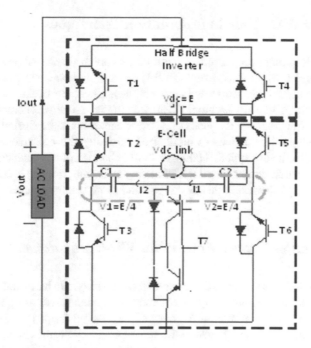

Fig. 1 Packed E cell inverter topology

levels at the output voltage as shown in Fig. 1. The packed E cell structure consists of six active bidirectional current devices T1, T2, T3, T4, T5, and T6; one DC source E, one four-quadrant switch S7, and two capacitors to form single-phase nine-level converter design.

The four-quadrant switch at the midway of two capacitors is forming DC link and AC terminal points of the inverter. In the packed E-Cell, nine-level configuration, capacitors are arranged in a horizontal row to produce only one secondary DC link and to make the multi-output voltage levels terminals due to the four-quadrant switch which makes it possible to attain five, seven, and nine-level at the output.

With the proper selection of switching sequences, each of C1, C2 capacitors voltages (V1, V2) is maintained to one-fourth of the voltage at the input (E) so that the packed E-Cell generates nine-level output voltage waveform. Table 1 depicts switching states of nine-level PEC inverter. According to Table 1, switches (T1, T4), (T2, T5) as well as (T3, T6, T7) are operating complementarily.

Table 1 Comparative analysis of results obtained

S. No.	Carrier wave used	Switching frequency (Hz)	Voltage THD %	Current THD%
1	Half parabolic	4000	7.28	0.98
2	Triangular	4000	10.92	0.89
3	Sinusoidal	4000	13.01	1.57

3 Carrier Wave Used in Modulation Techniques

There are various pulse programming methods that are available out of which carrier wave-based pulse width modulation (PWM) control strategies are found to be the most appropriate and preferred way in most of the applications because of some very significant features like low harmonic distortion in the waveform characteristics and a clear and distinct harmonic spectrum. Carrier waves could be shifted in phase or out of phase deposition and also a number of vertically shifted carriers changes as the number of the level required. Unlike hysteresis band control which has a sporadic operating frequency, carrier-based PWM having switching frequency fixed and also simple in the implementation makes this method stands out of others.

3.1 Triangular Carrier Wave-Pulse Width Modulation

The triangle intersection application approach which is used in hardware or software. In this modulation technique, high-frequency triangular waves are generated and compared with sinusoidal reference waves of the desired frequency. The pulses in this type change from being narrow at the staring of the cycle and end up being wide at the end. The pulses produced are given as the gate pulse to the switches of the inverter to obtain the desired output with low total harmonic distortion.

3.2 Sinusoidal Carrier Wave-Pulse Width Modulation

Sinusoidal carrier wave modulation technique is in which, for PWM generation, we use sine wave as a carrier wave of very high frequency and a sine wave of the fundamental frequency as a reference wave. These carriers could be shifted vertically in phase and also in inverse phase deposition as per the requirement of pulses. Sinusoidal carrier wave gives much error when used in inverter operation as compared with other carrier waves used in the latest inverter topologies.

3.3 Half Parabolic Carrier Wave-Pulse Width Modulation

An innovative carrier waveform for pulse width modulation has been designed to have better performance and to control the output voltage and to attain the lowest harmonic at the load voltage side with lowest harmonic distortion at the reduced switching frequency. The generation of half parabolic carrier wave is accomplished by using two waveforms which are rectangular pulses and sinusoidal waves, where the frequency of rectangular function is twice that of the sine function waveform f2.

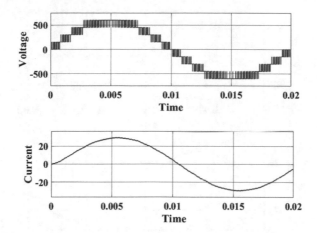

Fig. 2 Output voltage and output current waveforms for half parabolic carrier

It is the ratio of the frequency f1 and f2 which acts as the deciding factor for the shape of the parabolic waveform produced and by varying this ratio diverse waveforms can be obtained.

4 Results and Discussion

Different carrier waves for modulation have been used to analyze the inverter operation. The switching frequency has been set to 4000 Hz for all techniques, and load of resistance 20 Ω and inductor of 10 mH are used for simulation purposes. Output voltage and current waveforms have been investigated and the power factor is also monitored to check the power transferring and quality of power being generated by the application of these modulation techniques on nine-level PEC inverter topology (Figs. 2, 3, 4, 5, 6, 7, 8, 9 and 10).

5 Conclusions

In this chapter, comparative analysis and investigation of different modulation techniques on nine-level packed E cells have been presented. The half parabola carrier wave, sinusoidal carrier wave, and triangular carrier wave have been used, and simulation is done for fixed load and switching frequency. From the results, it has been concluded that the voltage and current THD% are maximum in the case of a sinusoidal carrier wave. The power factor is nearly around unity in all cases and comparatively higher in half the parabola carrier technique. Waveforms of current and voltages have not shown any significant change.

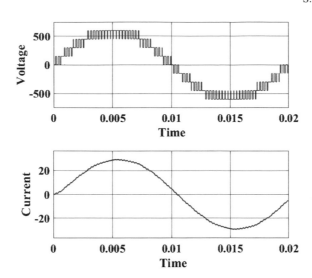

Fig. 3 Load voltage and current waveforms for sinusoidal carrier wave

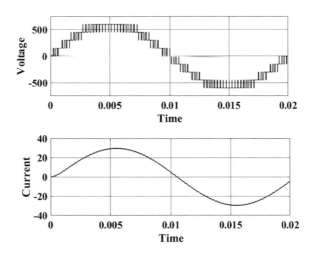

Fig. 4 Load voltage and current waveforms for triangular carrier wave

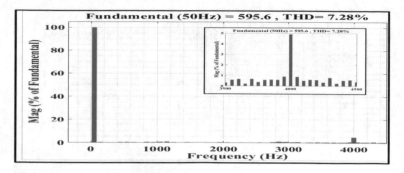

Fig. 5 Harmonic spectrum of voltage waveform for half parabola carrier wave

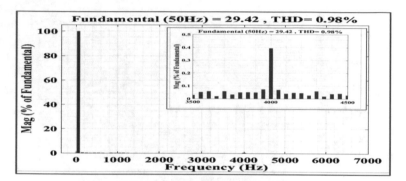

Fig. 6 Harmonic spectrum of load current waveform for half parabola carrier wave

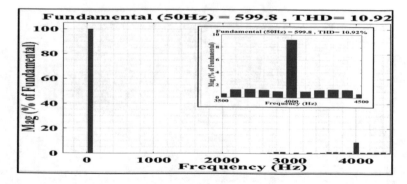

Fig. 7 Harmonic spectrum of voltage waveform for triangular carrier wave

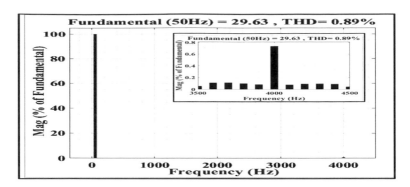

Fig. 8 Harmonic spectrum of current waveform in a triangular carrier wave

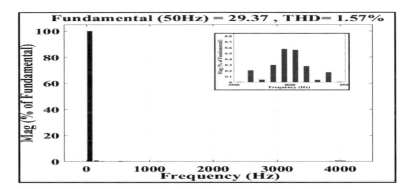

Fig. 9 Harmonic spectrum of current waveform in a sinusoidal carrier wave

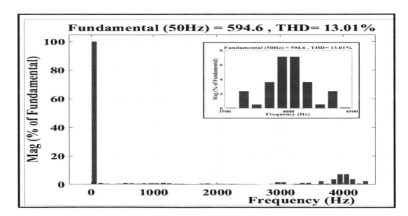

Fig. 10 Harmonic spectrum of voltage waveform in a sinusoidal carrier wave

References

1. Tariq, M., Maswood, A.I., Moreddy, A.C., Gajanayake, C.J., Lee, M.Y., Gupta, A.K.: Reliability, dead-time, and feasibility analysis of a novel modular tankless ZCS inverter for more electric aircraft. IEEE Trans. Transp. Electrif. **3**(4), 843–854 (2017). https://doi.org/10.1109/TTE.2017. 2704283
2. Asim, M., Tariq, M., Mallick M.A., Ashraf, I.: An improved constant voltage based MPPT technique for PMDC Motor. Int. J. Power Electroni. Drive Syst. **7**(4), 1330–1336 (2016). http:// doi.org/10.11591/ijpcds.v7.i4.pp1330-1336
3. Daher, S., Schmid, J., Antunes, F.L.M.: Multilevel inverter topologies for stand-alone PV systems. IEEE Trans. Industr. Electron. **55**(7), 2703–2712 (2008). https://doi.org/10.1109/TIE. 2008.922601
4. Bharatiraja, C., Selvaraj, R., Chelliah, T.R., Munda, J.L., Tariq, M., Maswood, A.I.: Design and implementation of fourth arm for elimination of bearing current in NPC-MLI-fed induction motor drive. IEEE Trans. Ind. Appl. **54**(1), 745–754 (2018). https://doi.org/10.1109/tia.2017. 2759204
5. Bharatiraja, C., Munda, J.L., Bayindir R., Tariq, M.: A common-mode leakage current mitigation for PV-grid connected three-phase three-level transformerless T-type-NPC-MLI. In: 2016 IEEE International Conference on Renewable Energy Research and Applications (ICRERA), Birmingham, 2016, pp. 578–583. https://doi.org/10.1109/icrera.2016.7884401
6. Khan, S.A., Upadhyay, D., Ali, M., Tariq, M., Rehman, K., Sarwar, A., Anees, M.A.: Integration of distributed PV system with grid using 9-level PEC inverter. In: International Conference on Modelling, Simulation & Intelligent Computing (MoSICom) 2020 Dubai, UAE
7. Wang, K., Zheng, Z., Wei, D., Fan, B., Li, Y.: Topology and capacitor voltage balancing control of a symmetrical hybrid nine-level inverter for high-speed motor drives. IEEE Trans. Ind. Appl. **53**(6), 5563–5572 (2017)
8. Vahedi, H., Sharifzadeh, M., Al-Haddad, K.: Modified seven-level packed U-cell inverter for photovoltaic applications. IEEE J. Emerg. Sel. TopicsPower Electron. **6**(3), 1508_1516 (2018)
9. Sharifzadeh, M., Al-Haddad, K.: Packed E-Cell (PEC) converter topology operation and experimental validation. IEEE Access **7**, 93049–93061 (2019)

PSO-Based Selective Harmonics Elimination Method for Improving THD in Three-Phase Multi-level Inverter

Nazia Rehman, Umme Aiman, Md Shahbaz Alam, Mohd Rizwan Khalid[iD]**, and Adil Sarwar**

Abstract Multi-level inverters (MLI) have improved power quality at output voltage as compared to conventional inverters. In MLI, number of switches increases with number of levels in output voltage. This increases the complexity and reduces the reliability of the MLI. In this chapter, a three-phase five-level MLI is proposed which involves lesser number of switches as compared with other topologies present in literature. The proposed MLI involves a single DC source and two capacitors along with 10 switches. For reducing total harmonic distortion (THD) in output voltage of the proposed MLI, a particle swarm optimization (PSO)-based selective harmonics elimination method is adopted. The proposed MLI topology is modeled in MATLAB®/Simulink. The simulation results obtained show the improved THD in output voltage and thus confirm the effectiveness of the proposed optimization method for the MLI. The proposed MLI can be used for the integration of renewable resources in the utility grid system.

Keywords Multi-level inverter (MLI) · Particle swarm optimization (PSO) · Power quality · Total harmonic distortion (THD) · Selective harmonic elimination

1 Introduction

Inverters have shown a dominating role in modern technological due to sudden increase in electrical vehicles demand and integration of renewable energy in the grid [1, 2]. They convert DC power into AC power with high power quality of output voltage waveform. Main applications include uninterruptable power supplies, drives, and active power filtering. Conventional inverter produces square wave output voltage which produces noise and also heat up equipment because of the large lower harmonic contents in it.

N. Rehman · U. Aiman · M. S. Alam · M. R. Khalid (✉) · A. Sarwar
Electrical Engineering Department, Aligarh Muslim University, Aligarh 202002, India
e-mail: mrk.rizwankhalid@gmail.com

© The Author(s), under exclusive license to Springer Nature Singapore Pte Ltd. 2021   429
H. Malik et al. (eds.), *AI and Machine Learning Paradigms for Health Monitoring System*, Studies in Big Data 86,
https://doi.org/10.1007/978-981-33-4412-9_28

Multi-level inverters (MLI) are preferred over conventional inverters because they are capable of generation output voltage with lower total harmonic contents (THD). They give better power quality performances, i.e., output waveform is closer to sinusoidal, low switching loss, and higher voltage capability. In literature, many different methods have been adopted to control the output voltage level.

Nowadays, in literature, numerous structures of MLI have been introduced with reduced number of active switches, driver circuits, and power supplies to reduce the complexity. One of such circuit is a switched capacitor multi-level inverter (SCMLI) [3]. This converter produces output with increased number of levels of voltage by incorporating lesser number of switches and power supplies. The conversation of DC power into AC power with stepped output voltage is done with SCMLI which mainly consist of capacitors and switches and reduces the harmonics contents [4]. For the better understanding of the PSO and related optimization technique implementation, the reader may refer [12–14].

2 Classification of Multi-level Inverter (MLI)

Multi-level inverters (MLI) are classified into various categories depending upon the components utilized in them. The idea of MLI was first evolved in 1975. MLI provides high power quality, low switching losses, and low conduction losses. MLI finds applications in electric vehicles, renewable energy integration, industrial drives, etc. [1]. Broadly, MLI are classified as diode clamped inverters, cascaded H-bridge inverters, and flying capacitor inverters [5].

First diode clamped/neutral point inverter was introduced in 1981. It has low problem of dynamic voltage, and it has good static voltage equalization without the increase of extra component [6]. In 1992, the first capacitor clamped MLI or flying capacitor MLI was proposed. Flying capacitor shows the improved results for medium voltage applications. The structure is so designed that it provides high power outage and lower down the switching state due to clamping capacitor. The main idea is to use capacitors in the inverter and to lower down the quantity of independent voltage sources. The flying capacitor has various applications which include no transformer, ability to naturally maintain the voltage level so there is self-balancing in topology which motivates its development [7].

In 1996, H-bridge multi-level inverter was proposed. The idea of this inverter is based on the cascaded connection of many H-bridges to obtain stepped output voltage [8, 9]. H-bridge contains four switches, and depending upon the switching condition, the output voltage changes its polarity depending on the circuit condition. The cascaded multi-level inverters have a large range of applications and have good flexibility over high power application and FACTs. Table 1 shows the comparison of different MLI present in the literature with the proposed MLI.

Table 1 Comparison of the proposed MLI with conventional MLI

Multi-level inverter structure	Switches	Diodes	Clamping diodes	Clamping capacitor	Total components
Diode clamped	18	18	12	0	48
Capacitor clamped	18	18	0	9	45
Cascaded H-bridge	18	18	0	0	36
Proposed inverter	10	10	0	2	22

Fig. 1 Proposed multi-level inverter

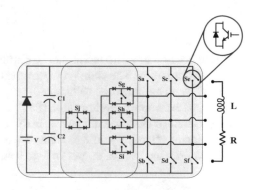

3 Proposed MLI Topology

The proposed MLI topology is shown in Fig. 1; it consists of conventional three-phase full-bridge configuration with four bidirectional switches. The circuit uses two capacitors with DC voltage source which reduce the number of sources for the generation of three-phase five-level stepped AC output voltage. Capacitors are considered to be initially discharged and are self-balanced by the single voltage source of 2 V DC. The three-phase stepped output voltage waveform of the proposed MLI is shown in Fig. 2.

The proposed MLI produces five different voltage levels in the line voltage having amplitudes: $2 \times V_{dc}$, $-V_{dc}$, V_{dc}, $2V_{dc}$, and 0. The different switching modes are shown in Fig. 3.

4 Selective Harmonic Elimination

Usually for wave shaping, the output waveform selective harmonic elimination-based pulse width modulation (SHEPWM) is adopted in MLI [10, 11]. SHEPWM have limitations and only eliminates four harmonics. Here any four harmonics are eliminated by solving different harmonic component of Fourier series except 3rd, 9th

Fig. 2 Three-phase
five-level modulated output
voltage of proposed MLI

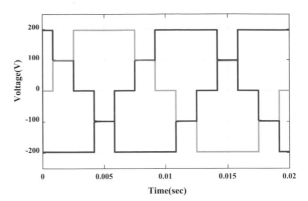

and 15th because these harmonic can be eliminated from line-to-line voltage by star delta transformation. The solution of different harmonic Fourier series components is solved by an optimization technique.

Here, particle swarm optimization (PSO) is used for solving the equation to find a different angle (α) for different pulses. In this case, 5th, 7th, 11th, and 13th harmonics are eliminated effectively. The modulated waveform is shown in Fig. 4.

The Fourier analysis of output voltage waveform with five levels is given by

$$V_0(\omega t) = \sum_{n=1,3,5\ldots}^{\infty} \frac{4V_{dc}}{n\pi}(\cos n\alpha_1 \pm \cos n\alpha_2 \ldots \pm \cos n\alpha_5 \pm \cos n\alpha_6)\sin(n\omega t) \quad (1)$$

where switching angles must meet

$$\alpha_1 < \alpha_2 < \alpha_3 < \alpha_4 < \alpha_5 < \alpha_6 < \frac{\pi}{3} \quad (2)$$

In (1), the negative sign indicates the falling edge and positive sign indicates the rising edge.

$$2M = (\cos\alpha_1 \pm \cos\alpha_2 \ldots \pm \cos\alpha_5 \pm \cos\alpha_6) \quad (3)$$

$$0 = (\cos 5\alpha_1 \pm \cos 5\alpha_2 \ldots \pm \cos 5\alpha_5 \pm \cos 5\alpha_6) \quad (4)$$

$$0 = (\cos 7\alpha_1 \pm \cos 7\alpha_2 \ldots \pm \cos 7\alpha_5 \pm \cos 7\alpha_6) \quad (5)$$

$$0 = (\cos 11\alpha_1 \pm \cos 11\alpha_2 \ldots \pm \cos 11\alpha_5 \pm \cos 11\alpha_6) \quad (6)$$

$$0 = (\cos 13\alpha_1 \pm \cos 13\alpha_2 \ldots \pm \cos 13\alpha_5 \pm \cos 13\alpha_6) \quad (7)$$

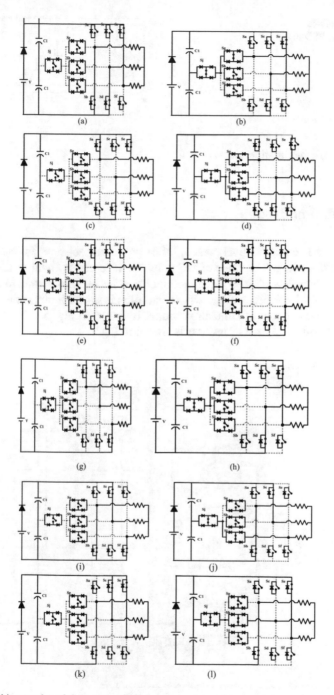

Fig. 3 Working modes of the proposed MLI

Fig. 4 Modulated
waveforms of PSO-based
SHEPWM

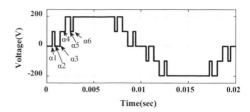

where *M* is the modulation index.

5   Simulation Results

To verify the computational result, the proposed scheme is modeled in
MATLAB®/Simulink. The value of DC source considered is equal to the value of
maximum voltage level (200 V). The modulation index (*M*) has certain range for the
proper SHEPWM implementation, whose variation is shown in the simulation. The
complete block diagram of simulation model is shown in Fig. 5. The three-phase
modulated five-level output of inverter is shown in Fig. 6.

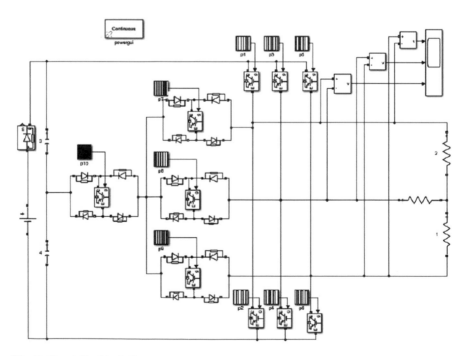

Fig. 5 Simulation block diagram

Fig. 6 Three-phase
five-level modulated output

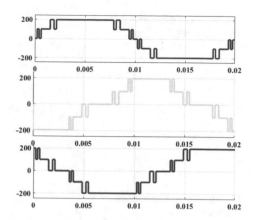

Selective harmonic elimination at modulation index 0.8 and 0.9 is shown in Figs. 7 and 8. The 5th, 7th, 11th, and 13th harmonics are completely eliminated from line voltage. These results show minimum THD of 22.14 and 22.92%. Figure 9 shows the variation of angle with modulation index, and harmonic is eliminated at every given point in the curve, but the plot of angle is constant as we have lower modulation index and at higher modulation index angle starts reducing. Figure 10 shows the plot between THD and modulation index, and the harmonic distortions decrease with the increasing modulation index.

Fig. 7 Eliminated
harmonics at $M = 0.8$

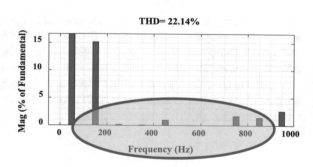

Fig. 8 Eliminated
harmonics at $M = 0.9$

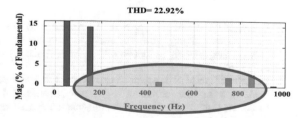

Fig. 9 Plot of firing angle versus modulation index

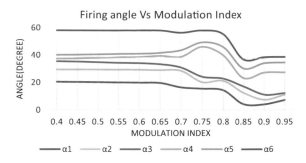

Fig. 10 Plot of THD versus modulation index

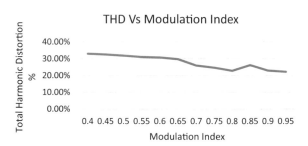

6 Conclusion

In this work, the MLI is proposed which requires lesser number of switches and DC sources. The proposed inverter gives three-phase five-level line-to-line voltage at the output. The circuit has two self-balancing capacitors. In order to remove lower-order harmonic SHEPWM was implemented. Multiple switching angles have been calculated using PSO algorithm. The lower-order harmonics were eliminated up-to 13th order for the proposed inverter. MATLAB®/Simulink environment was used to validate the concept.

References

1. Khalid, M.R., Alam, M.S., Sarwar, A., Asghar, M.S.J.: A comprehensive review on electric vehicles charging infrastructures and their impacts on power-quality of the utility grid. e-Transportation **1**, 100006 (2019). https://doi.org/10.1016/j.etran.2019.100006. ISSN 2590-1168
2. M. R. Khalid and M. S. J. Asghar, A new topology for single stage thyristor based grid connected single phase inverter for renewable energy systems. In: 2017 IEEE International Conference on Power, Control, Signals and Instrumentation Engineering (ICPCSI), Chennai, 2017, pp 724–731
3. Rawa, M., et al.: Dual input switched-capacitor-based single-phase hybrid boost multilevel inverter topology with reduced number of components. IET Power Electroni. **13**(4), 881–891 (2020)

4. Sandeep, N., Yaragatti, U.R.: A switched-capacitor-based multilevel inverter topology with reduced components. IEEE Trans. Power Electron. **33**(7), 5538–5542 (2018)
5. Koshti, A.K., Rao, M.N.: A brief review on multilevel inverter topologies. In: 2017 International Conference on Data Management, Analytics and Innovation (ICDMAI), Pune, 2017, pp. 187–193
6. Rasheed, M., Omar, R., Sulaiman, M., Aljanad, A., Ahmad, A.: Bridge and diode-clamped multilevel inverters. In: 2013 IEEE Conference on Clean Energy Technology, pp. 281–286, 2013
7. Siddique, M.D., et al.: A single DC source nine-level switched-capacitor boost inverter topology with reduced switch count. IEEE Access **8**, 5840–5851 (2020)
8. Khadse, S., Mendole, R., Pandey, A.: A 5-level single phase flying capacitor multilevel inverter, pp 348–352 (2017)
9. Boonmee, C., Somboonkit, P., Watjanatepin, N.: Performance comparison of three-level and multi-level for grid-connected photovoltaic systems. In: ECTI-CON 2015—2015 International Conference on Electrical Engineering/Electronics, Computer, Telecommunications and Information Technology
10. Siddique, M.D., Mekhilef, S., Shah, N.M., Ali, J.S.M., Blaabjerg, F.: A new switched capacitor 7L inverter with triple voltage gain and low voltage stress. IEEE Trans. Circuits Syst. II Express Briefs, pp. 1 (2019)
11. Khalid, M.R., Ahmad, B., Sarwar A., Jamil Asghar, M.S.: Review of thyristor based grid tied inverters for solar PV applications. In: 2019 IEEE 5th International Conference for Convergence in Technology (I2CT), Bombay, India, 2019, pp. 1–5
12. Iqbal, A. et al.: Metaheurestic algorithm based hybrid model for identification of building sale prices. in: Springer Nature Book: Metaheuristic and Evolutionary Computation: Algorithms and Applications, under book series "Studies in Computational Intelligence", 2020. https://doi.org/10.1007/978-981-15-7571-6_32
13. Fatema, N. et al.: Data-driven occupancy detection hybrid model using particle swarm optimization based artificial neural network. In: Springer Nature Book: Metaheuristic and Evolutionary Computation: Algorithms and Applications, under book series "Studies in Computational Intelligence", 2020. Doi: https://doi.org/10.1007/978-981-15-7571-6_13
14. Faiz Minai, A. et al.: Metaheuristics paradigms for renewable energy systems: advances in optimization algorithms. In: Springer Nature Book: Metaheuristic and Evolutionary Computation: Algorithms and Applications, under book series "Studies in Computational Intelligence", 2020. Doi: https://doi.org/10.1007/978-981-15-7571-6_2

Optimized Controller Design for Fast Steering Mirror-Based Laser Beam Steering Applications

Himanshu Chaudhary, Shahida Khatoon, Ravindra Singh, and Ashish Pandey

Abstract In last few decades, fast steering mirrors (FSMs) are predominantly used in steering and control of line of sight (LOS) in many applications which includes surveillance, tracking, pointing, photography, ground, space communication, and astronomy research. This chapter presents the dynamic modeling and control configuration design of FSM in azimuth direction. The ultimate objective of control configuration design is to obtain the faster input command response and isolate the line of sight movement from any kind of internal or external disturbances. Initially, a simplified model of FSM with suitable parametric values and adjustable gains is designed and that establishes the relationship between angular moment of LOS and applied torque. Then, a pre-existing proportional-integral-derivative (PID) controller configuration is developed, whose gains are further optimized using genetic algorithm (GA) and particle swarm optimization (PSO) algorithm. Integral time absolute error is considered as an objective function for both the algorithm. However, both GA and PSO tuned PID controller improves the performance of FSM system. But PSO tuned configuration certainly outperforms the existing controller in terms of desired characteristics.

Keywords Fast steering mirror (FSM) · Genetic algorithm (GA) · Particle swarm optimization (PSO) · Precision pointing · Disturbance attenuation

H. Chaudhary (✉) · S. Khatoon
Department of Electrical Engineering, Jamia Millia Islamia University, New Delhi, Delhi 110025, India
e-mail: himanshuchaudhary.h@gmail.com

R. Singh · A. Pandey
Defence Research and Development Organization, New Delhi, Delhi 110054, India

© The Author(s), under exclusive license to Springer Nature Singapore Pte Ltd. 2021   439
H. Malik et al. (eds.), *AI and Machine Learning Paradigms for Health Monitoring System*, Studies in Big Data 86,
https://doi.org/10.1007/978-981-33-4412-9_29

1   Introduction

Fast steering mirror is a mirror whose angular position can be controlled at a relatively higher bandwidth. Since mid-1980s, they become the integral part in almost every beam steering and pointing application [1, 2]. Initially, because of their less explored nature, complex design, and high cost they were only used in defense and aerospace application, but in last two decades, every commercial industry which involves beam steering and pointing, target tracking and acquisition, alignment, line of sight (LOS) stabilization, makes use of fast steering mirrors [3].

Although the use of FSM in acquisition, tracking, and pointing application offers several advantages in terms of precision, but in early phase of research, they also suffers with design limitation. First, FSM are usually suspended with metal flexures, which needs to be designed with utmost care to reduce stresses and save it from breaking. Second, FSM offers only limited travel capacity to system. Such restrictions were eliminated by Ball Aerospace System Group (BASG) team.

There are several types of tracking and pointing configuration developed so far other than fast steering mirror approach. Gimballed beam steering system [4–6] dominates any other form of electro-optical system in numerous applications. Gimballed mirrors or mass stabilized gimballed systems have been used to achieve stabilization and pointing performance in order of few micro-radians or better depending on field of view. They are generally larger in size and hence have much larger aperture than FSM. However, gimballed sensor system suffers from several disadvantages, which emphasize the researcher to develop the way for FSM in precise pointing applications.

In recent past, several FSM dynamics with different controller configurations have been proposed [7–9]. But still, the use of optimization algorithm [10–12] and intelligent controllers is very constrained with the proposed FSM dynamics so far. For the better understanding of the optimization technique implementation, the reader may refer [13–15].

2   Dynamic Modeling of FSM

Fast steering mirrors (FSMs) are the low inertia electro-optical device used to steer LOS of a sensor to the distant located target. These are actuated using piezoelectric (PZT) actuators [3]. The primary advantages of piezo actuators are unlimited resolution, less power consumption, and high force/mass ration. However, the limitations are: limited displacement range and limited operating temperature, i.e., below 100 °C. Figure 1 shows the elliptical FSM with two pairs of symmetrically placed piezo actuators for rotation about X and Y-axis.

Piezo-actuated FSM can be modeled as a simplified spring mass system as [16].Consider the azimuth rotation of FSM, as shown in Fig. 1b, due to piezo stiffness forces and spring forces. For small angle of rotation $\delta\theta_x$ of the mirror, the angular

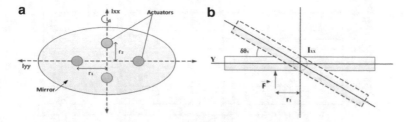

Fig. 1 **a** Sensor actuated FSM schematic, **b** FSM rotation about azimuth axis

rotation with respect to applied piezo force is represented in form of second-order transfer function as:

$$\frac{\delta\theta_x(s)}{F(s)} = \left(\frac{1}{I_{xx}S^2 + B.S + 2Kr_1^2}\right)$$
$$= \left(\frac{1}{6.4296e - 3S^2 + 2.03S + 2*80e6*0.05^\wedge2}\right) \quad (1)$$

Above numerical transfer function is calculated based on PZ T and FSM specifications in [16, 17]. The input is the voltage to the PZT in volts, and output is the angle of rotation of the mirror in radians. Above transfer function is modeled as (Fig. 2).

Figure 3 shows the compensated open loop Simulink model, followed by its bode plot characteristics as shown in Fig. 4.

Open loop FSM configuration has the advantages of simplicity, lower gain requirement, but not practically feasible in the presence of uncertainties and external disturbances. Hence, the closed loop design is always preferred as shown in Fig. 5.

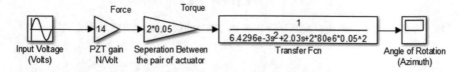

Fig. 2 Uncompensated FSM Simulink model

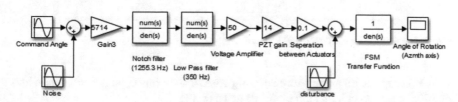

Fig. 3 Compensated open loop FSM Simulink model

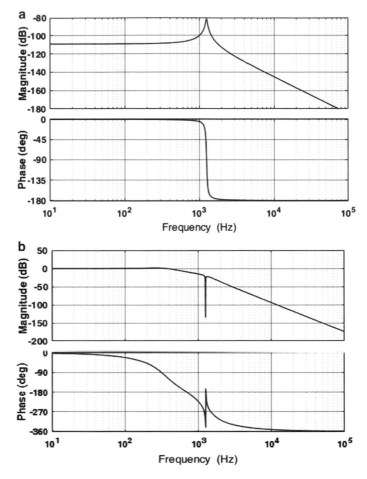

Fig. 4 **a** Open loop uncompensated bode plot, **b** open loop compensated bode plot

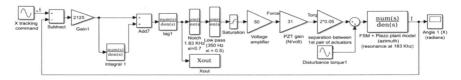

Fig. 5 Compensated closed loop FSM Simulink model

A PI compensator along with a lag compensator is designed, targeting a bandwidth of 100 Hz and open loop gain of 60 dB at 1 Hz (Fig. 6):

$$
\text{PI Compensator} = 2125 * \left(1 + \frac{1200}{s}\right); \quad \text{Lag Comensator} = \left(\frac{S + 2 * \text{pi} * 20}{S + 2 * \text{pi} * 1}\right)
$$

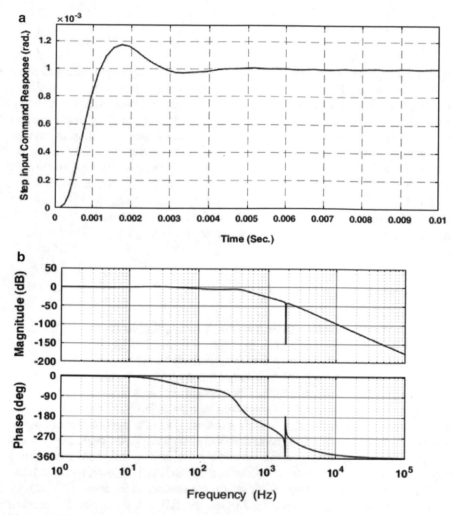

Fig. 6 **a** FSM open loop compensated step response, **b** closed loop frequency response

3 Optimized Controller Configuration Design

3.1 PID Controller

Standard form of the PID control algorithm in time and frequency domain is represented as:

$$u(t) = K_\mathrm{p}\left[e(t) + \frac{1}{T_\mathrm{i}} \int e(t)\mathrm{d}t + T_\mathrm{d}\frac{\mathrm{d}}{\mathrm{d}t}e(t)\right];$$

$$U(s) = K_p \left(1 + \frac{1}{T_i s} + \frac{s T_d}{1 + s \frac{T_d}{N}} \right) E(s)$$

where K_p represents proportional gain, T_i and T_d are the integral and derivative time constants, and N is the filter coefficient. The ultimate aim is the adjustment or tuning of K_c, T_i, and T_d for designing of PID controller. There are different tuning methods available, but it is noted that good gain method and Skogestad's method covers most of the practical cases [18]. Here, the good gain method is applied for determining the parameters of PID controller at the initial level. The parameters obtained with the fine-tuning of PID controller are: $K_{PGG} = 300$; $T_{ou} = 0.0025$; $T_i = 1.5 * 0.0025 = 0.00375$; $K_p = 0.8 K_{PGG} = 240$; $T_d = \frac{T_i}{4} = 0.0009375$.

Further, for fine-tuning of these PID controller parameters, i.e., K_p, T_i, T_d; GA and PSO algorithms are used with minimization of the integral time absolute error (ITAE) as the objective function. ITAE function is given as: $ITAE(t) = \int_{t=0}^{t=\infty} t * |e(t)| dt$.

3.2 Genetic Algorithm (GA)

GA based on the principle of Darwin mechanism, i.e., 'survival of fittest'. The basic foundation of simulation using GA depends on the natural biological property of evolution, which states that only that species tends to evolve which have highest probability of surviving [10, 19]. Individuals that do not have the capability to survive produces only few or no offspring and hence extinct after few generations. In engineering terms, GA assigned a fitness score to each individual based on nature of solution, and individual with very high score are given the opportunities to reproduce while the poorest score individuals will die out. Broadly, the evaluation process comprises of five stages, i.e., select the initial population, evaluate each member of population and select the fittest individuals, reproduction, crossover, and mutation.

Total number of chrosomes: 1000, maximum number of iteration: 100, number of optimization variables: 3 (K_p, T_i, T_d), ranges: [10 500; 0 100; 0 10], mutation rate: 0.15, fraction of population kept at 0.5, and total number of bits in a single chromosome is 32. Final obtained values of parameters are: K_p: 276.33, $T_i = 6.83$, $T_d = 0.5$.

3.3 Particle Swarm Optimization (PSO)

PSO is an optimization algorithm inspired by patterns of birds and fish population and was invented by Kennedy and Eberhart in 1995. In last few decades even after emergence of various optimization algorithms, PSO has always been proven to be most promising algorithm to get the global best value. The algorithm based on search of each individual particle by its own experience. Each particle needs to keep track of the coordinates of the target value which it has achieved so far while searching and this value is known as p-best or each particle individual best value. Out of these individual best which is closer to the targeted values is signified as the g-best or global best value [20].

Total number of population: 1000, number of iteration: 100, number of optimization variables: 3 (K_p, T_i, T_d), ranges: [10 500; 0 100; 0 10], velocity clamping factor: 2, c_1, c_2: 2, weight range: [0.4 0.9], and final obtained values of parameters are: K_p: 311.01, $T_i = 5.22$, $T_d = 0.075$.

4 Result and Discussion

The simulation and programming work has been performed in MATLAB environment. The analysis of the designed controllers is performed based on parameters such as rise time, settling time, percentage overshoot, tracking error, close loop bandwidth, and jitter reduction against angular disturbance of 0.2 rad/s. The output response characteristics in terms of step input command response and jitter reduction are shown in Fig. 7 and their comparative analysis is shown in Table 1.

5 Conclusion

FSM dynamic model is created using compensation approach that not only validates the chosen parametric values of electrical components but also satisfied the minimum required level of accuracy. Then, a PID controller is designed based on good gain method approach to achieve the desired closed loop time response characteristics. Further, the gains of PID controllers are tuned using GA and PSO algorithm within the defined range. The aim of the optimization algorithm is to minimize the chosen objection function ITAE. Numerical simulation runs validates the performance characterisitics of the designed controller configurations. PSO tuned controller completely outperforms the other two configurations in terms of both input command response and disturbance rejection ability.

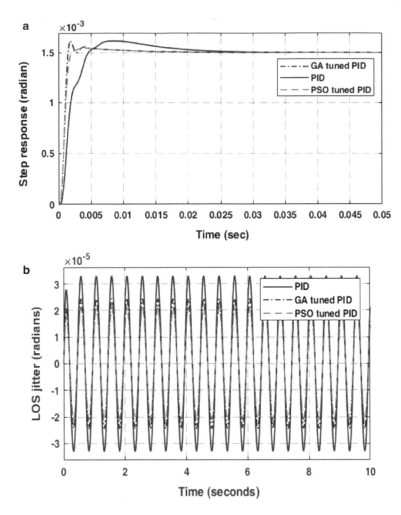

Fig. 7 **a** Step input command response, **b** line of sight jitter for disturbance signal

Table 1 Output characteristics comparative analysis

Characteristics	PID controller	GA tuned PID	PSO tuned PID
Rise time	0.009	0.006	0.003
Settling time (s)	0.03	0.015	0.005
% Overshoot	32. 56%	30%	15%
Steady-state error	Zero or minimal	Zero or minimal	Zero or minimal
Angular disturbance (rad/s)	0.2	0.2	0.2
Jitter attenuation	35 microradian	26 microradian	20 microradian

References

1. Chaudhary, H.: Fast steering mirror for optical fine pointing applications : a review chapter. In: IEEE Conference (CIPECH-2018), pp. 102–106 (2018)
2. Hilkert, J.M., Kanga, G., Kinnear, K.: Line-of-sight kinematics and corrections for fast-steering mirrors used in precision pointing and tracking systems. SPIE **9076**, 1–15 (2014). https://doi.org/10.1117/12.2049857
3. Zhou, Q., Ben-Tzvi, P., Fan, D.: Design and analysis of a fast steering mirror for precision laser beams steering. Sens. Transducers J. **5**, 104–118 (2009)
4. Hilkert, J.M.: Platform technology—concepts and principles. IEEE Control Syst. magz. 26–46 (2008). https://doi.org/10.1109/mcs.2007.910256
5. Arefi, M.M., Khayatian, M.: Adaptive dynamic surface control of a two-axis gimbal system. IET Sci. Meas. Technol. **10**, 607–613 (2016). https://doi.org/10.1049/iet-smt.2016.0005
6. Xia, K., Li, H., Li, Z.: Panoramic shot device of 720-degree VR for hexacopter UAV based on three-axis gimbal. **55**, (2019). https://doi.org/10.1049/el.2018.5387
7. Zhang, B., Zhang, L., Huang, G., Shu, R.: Research on pointing of piezoelectric fast steering mirror under vibration condition. In: Proceedings of SPIE (Soc. Photo Instrum. Eng. **8191**, 1–7 (2011)
8. Li, Q., Liu, L., Ma, X., Chen, S., Yun, H., Tang, S.: Development of multitarget acquisition, pointing, and tracking system for airborne. IEEE Trans. Ind. Inf. **15**, 1720–1729 (2019). https://doi.org/10.1109/TII.2018.2868143
9. Tian, J., Yang, W., Peng, Z., Tang, T.: Inertial sensor-based multiloop control of fast steering mirror for line of sight stabilization. SPIE Opt. Eng. **55**, 1–6 (2019). https://doi.org/10.1117/1.OE.55.11.111602
10. Jin, Z., Hou, Z., Yu, W., Wang, X.: Target tracking approach via quantum genetic algorithm. IET Comput. Vis. **12**, 241–251 (2018). https://doi.org/10.1049/iet-cvi.2017.0176
11. Fatihu, M., Jen, H., Ahmed, I.: Engineering applications of artificial intelligence Cuckoo search algorithm based design of interval Type-2 fuzzy PID controller for Furuta pendulum system. Eng. Appl. Artif. Intell. **62**, 134–151 (2017). https://doi.org/10.1016/j.engappai.2017.04.007
12. Yu, Z., Cui, N., Chen, X., Xu, C., Cao, K.: H ∞ control for fast steering mirror based on the incremental PI controller. In: Proceedings of SPIE **9521**, 95210G–1–95210G–5 (2015). https://doi.org/10.1117/12.2087306
13. Iqbal, A. et al.: Metaheurestic algorithm based hybrid model for identification of building sale prices. In Springer Nature Book: Metaheuristic and Evolutionary Computation: Algorithms and Applications, under book series "Studies in Computational Intelligence", 2020. https://doi.org/10.1007/978-981-15-7571-6_32
14. Fatema, N. et al.: Data-driven occupancy detection hybrid model using particle swarm optimization based artificial neural network. In: Springer Nature Book: Metaheuristic and Evolutionary Computation: Algorithms and Applications, under book series "Studies in Computational Intelligence", 2020. https://doi.org/10.1007/978-981-15-7571-6_13
15. Faiz Minai, A. et al.: Metaheuristics paradigms for renewable energy systems: advances in optimization algorithms. In: Springer Nature Book: Metaheuristic and Evolutionary Computation: Algorithms and Applications, under book series "Studies in Computational Intelligence", 2020. https://doi.org/10.1007/978-981-15-7571-6_2
16. Chaudhary, H., Khatoon, S., Singh, R., Pandey, A.: Modeling and simulation of fast steering mirror plant for laser beam pointing application. In: 2018 3rd International Innovative Applications of Computational Intelligence on Power, Energy and Controls with their Impact on Humanity (CIPECH). pp. 102–106. IEEE (2018)
17. Chaudhary, H., Khatoon, S., Singh, R., Pandey, A.: Grey wolf optimizer based PID controller design for LAser beam pointing Application. In: Lecture notes in mechanical engineering. p (in press, 2019)
18. Basilio, J.C., Matos, S.R.: Design of PI and PID controllers with transient performance specification—Education. IEEE Trans.—ieee-edu2002.pdf **45**, 364–370 (2002)

19. Gaur, M., Chaudhary, H., Khatoon, S., Singh, R.: Genetic algorithm based trajectory stabilization of quadrotor. In: 2nd IEEE International Conference on Innovative Applications of Computational Intelligence on Power, Energy and Controls with their Impact on Humanity CIPECH 2016. (2017). https://doi.org/10.1109/cipech.2016.7918731
20. Qi, Z., Shi, Q., Zhang, H.: Tuning of digital PID controllers using particle swarm optimization algorithm for a CAN-based DC motor subject to stochastic delays. IEEE Trans. Ind. Electron., pp. 1 (2019). https://doi.org/10.1109/tie.2019.2934030

Comparison of Metaheuristic and Conventional Algorithms for Maximum Power Point Tracking of Solar PV Array

Mohammad Asfar Khan, Monaem Ibn Nasir, Syed Mohd Subhan, and Imran Pervez

Abstract The use of solar power is on the rise as energy demand increases and fossil fuels are under increasing stress. Solar energy is an eco-friendly and cheap source of energy as opposed to traditional energy sources. The solar photovoltaic (PV) cells utilize solar radiation to harness energy, but not in all cases the solar PV array operates in ideal conditions. The sun may not always be in direct line-of-site of the solar PV array as the direction of sun changes both annually and diurnally coupled with local blockade from nearby trees, buildings, natural barriers, clouds, etc. which ultimately leads to partial shading. The bypass diodes that are inculcated in order to reduce this partial shading effect create different power points in the *P–V* curve. The PV array cannot harvest the maximum power out of all available peaks. The conventional algorithms although worked well under full insolation conditions and failed under partial shading conditions. Hence, in this chapter the metaheuristic algorithms have been used in order to track the maximum power among various available peaks. Also, the comparison between different metaheuristic algorithms is done to show the best algorithm for Maximum Power Point Tracking (MPPT) applications.

Keywords MPPT · P&O · PSO · Bat · Jaya · GMPP · LMPP · Solar PV

1 Introduction

Solar power is quickly growing in popularity as it is cheap, inexpensive and requires little maintenance. Solar radiation is abounding and can be harnessed easily using currently available technology. For these reasons, the use of solar power has increased even in common household applications as well in rural areas. Solar PV arrays trap solar energy and convert it into electricity. Solar panels are easily available and do not require continuous monitoring and maintenance to remain operational. A solar PV array will generate energy constantly as long as sunlight is incident upon the

M. A. Khan · M. I. Nasir · S. M. Subhan · I. Pervez (✉)
Department of Electrical Engineering, ZHCET, Aligarh Muslim University, Aligarh, India
e-mail: imranpervez7@gmail.com

© The Author(s), under exclusive license to Springer Nature Singapore Pte Ltd. 2021   449
H. Malik et al. (eds.), *AI and Machine Learning Paradigms for Health Monitoring System*, Studies in Big Data 86,
https://doi.org/10.1007/978-981-33-4412-9_30

entirety of the PV array. However, if even a part of the solar panel is shaded, the power output of the shaded array drops drastically due to reverse current flow to the shaded PV panel from the non-shaded panels. To redress this, we used bypass diodes at the terminals of PV module to stop reverse current flow. This mitigated the power losses but produced multiple local maxima at the output. It made difficult to track the maximum power point (MPP) of the solar panel. Traditional MPPT methods like hill climbing [1] get stuck at one of the local maxima as insolation is varied and do not track the entire range of operation to find maximum power point. Artificial intelligence (AI)-based techniques like fuzzy logic [2] are applied, and they are successful at tracking the MPPT, but these require large amount of training data which put large stress on the computer. Metaheuristic algorithms like PSO [3, 4], Jaya [5], bat [6], etc. are used in place of AI-based algorithms as they track the MPPT correctly in little time and do not require large amount of training data. In this research, we have compared the conventional P&O algorithm against metaheuristic algorithms PSO, Jaya [5] and bat [6] available in the literature. For the better understanding of the optimization technique implementation, reader may refer [7–12].

2 Partially Shaded Solar PV Array

Partial shading happens when sunlight is blocked to a part of PV array due to blockage from clouds or nearby buildings. This partial shaded condition causes huge power losses. Bypass diodes are connected to the terminals of the module to mitigate the high reverse current, but this also reduces power output significantly. Also, multiple peaks of maximum power are seen at the output which makes it difficult to determine the MPP of the PV array (Fig. 1).

Fig. 1 A cloud blocking the sun and putting the panel under partial shaded condition

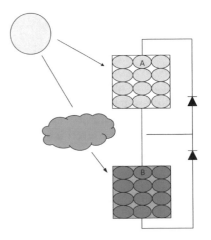

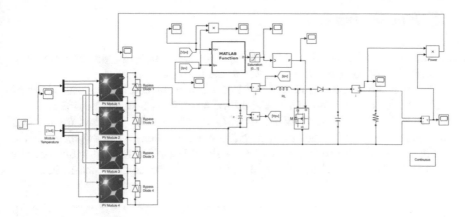

Fig. 2 Simulink model of solar PV array

3 Metaheuristic Algorithms for Maximum Power Point Tracking

To deliver maximum power from the solar panel, a boost converter is used. The duty ratio of the boost converter is calculated using various algorithms. These algorithms can be developed in MATLAB or any other programming language and can then be deployed on a microprocessor. The microprocessor controls the duty ratio of the boost converter and delivers maximum power in all possible conditions.

Figure 2 shows the Simulink model used to obtain the results under various shading conditions. A DC-DC boost converter is used as a medium to adjust the voltage between the PV array and the output. MATLAB function represents a microcontroller which can be used to implement MPPT algorithms such as BAT and Jaya. This microcontroller controls the duty ratio of boost converter and tries to provide maximum power at the output.

We have used this MATLAB function to implement the algorithms which are compared in this research, namely P&O, PSO, BAT and Jaya.

4 Results

The results are taken for two different insolation conditions to show the superiority of metaheuristic algorithms over conventional algorithms.

4.1   Shading Pattern I

Insolation was distributed as 1000, 900, 400 and 300 W/m² on four modules, respectively, for this case. The peak was at the leftmost position

Figure 3 shows the performance of P&O which tracked the optimal power of 33.46 W with an efficiency of 99.28 and time taken for convergence 0.482 s.

Figure 4 shows the performance of PSO algorithm which tracked the optimal power of 33.54 W with an efficiency of 99.70 and time taken for convergence 1.201 s.

Figure 5 shows the performance of Jaya algorithm which tracked optimal power of 33.43 W with an efficiency of 99.43 and time taken for convergence 1.293 s.

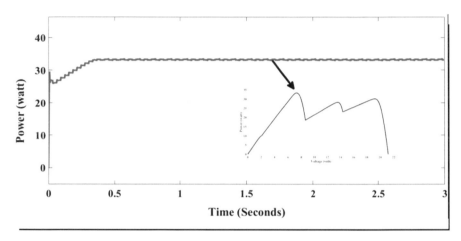

Fig. 3   P&O

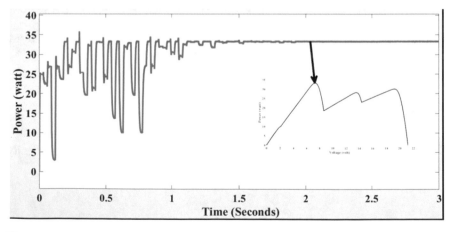

Fig. 4   PSO

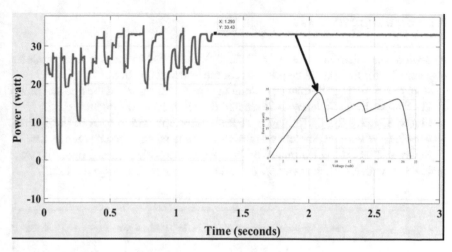

Fig. 5 Jaya

Figure 6 shows the performance of bat algorithm which tracked the optimal power of 32.22 W with an efficiency of 96.49 and time taken for convergence 1.191 s.

Above comparisons unequivocally prove that P&O algorithm tracked MPP in the minimum amount of time. On the other hand, PSO algorithm tracked MPP with highest efficiency. PSO tracked the highest power, but all the algorithms tracked power almost identically under full insolation condition. There is virtually no difference in all algorithms except P&O which takes very little time, but these results do not hold as we will see in the next section.

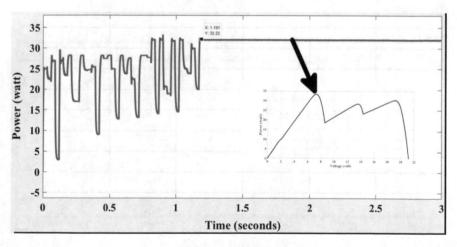

Fig. 6 Bat

4.2 Shading Pattern II

Insolation was distributed as 1000, 900, 300 and 400 W/m² on four modules, respectively, for this case. The peak was at the leftmost position.

Analysis of P&O performance is done in Fig. 7 which tracked the optimal power of 41.15 W with an efficiency of 99.86 and time taken for convergence 0.369.

Figure 8 shows the performance of PSO algorithm which tracked the optimal power 49.21 W with an efficiency of 99.86 and time taken for convergence 1.927.

Figure 9 shows the performance of Jaya algorithm which tracked optimal power of 49.08 W with an efficiency of 99.86 and time taken for convergence 1.023.

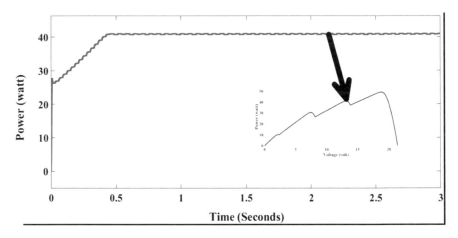

Fig. 7 P&O

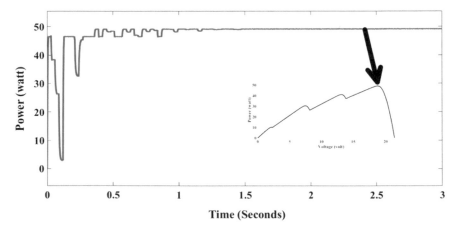

Fig. 8 PSO

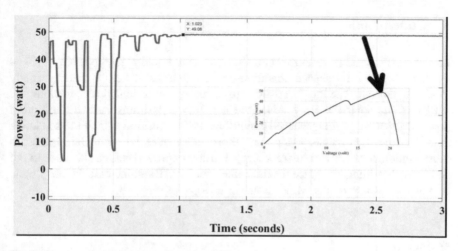

Fig. 9 Jaya

Figure 10 shows the performance of bat algorithm which tracked the optimal power of 48.85 W with an efficiency of 99.86 and time taken for convergence 1.185.

From the above comparison, it can be seen that P&O algorithm tracked MPP in the minimum amount of time but did not properly track the MPP and got stuck at local maxima. PSO and Jaya tracked the MPP correctly; all algorithms tracked MPP with highest efficiency.

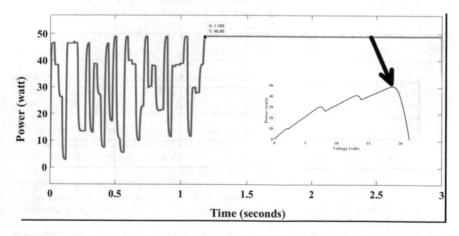

Fig. 10 Bat

5 Conclusion

As can be observed from above analysis, traditional tracking methods have tracked the MPP under fully shaded conditions, wherein stuck at LMPP under partially shaded condition. The metaheuristic algorithms are more reliable for tracking the MPPT of the solar PV array. Also, Bat and Jaya algorithms tracked the highest power even under partially shaded conditions. PSO algorithm is found to be slower than the other two metaheuristic algorithms; this makes Jaya and Bat algorithms more suitable for MPPT of solar PV array. Further improvements can be made to Bat and Jaya algorithms to reduce the time taken for MPPT and increase the magnitude of power output, and thus, MPPT is an active topic of research.

References

1. Nejila, V.P., Immanuel Selvakumar, A.: Fuzzy-logic based hill-climbing method for maximum power point tracking in PV systems. In: 2013 International Conference on Power, Energy and Control (ICPEC)
2. Syafaruddin, Karatepe, E., Hiyama, T.: Artificial neural network polar coordinated fuzzy controller based maximum power point tracking control under partially shaded conditions. IET Renew. Power Gener. 3(2), 239–253 (2009)
3. Miyatake, M., Veerachary, M., Toriumi, F., Fujii, N., Ko, H.: 'Maximum power point tracking of multiple photovoltaic arrays: a PSO approach'. IEEE Trans. Aerosp. Electron. Syst. 47(1), 367–380 (2011)
4. Lian, K.L., Jhang J.H., Tian, I.S.: A maximum power point tracking method based on Perturb-and-Observe combined with particle swarm optimization. IEEE J. Photovolt. 4(2), 626–633 (2014)
5. Huang, C., Zhang, Z., Wang, L., Song Z., Long, H.: A novel global MPPT for PV system using Jaya algorithm. In: 2017 IEEE Conference on Energy Internet and Energy System Integration (EI2), Beijing, 2017, pp. 1–5
6. Tey, K.S., Mekhilef S., Seyed Mahmoudian, M.: Implementation of BAT algorithm as maximum power point tracking technique for photovoltaic system under partial shading conditions. In: 2018 IEEE Energy Conversion Congress and Exposition (ECCE), Portland, 2018, pp. 2531–2535. https://doi.org/10.1109/ecce.2018.8557460
7. Fatema, N. et al.: Data-driven occupancy detection hybrid model using particle swarm optimization based artificial neural network. In: Springer Nature Book: Metaheuristic and Evolutionary Computation: Algorithms and Applications, under book series "Studies in Computational Intelligence", 2020. https://doi.org/10.1007/978-981-15-7571-6_13
8. Iqbal, A. et al.: Metaheurestic algorithm based hybrid model for identification of building sale prices. In: Springer Nature Book: Metaheuristic and Evolutionary Computation: Algorithms and Applications, under book series "Studies in Computational Intelligence", 2020. https://doi.org/10.1007/978-981-15-7571-6_32
9. Faiz Minai, A. et al.: Metaheuristics paradigms for renewable energy systems: advances in optimization algorithms. In: Springer Nature Book: Metaheuristic and Evolutionary Computation: Algorithms and Applications, under book series "Studies in Computational Intelligence", 2020. https://doi.org/10.1007/978-981-15-7571-6_2
10. Vinoop, P. et al.: PSO-NN-based hybrid model for long-term wind speed prediction: a study on 67 cities of India. In: Book chapter in Applications of Artificial Intelligence Techniques in Engineering, Advances in Intelligent Systems and Computing vol. 697, pp. 319–327 (2018). https://doi.org/10.1007/978-981-13-1822-1_29

11. Mukherji, V. et al.: Fractional order control and simulation of wind-biomass isolated hybrid power system using particle swarm optimization. In: Book chapter in Applications of Artificial Intelligence Techniques in Engineering, Advances in Intelligent Systems and Computing vol. 698, pp. 277–287 (2018). https://doi.org/10.1007/978-981-13-1819-1_28
12. Mahto, T., et al.: Load frequency control of a solar-diesel based isolated hybrid power system by fractional order control using particle swarm optimization. J. Intell. Fuzzy Syst. **35**(5), 5055–5061 (2018). https://doi.org/10.3233/JIFS-169789
13. Chao, K.-H., Wu, M.-C.: Global maximum power point tracking (MPPT) of a photovoltaic module array constructed through improved teaching-learning-based optimization. Energies **9**, 986 (2016)

Artificial Neural Network-Based Maximum Power Point Tracking Method with the Improved Effectiveness of Standalone Photovoltaic System

Asim Iqbal Khan, Rashid Ahmed Khan, Shoeb Azam Farooqui, and Mohammad Sarfraz

Abstract The application of the solar photovoltaic (SPV) power has been expanding speedily due to its numerous advantages. However, it has a few limitations. PV system shows nonlinear behavior, very low power conversion efficiency, a high initial investment in installation and depends totally on natural conditions, that is, solar insolation and ambient temperature. So, to take out maximum permitted power from the PV system, maximum power point tracker (MPPT) is employed. Various algorithms have been introduced for tracking the maximum power point, but many of these algorithms do not perform well under varying environmental conditions, while few among them track maximum power point efficiently. In this paper, ANN-based algorithm has been utilized as this method is fast and precisely tracks the MPP. The result is validated by simulation using MATLAB/Simulink.

Keywords Solar photovoltaic (SPV) system · Partial shading conditions (PSC) · Maximum power point tracking (MPPT) · Artificial neural network (ANN)

1 Introduction

The electrical energy demand is increasing rapidly due to population explosion. Due to alarming environmental concerns and depleting fossil fuels, the production of electrical energy from coal is going to end in a few decades. Switching to renewable energy sources for major portion of electrical energy generation lessens

A. I. Khan (✉) · R. A. Khan · S. A. Farooqui · M. Sarfraz
Department of Electrical Engineering, Aligarh Muslim University, Aligarh, India
e-mail: aasimiqbal3d@gmail.com

R. A. Khan
e-mail: rashidkhan6417@gmail.com

S. A. Farooqui
e-mail: shoebazam6331@gmail.com

M. Sarfraz
e-mail: m.sarfraz@zhcet.ac.in

© The Author(s), under exclusive license to Springer Nature Singapore Pte Ltd. 2021   459
H. Malik et al. (eds.), *AI and Machine Learning Paradigms for Health Monitoring System*, Studies in Big Data 86,
https://doi.org/10.1007/978-981-33-4412-9_31

these concerns. Out of renewable energy resources, solar energy is the best alternative for producing electrical power [1–3]. Solar energy extraction using solar PV panels shows an appreciable ability in completing the global demand for energy. This renewable energy can provide security to our future development.

Advantage of photovoltaic power generation system includes long-term benefits, negligible maintenance, absence of fuel cost, and environmentally friendly [3, 4]. However, the main problem in the implementation and integration of the PV system is higher initial cost and low power transformation efficiency of solar insolation into electricity [4]. Moreover, the power produced from the solar PV module highly relies on the level of solar insolation and the temperature [5]. The insolation received by the PV module varies due to continuous change in orientation of earth and due to partial shading because of passing clouds, shade of neighboring buildings, and trees. By the application of photovoltaic (PV) cells, solar energy is trapped. Therefore, the power-voltage characteristic of solar PV system is not linear [6]. For ensuring optimum utilization of incident light, MPPT is employed.

PV technology works on the principle of the photoelectric effect and utilizes solar radiation to generate electricity [6]. Due to its economic and environmental benefits, the PV system is widely employed. The shortcoming of the PV panel encourages the researches to find some techniques to take out the maximum permitted power from PV system to optimize the efficiency of the solar panel. The energy produced from the PV module is entirely dependent on surrounding conditions like ambient temperature and irradiance, which are not constant. It keeps on changing with time [7]. So, certain MPPT algorithms have been evolved to get maximum output from the PV system even in varying environmental conditions. Figure 1 shows a general layout of MPPT for the PV system.

The power capacity of the panel could be increased by connecting the module in series and parallel arrangement. If some part of the module receives less intensity of light than the other, it is partial shading condition. This may occur due to clouds, shadows of high-rise buildings, trees, and other neighboring objects [7]. A hotspot is formed because of non-uniform solar insolation throughout the string due to the partial shading of the module. To overcome the disadvantage of the hotspot, a diode is

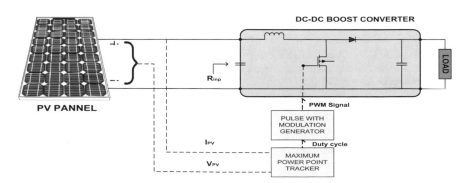

Fig. 1 General configuration of the MPPT for the PV system

used for bypassing the current and is connected across each module, thus, protecting the PV module. PSC results in more complex PV characteristics and exhibiting multiple peaks [8].

Many techniques have been introduced for MPPT which are categorized as a conventional technique, artificial intelligence technique, and stochastic-based technique. Conventional methods of MPPT are perturbation and observation method (P & O), method of fractional open-circuit voltage, and short circuit current and incremental conductance method, which are based on hill-climbing techniques [4–8]. These techniques are simple and are generally employed for uniform irradiance. Under PSC, the tracking efficiency of these techniques is very poor due to the presence of multiple peaks of its PV characteristics. Disparate artificial intelligence technique and stochastic-based algorithm have been proposed due to the interfacing of conventional methods. These techniques are inspired by nature and biological structure. It includes cuckoo search algorithm (CSA), particle swarm optimization (PSO), firefly algorithm (FA), ant colony specialization, artificial neural network (ANN), differential evolution (DE), and Jaya algorithm [9, 10]. These strategical algorithms or methods can be utilized to take the maximum power under the varying and partially shaded condition [11]. Among the numerous MPPT methods, the method with low complexity, minimum output power fluctuation, and quick tracking speed under partially shaded conditions are preferred. The artificial neural network method does well under rapidly varying environmental conditions in terms of tracking time and number of iterations [12]. So, the ANN-based MPPT technique has been used in this work. The ANN is the most effective and accurate soft computing techniques to locate the MPP, and it is inspired by the biological phenomenon. An ANN has three layers, which are connected to each other [13]. The neural network works on three steps: building training and testing. The backpropagation algorithm is very common to train the neural network [14]. The input may be atmospheric data like temperature irradiance or PV array parameters like panel voltage and current or any combinations of these. The output may be the duty cycle or the voltage at MPP [15].

2　PV Module Modeling

The energy conversion in solar modules or cells is done by the photoelectric effect. A PV module is made up of many photovoltaic cells. An arrangement is made by connecting these cells in parallel and series to increase the output current and module voltage, respectively. Different equivalent models of the solar PV cell have been proposed by the researchers, but single diode model of PV cell is used here which has been illustrated in Fig. 2. PV cells are neither a current source nor a constant voltage source. It can be considered as a current generator with dependent voltage sources. The circuit consists of a diode in parallel with current source, a shunt resistance, and a series resistance in parallel. Iph is a PV generated current that relies on temperature and solar radiation. The stronger irradiance will generate greater Iph. The nonlinear $I-V$ characteristic of the solar PV module is due to the current I_d. The

Fig. 2 Single diode model
of the PV cell

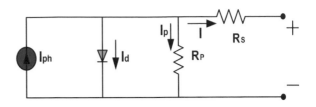

output current is given by applying the KCL.

$$I = I_{ph} - I_d - I_p \tag{1}$$

Which can be written as

$$I = I_{ph} - Io\left[e^{\left(\frac{q(V+I*Rs)}{akT}\right)} - 1\right] - \frac{V + I * Rs}{Rp} \tag{2}$$

where

I PV cell current,
I_{ph} Insolation current,
I_d Diode current,
I_p Current through R_P,
V PV module output voltage,
R_P Parallel resistance and,
R_S Series resistance,
q Charge on electron [1.602×10^{-19} C],
K Boltzmann constant [1.380×10^{-23} J/K],
T Temperature of cell (Kelvin),
a Ideality factor of the diode.

PV current is expressed as below if we consider the effect of irradiance and temperature

$$I_{ph} = \left(I_{ph}, n + K * \Delta T\right)\frac{G}{Gn} \tag{3}$$

where G and Gn are irradiance at the operating condition and nominal condition, respectively.

ΔT is the temperature difference of the nominal and actual temperature.

Figure 3 illustrates the I–V curve of the solar module for various values of solar insolation. Figure 4 depicts the temperature effect on the I–V curve of the solar module. If some part of the module receives less intensity of light than the other, it is partial shading conditions. This may appear due to the presence of clouds, shadows of high-rise building, trees, and other neighboring objects. PSC results in more complex PV characteristics and exhibiting multiple peaks. These techniques can be employed

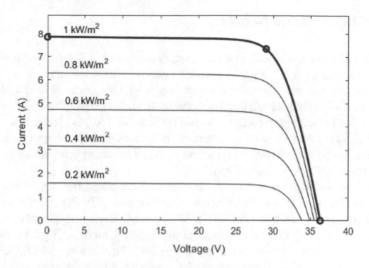

Fig. 3 Effect of the insolation on $I–V$ characteristic

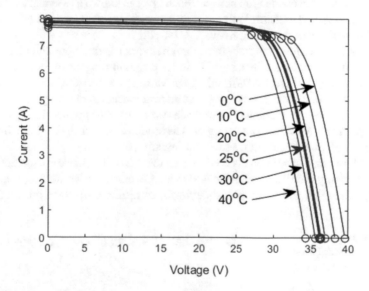

Fig. 4 Effect of the temperature on $I–V$ characteristic

under rapidly varying and partially shaded atmospheric conditions to take out the maximum permitted power.

3   Artificial Neural Network

The ANN is a computational method which is commonly inspired by the working of a human being. It is an interconnected system of neurons and can be used to approximate or estimate the function depending on a large number of inputs. Neurons are the handling unit that initially gauges the information directly. These coordinates to each other by sending messages. Activation function (AF) is used to evaluate the sum which is a nonlinear function. The result is finally sent to the respective neurons. A directed graph may be used to represent an ANN in which synapses and neurons are the edges and nodes, respectively.

Based on the interconnection of neurons to each other, the ANN structure is mainly of two types first is the recurrent neural network (RNN) and the second is the feed-forward neural network (FNN). ANN can quickly and accurately locate the maximum power point by different sets of input data without falling trap into local maxima. A common ANN is commonly comprised of three layers which are named as input layer, hidden layer, and output layer, which are identical to the neurons of the nervous system. A multilayer FNN is shown in Fig. 5. These layers are interconnected to each other and the connection between each layer is known as a synapse. Random weights are assigned to them. Training, validation, and testing are the three steps on which the working of the neural network is based.

Some data are required to train the neural networks as the input and output variables. It can be obtained either by PV model programming or by developing PV model simulation in MATLAB/Simulink for various solar insolation and temperature values. The input may be the temperature, irradiance, panel voltage, and current, i.e., V_{OC} or I_{SC} or any combination of these can be used to predict the V_{MPP}. Duty cycle or voltage at MPP may be the output. The hidden layer consists of basic function which is a weighted linear sum, activation function, and tansig.

Several methods have been evolved to train the ANN. The backpropagation algorithm is generally used for training the ANN with Levenberg–Marquardt optimization method, which is mainly used in a supervised learning for ANN. In this method, a

Fig. 5 Multilayer
feed-forward neural network

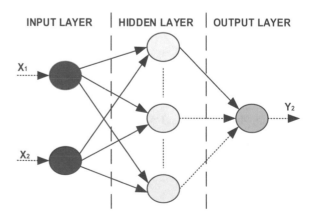

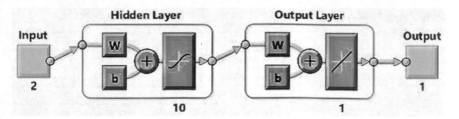

Fig. 6 Neural network model

few combinations of input values and related desired solutions are used to train the ANN. ANN progressively learn and minimizes the error by making a comparison in the reference with the actual output. The error function is evaluated with each epoch (iteration) between the actual and targeted value. To reduce the error between the two values, a supervised learning technique is properly used to manipulate the weights, which are set randomly at initial. ANN design is complicated and it requires high processing time and training as well.

Training time can be reduced by avoiding the identical PV curve. At every stage of the learning process, V_{PV} and I_{PV} are the inputs at n different points and the desired output are the voltage corresponding to global maximum power point. Figure 6 shows a neural network model with two input layers, one output, and ten hidden layer.

4 Proposed MPPT Method

The simulation of solar PV system with artificial neural network-based MPPT is done through MATLAB/Simulink, whose schematic representation is shown in Fig. 7. In this approach, temperature and irradiance are the inputs while output is the duty cycle. Voltage and current sensor are employed for sensing the voltage and current. It is fed to the ANN-based algorithm which is already trained with a sufficient amount

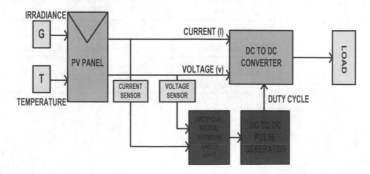

Fig. 7 Schematic representation of solar PV system with the proposed MPPT technique

Table 1 Specification of the solar PV module

Parameters	Value
Maximal power (W)	249
Voltage at open circuit V_{oc} (V)	36.8
MPP voltage V_{mp} (V)	30
Temp. coeff. of V_{oc} (%/ °C)	-0.33
No. of cells in a module (N_{cell})	60
Current at short circuit I_{sc} (A)	8.83
MPP current I_{mp} (A)	8.3
Temp. coeff. of I_{sc} (%/ °C)	0.063805

of data. This algorithm will optimize the duty ratio for the DC to DC converter to make system works at the MPP for maximum permitted power extraction.

The real-life condition is achieved with simulation by randomly generating the temperature from 25 to 35 °C and irradiance differing between 100 and 1200 (W/m^2). It is same as the solar radiation receives on the surface of module. The simulation is run for a total of 0.9 s. In the simulation, solar PV module fabricated by Tata power, TP250MBZ is used and its estimated maximum power is 249 W.

For the switching purpose of MOSFET or IGBT in the converter, the ANN algorithm optimizes the duty ratio and then the PWM generator is employed to produce the pulses. Then, for switching the MOSFET/IGBT employed in the converter, these pulses are used.

The dataset is generated for 65,522 data points. A three-layered feed-forward network with 2 inputs, 10 hidden layers, and 1 output layer is employed. Out of 65,522 samples, 45,866 (70%) samples are considered for training, 9828 (15%) samples are utilized for validation, and 9828(15%) are utilized for the testing process. In this model of ANN, the Levenberg–Marquardt algorithm is adopted for training purposes. PV module specifications are displayed in Table 1 and the proposed method system specifications are displayed in Table 2.

Table 2 Standalone PV system specifications

Parameter	Value
Inductance	1.1478 mH
Capacitance	0.4676 μF, 10 μF
Resistance	53
Switching frequency	10 kHz

5 Simulation Results

The simulated model of the standalone solar PV system with ANN-based MPPT has been shown in Fig. 8. It is done in three parts (a) under the nominal condition which means 1000 W/m^2 and 25 °C, (b) under varying solar insolation or irradiation keeping nominal temperature, and (c) under varying temperature keeping nominal irradiation.

In Fig. 9a, ANN-based MPPT tracks the maximum power point in 0.1 s under the nominal condition and maximum power is found to be 249 watts. The simulation time for the proposed PV system is 0.9 s, as shown in Fig. 9b, solar insolation is 1000 W/m^2 for 0.3 s, 900 W/m^2 for next 0.3 s, and 800 W/m^2 for another next 0.3 s keeping nominal temperature. Maximum power decreases as solar insolation decreases which clear from the given figure. In Fig. 9c, temperature is changing with a step of 25, 30, and 35 °C for 0.3 s each respectively keeping nominal solar insolation. Maximum power decreases as temperature decreases. Tracking time is similar in all conditions.

Pulses from ANN under nominal condition are depicted in Fig. 10a, and the duty ratio is always varying from 0 to 1 but some numerical value of duty ratio is not in between 0 and 1. After saturation from 0 to 1, pulses are modified as shown in Fig. 10b. Pulse width modulation is done through DC to DC pulse generator which is given to the MOSFET/IGBT having a frequency of 10 kHz and pulses width modulated waveform is shown in Fig. 10c. Solar insolation and temperature are varying according to the given waveform as shown in Fig. 10d, e, respectively.

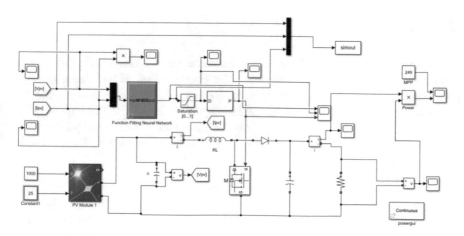

Fig. 8 Simulation of the proposed PV system

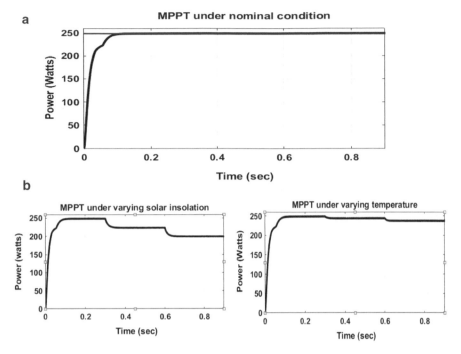

Fig. 9 **a** MPPT under varying solar insolation keeping nominal temperature, **b** MPPT under varying temperature keeping nominal solar insolation

6 Conclusion

This paper presented an ANN-based MPPT method which works satisfactorily under constant and rapidly varying condition. This configuration of the neural network is upfront with no computational burden. Results of simulation showed that the proposed method of ANN tracks the maximum power within 0.1 s. Consequently, the ANN-based MPPT demonstrates in this paper has a good accuracy and performance in terms of number of iteration and tracking time which is suitable for household applications.

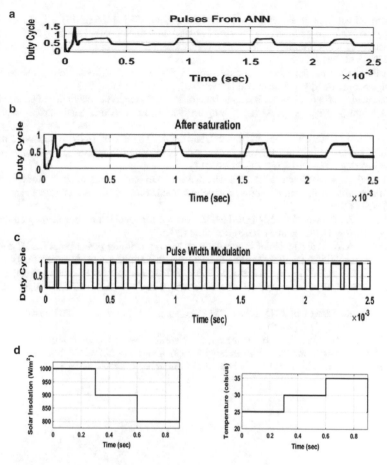

Fig. 10 **a** Pulses from ANN under the nominal condition, **b** pulses after saturation from ANN under nominal condition, **c** pulse width modulation of duty cycle waveform under nominal condition, **d** solar insolation waveform, **e** temperature waveform

References

1. Mandour, R., Elamvazuthi, I.: Optimization of maximum power point tracking (MPPT) of photovoltaic system using artificial intelligence (AI) algorithms. J. Emerg. Trends Comput. Inf. Sci. **4**(8), 662–669 (2013)
2. Bouselham, L., Hajji, M., Hajji, B., Bouali, H.: A New MPPT-based ANN for photovoltaic system under partial shading conditions. Energy Procedia **111**(September 2016), 924–933 (2017)
3. Sreedhar, S., Jagadeesh, D.: A review on optimization algorithms for MPPT in solar PV system under partially shaded conditions, pp. 23–32 (2016)
4. Johnson, J., Professor, A.: Analysis of different MPPT techniques. Int. J. Adv. Res. Electr. Electron. Instrum. Eng. (An ISO, **3297**, 1694–1698 (2007)
5. Sher, H.A., Murtaza, A.F., Al-Haddad, K.: A hybrid maximum power point tracking method for photovoltaic applications with reduced offline measurements. In: Proceedings of the IEEE

International Conference on Industrial Technology, pp. 1482–1485 (2017)

6. Attia, H.A.: High performance PV system based on artificial neural network MPPT with PI controller for direct current water pump applications. Int. J. Power Electron. Drive Syst. **10**(3), 1329–1338 (2019)

7. Beriber, D., Talha, A.: MPPT techniques for PV systems. International Conference on Power Engineering, Energy and Electrical Drives, May, pp. 1437–1442 (2013)

8. Sedaghati, F., Nahavandi, A., Badamchizadeh, M.A., Ghaemi, S., Abedinpour Fallah, M.: PV maximum power-point tracking by using artificial neural network. Math. Probl. Eng. **2012** (2012)

9. Al-Gizi, A.G., Craciunescu, A., Al-Chlaihawi, S.J.: The use of ANN to supervise the PV MPPT based on FLC. In: 2017 10th International Symposium on Advanced Topics in Electrical Engineering ATEE 2017, pp. 703–708 (2017)

10. Khanaki, R., Mohd Radzi, M.A., Marhaban, M.H.: Artificial neural network based maximum power point tracking controller for photovoltaic standalone system. Int. J. Green Energy **13**(3), 283–291 (2016)

11. Rizzo, S.A., Scelba, G.: ANN based MPPT method for rapidly variable shading conditions. Appl. Energy **145**(September 2018), 124–132 (2015)

12. Ibrahim, A.W. et al.: Artificial neural network based maximum power point tracking for PV system. In: Chinese Control Conference CCC, vol. 2019-July, pp. 6559–6564 (2019)

13. Phan, Q.D., Le, D.K., Hong, H.L., Le, M.P., Vu, N.T.D.: The new MPPT algorithm using ANN-based PV. In: 2010 International Forum on Strategic Technologies IFOST 2010, pp. 402–407 (2010)

14. Duwadi, K.: Design of ANN based MPPT for solar panel design of ANN based MPPT for solar panel. July, 0–4 (2015)

15. Allahabadi, S., Iman-Eini, H., Farhangi, S.: Neural network based maximum power point tracking technique for PV arrays in mobile applications. In: 2019 10th International Power Electronics, Drive Systems and Technologies Conference PEDSTC 2019, pp. 701–706 (2019)

Analysis on Various Optimization Technique Used for Load Frequency Control

Mohammed Asim, Archana Verma, and Ahmed Riyaz

Abstract In modern energy system, the load frequency control (LFC) is the main operation which is done at system at daily basis. The purpose of the load frequency control is to maintain the power balance between the interconnected systems and to control the tie lines power flow. In this chapter, we provide an overview of the different LFC technique which is based on different controllers. The conventional and soft computing techniques of load frequency control techniques have been compared for reheat turbine system and non-reheat turbine system.

Keywords LFC · Controllers · Settling time

1 Introduction

One of the most important works of any power system is to maintain the balance between the demand and generation. Tie line power flow and frequency are affected by small change in power demand. Based on area control error (ACE), the adjustment of active power is done, so that the generation and load demand matches. Hence, the main objectives of load frequency control are achieved.

The automatic load frequency control (ALFC) technique is a closed loop technique. Due to the dynamic nature of the power system, change in load always occurs a change in active power and reactive power flow.

A system in which two or more generating units are interconnected through a tie line. This type of system is called a multi-area connected power system. Various similar or different power systems like thermal–thermal, hydro–hydro or plant-like thermal hydro–thermal-wind share power via tie line. For the better understanding of the optimization technique implementation, reader may refer [1–6].

M. Asim (✉) · A. Verma
Department of Electrical Engineering, Integral University, Lucknow, India
e-mail: asimamu@gmail.com

A. Riyaz
Department of Electrical Engineering, BGSB University, Rajouri, India

© The Author(s), under exclusive license to Springer Nature Singapore Pte Ltd. 2021   471
H. Malik et al. (eds.), *AI and Machine Learning Paradigms for Health Monitoring System*, Studies in Big Data 86,
https://doi.org/10.1007/978-981-33-4412-9_32

1.1 Aims of LFC

The power quality of the system depends then on the performance of the complex power system falls down which results in fluctuations in area frequency and disturbance in tie line. Thus, by the use of the LFC techniques, we can reduce the undesirable effects on the system due to load disturbance, parameter uncertainties, and nonlinearities [7]. The main aim of LFC is given below:

(a) Maintaining a constant frequency.
(b) To manage load disturbance.
(c) Maintaining scheduled power flow between neighboring areas.
(d) To make a power system robust for uncertainties.
(e) Maintaining time response specifications.

2 Control Strategies

The primal objective of LFC is the minimization of frequency deviation and unwanted line interchange. There are different types of controllers available which are broadly classified as conventional control techniques and soft computing techniques.

2.1 Classical Control Techniques

There are various types of LFC discussed in the literature, but the PI controller is frequently used for the speed-governing system for most of the LFC scheme. PI controller is most popularly used controller for industrial applications because proportional controller delivers a relatively more stable system with better frequency response. On the basis of its performance and robustness, PID controller is mostly used for industrial applications. In PID, derivative component creates noise because of this it is not used. So PI controller is preferred than PID controller. The modern control power system has seen development in the field of optimal control [8, 9].

Nowadays, adaptive control methods are used for designing the AGC regulators. The addition of self-tuning feature in conventional PID controller results in the increased controlled performance of the controller. Self-tuning PID controller delivers much improved performance compared to the conventional PID controller. When the system order increases the order of the controller will also increase. This leads to a complex control system for solving, where genetic algorithm (GA) is used to design well-tuned PI controller for multi-area power system. By the use of artificial intelligence techniques, faults are detected within very short time because they had capability to process complex information [10].

2.2 Soft Computing Technique

2.2.1 Fuzzy Control Optimization

In fuzzy control optimization technique, the controller is based on fuzzy logic. Whenever the source of information is not exact, at this place, fuzzy technique plays a very important role. This technique provides algorithm that converts linguistic-based control strategy on expert knowledge into an automatic control. This technique contains mainly four parts:

- Fuzzification
- Knowledge base
- Fuzzy interference system
- A membership function.

Fuzzification is the process of changing crisp value to a fuzzy value. This fuzzy value carries uncertainty in it. This value is represented by membership function. Fuzzy control loop consists of fuzzy reasoning and rule base to give decision. Knowledge base defines parameter and variable of fuzzy set. Defuzzification is the process of changing the fuzzy value into crisp values. It is basically interpreting fuzzy set membership degree into decision or real value.

Fuzzy logic is one of the latest soft computing techniques being used for LFC. Here, when we do not have exact input or do not have a mathematical model or relationship, then fuzzy logic controller helps.

For a multi-area system, fuzzy PI controller is adopted which results in better performance of the system [11].

An indirect adaptive fuzzy logic control for multi-area system with unknown parameter like wear and tear of equipment and unknown parameter of interconnected like variation in synchronous power is used. The parameter of controller is obtained from formulating by updating the procedure and also appropriating adopted control low. The fuzzy controller will ensure the limits of all parameter in tracking error for closed loop system.

In the power system, fuzzy logic technique is most wildly used in recent year. This becomes a very important method for the modern power system. There are various type of conventional controller which are used in the power system but they have various disadvantage related to efficiency and stability, so we use fuzzy type controller to overcome these problems based on experience and knowledge about system. Some new intelligence control technique based on polar fuzzy sets also introduce in 1990. Polar fuzzy sets methods are slightly different from standard fuzzy sets technique. Stability and dynamic performance are improved by the polar fuzzy control method.

2.2.2 Genetic Algorithm-Based Technique

J. H. HOLLAND in 1970 developed genetic algorithm which is a heuristic algorithm based on natural genetic. Optimal solution and satisfactory solution are solved by the generational evaluation of population. Basically, there are three phases in GA, i.e., creation of initial population, evaluation of fitness function, and production of new population.

After iteration which is also called generation, we get the optimum solution. The chromosome length and population size govern the speed of the iteration. By generational and steady-state methods, GA generates itself. The whole population is swapped after iteration in generational method. In steady-state, small member of population is rejected after each iteration and the total size of population remains fixed. There are some drawbacks in this method which are given below:

- For initial population, it is very sensitive.
- Sub-optimal solution is obtained in some cases.

In the area of AGC of power system, GA has been extensively used. A different system like hydroplant has been studied. GA combined with fuzzy has also been implemented. The GA-based LFC is implemented for multi-area system.

2.2.3 PSO Algorithm-Based Technique

The particle swarm optimization method is basically based on the intelligence of the bird swarm. PSO method is based on the behavior of flock of bird and fish.

PSO works on the process that is particle moves along the direction, according to its current direction, personal best position, and best position. In order to achieve the best position, i.e., to reach the objective, continuous iteration is done. Results are best when we achieve the target or the objective in minimum number of iteration.

PSO give better result than GA in the designing of the controller as PSO is not restricted to load minima as GA. Several multi-objective controllers are discussed in the literature using PSO-based design for two-area power system having good performance [12].

2.2.4 Artificial Neural Network (ANN)-Based Technique

Artificial neural network is the human brain's neural system-based computing system. The main motive of ANN system to solve any problem in the same way like brain in the ANN system activation function plays a very important role for something complicated. For large-scale deregulated power system, flexible ANN techniques gives better result.

3 Comparative Analysis of Different Control Systems

Figure 1 shows a general block diagram of a single area control system.

Here, we have considered two examples to compare the result of single area power system one with non-reheat turbine and another with reheat turbine whose parameters are as:

System parameters: $K1_P = 120, T1_P = 20, T1_T = 0.3, T1_G = 0.08, R1 = 2.4$.

System parameters: $K2_P = 1.25, T2_P = 12.5, T2_T = 0.5, T2_G = 0.2, R2 = 0.05$.

where $K1p$ and $K2p$ are system gain for reheat and non-reheat turbine, respectively, and $T1_P, T2_P, T1_T, T2_T, T1_G$, and $T2_G$ are time constant of system, turbine, and governor for reheat and non-reheat turbine, respectively.

The performance of the controller is studied by applying a step load of $\Delta P_D = 0.01$ p.u at $t = 1$ s. The robustness of the system is also checked by varying system constant and time constant of the system.

The performance analysis for different optimization techniques was done and is plotted in Figs. 2 and 3, respectively. Figure 2 shows the frequency regulation performance of reheat turbine and Fig. 3 shows the non-reheat turbine. The results show that PSO gives better result compared to other techniques and use of soft computing methods improve the result compared to conventional techniques.

The settling time of PSO-based LFC is 4.3 s which has increased from 9.5 s in case of PID-based LFC for reheat turbine and result of peak value and integral square error also improves. Similarly, in case of non-reheat turbine, PSO gives better result and all the parameters improve.

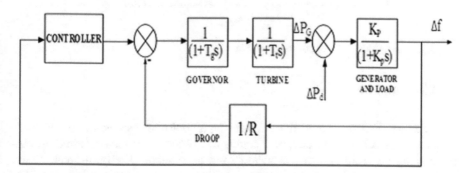

Fig. 1 LFC for single area system

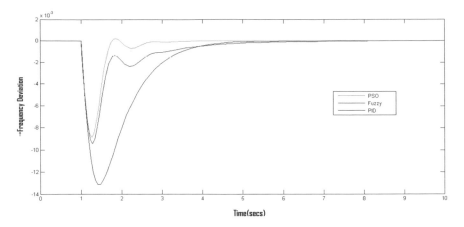

Fig. 2 Frequency deviation for reheat turbine

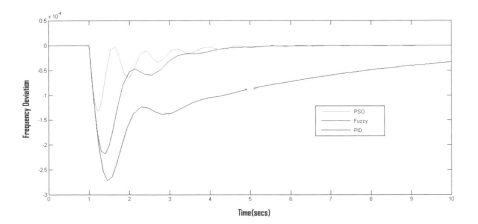

Fig. 3 Frequency deviation for non-reheat turbine

4 Conclusions

This chapter discusses about the different type controller technique for the load
frequency control. The system performance was observed on the basis of dynamic
parameters, i.e., settling time, overshoot, and undershoot. The performance was
analyzed for both reheat and non-reheat turbine. It is seen that modern-day soft
computing techniques give better result compared to conventional techniques for a
load frequency control system.

Acknowledgements The authors would like to acknowledge Integral University for providing the
MCN number IU/R&D/2020-MCN000839.

References

1. Fatema, N. et al.: Data-driven occupancy detection hybrid model using particle swarm optimization based artificial neural network. In: Springer Nature Book: Metaheuristic and Evolutionary Computation: Algorithms and Applications, under book series "Studies in Computational Intelligence", 2020. https://doi.org/10.1007/978-981-15-7571-6_13
2. Iqbal, A. et al.: Metaheurestic algorithm based hybrid model for identification of building sale prices. In: Springer Nature Book: Metaheuristic and Evolutionary Computation: Algorithms and Applications, under book series "Studies in Computational Intelligence", 2020. https://doi.org/10.1007/978-981-15-7571-6_32
3. Shahabuddin, M., Asim, M., Sarwar, A.: Parameter extraction of a solar PV cell using projectile search algorithm. In: 2020 International Conference on Advances in Computing, Communication & Materials (ICACCM), Dehradun, India, pp. 357–361 (2020). https://doi.org/10.1109/ICACCM50413.2020.9213005
4. Vinoop, P. et al.: PSO-NN-based hybrid model for long-term wind speed prediction: a study on 67 cities of India. In: Book chapter in Applications of Artificial Intelligence Techniques in Engineering, Advances in Intelligent Systems and Computing, vol. 697, pp. 319–327 (2018). https://doi.org/10.1007/978-981-13-1822-1_29
5. Mukherji, V. et al.: Fractional order control and simulation of wind-biomass isolated hybrid power system using particle swarm optimization. In: Book chapter in Applications of Artificial Intelligence Techniques in Engineering, Advances in Intelligent Systems and Computing, vol. 698, pp. 277–287 (2018). https://doi.org/10.1007/978-981-13-1819-1_28
6. Mahto, T., et al.: Load frequency control of a solar-diesel based isolated hybrid power system by fractional order control using particle swarm optimization. J. Intell. Fuzzy Syst. 35(5), 5055–5061 (2018). https://doi.org/10.3233/JIFS-169789
7. Asim, M., Riyaz, A., Tiwari, S., Verma, A.: Performance evaluation of fuzzy controller for boost converter with active PFC, Journal of Intelligent & Fuzzy Systems (JIFS) 35, 5169–5175 (2018)
8. Chidambaram, M., Sree, R.P.: A simple method of tuning of PID controller for integrating/dead time processes. Comput. Chem. Eng. 27, 211–215 (2003)
9. Shamsuzzoha, M.: A unified approach for proportional–integral–derivative controller design for time delay processes. Korean J. Chem. Eng. https://doi.org/10.1007/s11814-014-0237-6
10. Zhang, W., Xi, Y., Yang, G., Xu, X.: Design PID controllers for desired time-domain or frequency-domain response. ISA Trans. 41, 511–520 (2002)
11. Bhatt, Ghoshal, S.P., Roy, R.: Coordinated control of TCP Sand SMES for Frequency regulation off interconnected restructured Power systems with dynamic participation from DFIG based wind farm. Renew. Energy 40(1), 40–50 (2012)
12. Dhillon, S.S., Lather, J.S., Marwaha, S.: Multi objective load frequency control using hybrid bacterial foraging and particle swarm optimized PI controller. Electr. Power Energy Syst. 79, 196–209 (2016)

Optimal Design of Permanent Magnet Brushless DC (PMBLDC) Motor Using PSO Algorithm

Raj Kumar and Md Nishat Anwar

Abstract In this paper, the optimal design of permanent magnet brushless DC (PMBLDC) motor has been described. For optimal design of PMBLDC, particle swarm optimization (PSO) algorithm was used. The motor characteristic is expressed as its geometrical functions. The optimal function is the combination of its cost, losses and volume. In this optimization procedure, mainly four design variables, i.e., axial length of stator/rotor (l_{sr}), radius of rotor (r_{ro}), thickness of magnet (l_{mag}) and thickness of winding (l_{wd}) are given. The optimization technique was done using MATLAB program and designing of PMBLDC Ansys Maxwell was used.

Keywords Permanent magnet brushless DC (PMBLDC) motor · Ansys Maxwell · Particle swarm optimization (PSO) · Optimization · MATLAB

1 Introduction

The motor which has gained popular these days is permanent magnet brushless DC (PMBLDC) motor. PMBLDC motors are electronically commuted because it does not have brushes. PMBLDC motors have many advantages like heavy duty operation, ratio of speed to torque is more, less noisy, dynamic response is more, range of speed is high and robust construction, where their size, weight and shape are the major factors that PMBLDC motor use. With these advantages, PMBLDC motor finds numerous applications in automotive.

In the paper, Rahides [1] had proposed the optimal design of slotless PMBLDC motor genetic algorithms. The paper was presented by Markovic [2], and this paper shows the use of MATLAB optimization to a slotless PMBLDC motor design. In this paper, seven design parameters and for optimization genetic algorithms (GA)

R. Kumar (✉) · M. N. Anwar
Department of Electrical Engineering, National Institute of Technology Patna, Patna 800005, India
e-mail: raj.ee18@nitp.ac.in

M. N. Anwar
e-mail: nishat@nitp.ac.in

© The Author(s), under exclusive license to Springer Nature Singapore Pte Ltd. 2021   479
H. Malik et al. (eds.), *AI and Machine Learning Paradigms for Health Monitoring System*, Studies in Big Data 86,
https://doi.org/10.1007/978-981-33-4412-9_33

were used. The paper is presented by Hwang [3], and the main aim of this paper is to design more efficient and more power density PMBLDC motor.

In this paper, we have described the optimum strategy for designing of permanent magnet brushless direct current (PMBLDC) motor. For optimal design, we have used [4] particle swarm optimization (PSO) and the motor characteristic expressed as its geometrical function. The optimal function is combined of its cost, losses and volume, and this paper objective is to design a 2.1 KW, 310 V, 2500 rpm PMBLDC motor using Ansys Maxwell. For the better understanding of the PSO and its recent optimization technique implementation, reader may refer [8–13].

2 Problem Formulation

The objective function consists of overall motor volume, losses that are incurred and cost that is to be minimized. As the constraints on electromagnetic developed torque, flux density of stator yoke and speed had to be fulfilled, these should also be incorporated in objective function. The independent variable that is taken in objective function is the ratio of pole-arc to pole-pitch (β), radius of rotor (r_{ro}), thickness of magnet (l_{mag}), number of pole pairs (p), current density (j), thickness of stator/rotor core (l_c), thickness of winding (l_{wd}), air gap (l_a) and axial length of stator/rotor (l_{sr}), which can be defined by form factor of the machine ($\lambda = d_b/l_c$, where $d_b = 2(r_{ro} + l_a)$ is diameter of bore). The objective function that is formulated depends on following variables (Fig. 1).

2.1 Electromagnetic Torque

The MMF of the winding is [1]

Fig. 1 Motor geometric parameter

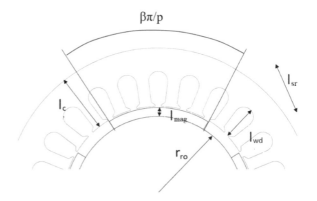

$$NI = A_{wd} J k_{fi} k_{co} \tag{1}$$

where $A_w = \pi l_w (2r_{ro} + 2l_a + l_{wd})$, k_{co} denotes the correction factor based on the control system employed (This is defined as the ratio of the no. of coils that is energized to the total no. of coils.), N denotes number of conductor, A_{wd} denotes the cross-sectional area of winding, I denotes the current carried by the conductor, and k_{fi} denotes winding filling factor. $k_{co} = 2/3$. In the air gap, magnetic flux density on the winding surface is

$$B_a = \frac{F_m}{A_g R} \tag{2}$$

$$F_m = \frac{B_r l_{mag}}{\mu_o \mu_{r1}}, \tag{3}$$

$$A_g = l_{sr} \frac{\beta \pi}{p} (r_{ro} + l_a). \tag{4}$$

A_g and F_m are area under individual pole and MMF developed by individual magnet at the winding surface. Then, Eq. (2) can be rewritten as

$$B_g = \frac{B_r l_{mag}}{(r_{ro} + l_a) \ln \left(\frac{r_{ro} + l_a + l_{wd}}{r_{ro} - l_{mag}} \right)} \tag{5}$$

Electromagnetic torque produced can be written as

$$T_{em} = \frac{\pi k_{fi} k_{co} k_1 k_\beta B_r l_{mag} l_{sr} l_{wd} (2r_{ro} + 2l_a + l_{wd}) J}{\ln \left(\frac{r_{ro} + l_a + l_{wd}}{r_{ro} - l_{mag}} \right)} \tag{6}$$

where k_1 denotes leakage factor and k_β denotes span contribution of active winding and magnet.

2.2 EMF and Voltage

The equation for EMF is obtained assuming all coils are attached back to back, i.e., the winding is in star connection and is given by

$$E = \frac{(r_{ro} + l_a) k_\beta k_1 B_g \omega_r l_{sr} k_{fi} k_{co} A_{wd}}{A_c} \tag{7}$$

The terminal voltage can be found out by equation $V = E + IR$, where R is the resistance of the active winding and is given by

$$V = \frac{l_{sr}k_{fi}k_{co}A_{wd}}{A_c}\left(\rho k_{edt}J + \frac{k_\beta k_1 B_{rl}l_{mag}\omega_r}{\ln\left(\frac{r_{ro}+l_a+l_{wd}}{r_{ro}-l_{mag}}\right)}\right) \tag{8}$$

where k_{edt} is a factor for compensation of end turn winding and ρ is wire resistivity.

2.3 Constraint on Rotational Velocity

For maximum electromagnetic torque generation, the following relationship between time constant and motor speed must be satisfied

$$\omega_r \leq \frac{\pi}{4p\tau} \tag{9}$$

where $\tau = L/R$, L is the inductance, and R is resistance.

2.4 Cost of Materials

Since objective function has to incorporate cost of materials, it must be formulated such that it depends on motor geometric parameters. We can express cost as

$$\begin{aligned} C = & c_{mat1}\rho_{mag}V_{mag} + c_{mat2}p \\ & + c_{wd}A_c k_{fi}\rho_{wd}V_{wd} + c_c\rho_c V_{th} \end{aligned} \tag{10}$$

where ρ_{wd}, ρ_{mag} and ρ_c are winding mass density, magnet mass density and rotor or stator core mass density; c_{wd}, c_c and $c_{mat1(2)}$ are the cost of wire, magnet and core materials per unit mass. V_{wd}, V_{th} and V_{mag} are the winding, stator or rotor core and magnet volumes.

In punching and pressing process, materials are wasted, so the volume of material consumed in the core can be written as

$$V_{th} = \pi l_{sr}(r_{ro} + l_a + l_{wd} + l_c)^2 \tag{11}$$

2.5 Power Loss

Losses in electrical machine mostly comprise electrical loss, i.e., copper loss and magnetic loss (hysteresis and eddy current loss), and copper loss is given by,

$$P_{cu} = \rho \, k_{fi} k_c k_{edt} A_{wd} l_{sr} J^2 \tag{12}$$

Hysteresis and eddy current loss can be written as

$$P_h = k_h \rho_c V_{sy} \, B_{sy}^2 f \tag{13}$$

$$P_e = k_e \rho_c V_{sy} B_{sy}^2 f^2 \tag{14}$$

where B_{sy} is maximum flux density in the stator core due to permanent magnets and is given by [1]

$$B_{sy} = \frac{\pi k_1 \beta B_r l_{mag}}{2 p l_c \ln\left(\frac{r_{ro} + l_a + l_{wd}}{r_{ro} - l_{mag}}\right)} \tag{15}$$

2.6 Defining Objective Function and Constraint

Constraint formation can be split into four parts. First is the electrical constraint which is the magnitude of the source voltage, V^* for motor. In the same way, there are mechanical constraints like torque, T_{em}, and speed, ω_r^{max}.

These constraints are defined by

$$T_{em} \geq T_{em}^* \tag{16}$$

$$\omega_r^{max} \geq \omega_r^* \tag{17}$$

T_{em}^* and ω_r^* are the required torque and speed, respectively.

The magnetic core can be expressed as

$$B_{sy} \leq B_{sy}^{knee} \tag{18}$$

$$k_{fi} l_{wd} J^2 \leq k \tag{19}$$

where k is the maximum heat capacity of the winding.

The most pivotal section of any optimization problem is formulation of the objective function. The first step is to define the independent variables, and it is represented in the form of a vector $X = \{l_{mag} l_c \, l_{wd} l_a r_{ro} \beta \lambda\}$. The objective function that is formed incorporating electromagnetic torque, speed and maximum stator flux density requirement is

Table 1 Given parameters and their respective values

Parameters	Value	Parameters	Value
$B_{sy}^{knee}(T)$	1.5	F	0.2
$B_r(T)$	1.0	Σ	1000
k $(A^2\ m^{-3})$	10^{11}	ρ_{mag} (kgm^{-3})	7400
ρ $(\Omega\ m)$	1.8×10^{-8}	ρ_{wd} (kgm^{-3})	8900
k_h $(Ws\ kg^{-1}\ T^{-n})$	0.018	ρ_c (kgm^{-3})	7700
k_e $(Ws^2 kg^{-1}\ T^{-2})$	0.00008	$C_{mat1}(£kg^{-1})$	20
N	1.92	C_{mat2} $(£kg^{-1})$	1
w_p	0.02	C_y $(£kg^{-1})$	3
w_v	2000/3	C_1 $(£\ mm^2\ kg^{-1})$	0.045
w_c	0.0125	C_2 $(£\ mm^2\ kg^{-1})$	5.42
k_{fi}	0.7		
K_{co}	2/3	T_{em}^* (Nm)	261.8
		ω_r^* $(rads^{-1})$	261.8
k_s	0.95	$V^*(V)$	310

$$f_0(x) = w_{pow} P_{loss}(x) + w_{vo} V_v(x) + w_{co} C(x) + \frac{1}{\varepsilon}\Big[f_n\big(1 - T_{em}/T_{em}^*\big)$$
$$+ f_n\big(1 - \omega_r^{max}/\omega_r^*\big) + f_n\Big(B_{sy}/B_{sy}^{knee} - 1\Big)\Big] \tag{20}$$

where w_{vo}, w_{pow} and w_{co} are weighing factors for volume, power loss and cost, respectively, and ε is a small constant. P_{loss} is the total magnetic, electrical and mechanical losses (i.e., $P_{loss} = P_e + P_h + P_{cu}$), C is the whole material cost, V_t is volume, $f_n(x) = \frac{1}{1+e^{-\sigma x}}$, and σ is a constant (Table 1).

For optimization, here we use particle swarm optimization (PSO). Particle swarm optimization (PSO) [4] algorithm is an associate of the widespread category of swarm intelligence approaches for puzzle out global optimization difficulties. It is a population-based optimization tool, got inspiration from the fish schooling or birds flocking how they behave in social. In search space, all of the solutions are "birds", which we called "particle". All of the particles had their fitness standards, which is estimated by the function of fitness, which have to be improved, i.e., optimized, and had their velocities which give the direction of the particles for flying. In each reiteration, every particle is updated by two "best" values. The first value is the best solution (fitness) which has achieved so far, i.e., personal best (P_{best}). Second "best" result obtained by any particle and detected by PSO is the best global value which is known as G_{best}.

For the updation of velocities of every particle and positions of the all particle, following formulas are used:

$$V_n(z + 1) = \omega V_n(z) + C_1 r_1(z)\big(P_{best(n)} - X_n(z)\big) + C_2 r_2(z)\big(G_{best(n)} - X_i(z)\big) \tag{21}$$

$$X_n(z + 1) = X_n(z) + V_n(z + 1) \tag{22}$$

where $V_n(z)$ is the velocity of the particle, $X_n(z)$ is the position of the particle, $P_{best(n)}$ is personal best, $G_{best(n)}$ is global best of the particle, ω is inertia weight, C_1 and C_2 are the learning factor (usually, $C_1 = C_2 = 2$), and $r_1(z)$ and $r_2(z)$ are the random number between $(0, 1)$ (Fig. 2).

3 Design of PMBLDC Motor

For designing of permanent magnet brushless DC motor (PMBLDC), we use Ansys Maxwell [5].

3.1 Machine Properties

It includes general information about machine like position of rotor, type of machine, number of poles, frictional loss, windage loss and circuit type.

3.2 Stator Properties

This window includes stator data like its inner and outer diameters, length, number of stator slots, slot type and steel type. Several categories of steel can be defined by the software, correspondingly steel categories can be added and exhibited if their constraints are approved which is known, laterally with coefficients of core loss K_c, K_h and K_e. In Rotating Machine Expert (RMxprt), there are six categories of slots given for rotating machines (Table 2).

3.3 Rotor Properties

In rotor properties window, it includes the data about rotor outer diameter and rotor inner diameter of rotor, rotor core length and pole property (like magnet thickness, magnet type) (Table 3).

Fig. 2 Flow-chart of PSO

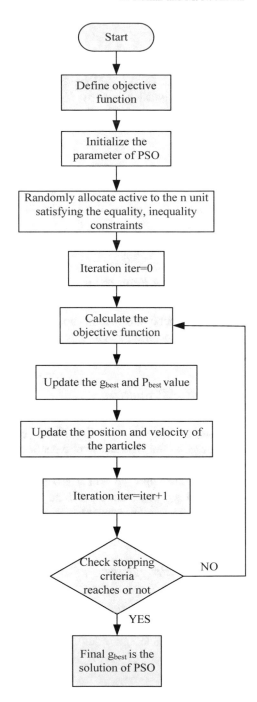

Table 2 Optimal stator geometric parameters

Name	Value
Diameter (outer in mm)	130
Length of core (in mm)	145
Diameter (inner in mm)	80
Steel type	M15_26G
Total slots	30

Table 3 Optimal rotor geometric parameters

Name	Value	Unit
Diameter (outer)	77.5	mm
Core length	145	mm
Diameter (inner)	26	mm
Steel type	M19_26G	

4 Results and Discussion

4.1 Design Sheet

See Table 4.

Table 4 Data at full-rated load

Name	Value
I/P current (avg. in A)	7.36795
Armature current (rms in A)	5.95209
Loss (diode in W)	0.665508
Loss (stray in W)	47.533
Efficiency (%)	87.6068
Loss (copper in W)	86.1044
Loss (transistor in W)	28.5733
Loss (total in W)	283.07
O/P power (W)	2100.99
I/P power (W)	2284.06
Loss (core in W)	120.194
Speed (rated in rpm)	2572.98
Torque (rated in N.m)	7.42644

4.2 Different Plots

The plot shows that when PMBLDC motor reaches its rated speed, i.e., 2500 rpm, then the input current is approximately 8A (Fig. 3).

This plot shows the response between efficiency and speed [6]. The efficiency of the PMBLDC motor is more than the other DC motor. As Fig. 4 shows when the motor is at its rated speed, the efficiency is about 87%.

As Fig. 5 shows at speed around 1100 rpm, then the motor reaches its maximum output power, and when motor is at rated speed, motor power is 2.1 KW.

In PMBLDC motor, cogging torque [7] is an unwanted effect, because of this motor vibrates and it gives more audible noise. Figure 6 shows response of cogging torque and electrical degree. In this paper, peak cogging torque is about ±0.07 N m.

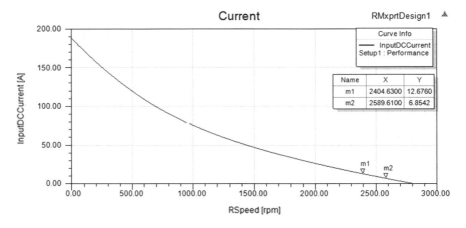

Fig. 3 Response of input DC versus speed

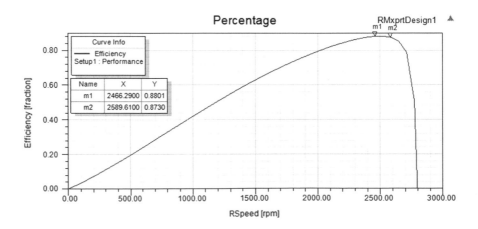

Fig. 4 Response of efficiency versus speed

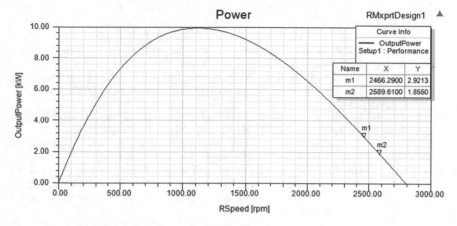

Fig. 5 Response of output power versus speed

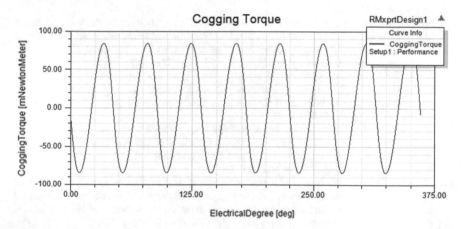

Fig. 6 Response of cogging torque vs electrical degree

5 Conclusion

PMBLDC motor geometric parameters are optimized using PSO, and geometric specifications are designed in Ansys Maxwell. The objective function is designed such that cost of materials, losses, volume, speed and torque requirement, flux density requirement and thermal limitations are considered. The higher and lower boundaries of all the motor geometric specifications are also specified. Different plots are presented, i.e., efficiency versus speed, output torque versus speed and cogging torque versus electrical degree in the result section. In this paper, maximum cogging torque of designed PMBLDC is about 0.07 N m.

References

1. Rahideh, A., Korakianitis, T., Ruiz, P., Keeble, T., Rothman, M.T.: Optimal brushless DC motor design using genetic algorithms. J. Magn. Magn. Mater. **322**(22), 3680–3687 (2010)
2. Markovic, M., Ragot, P., Perriard, Y.: Design optimization of a BLDC motor: a comparative analysis. In: Proceedings of IEEE International Electric Machines and Drives Conference, IEMDC 2007, 2007
3. Hwang, C.C., Chang, J.J.: Design and analysis of a high power density and high efficiency permanent magnet DC motor. J. Magn. Magn. Mater. **209**(1–3), 234–236 (2000)
4. AlRashidi, M.R., El-Hawary, M.E.: A survey of particle swarm optimization applications in electric power systems. IEEE Trans. Evol. Comput. **13**(4), 913–918 (2009)
5. Singh, V.K., Marwaha, S., Singh, A.K.: Design and analysis of permanent magnet brushless DC motor for solar vehicle using Ansys Software. Int. J. Eng. Res. **V6**(04), 79–84 (2017)
6. Jang, S.M., Cho, H.W., Choi, S.K.: Design and analysis of a high-speed brushless DC motor for centrifugal compressor. IEEE Trans. Mag (2007)
7. Nizam, M., Waloyo, H.T., Inayati, Design of optimal outer rotor brushless DC motor for minimum cogging torque. In: Proceedings of the 2013 Joint International Conference on Rural Information and Communication Technology and Electric-Vehicle Technology, rICT and ICEV-T 2013, 2013
8. Fatema, N. et al.: Data-driven occupancy detection hybrid model using particle swarm optimization based artificial neural network. In: Springer Nature Book: Metaheuristic and Evolutionary Computation: Algorithms and Applications, under book series "Studies in Computational Intelligence", 2020. https://doi.org/10.1007/978-981-15-7571-6_13
9. Iqbal, A. et al.: Metaheurestic algorithm based hybrid model for identification of building sale prices. In: Springer Nature Book: Metaheuristic and Evolutionary Computation: Algorithms and Applications, under book series "Studies in Computational Intelligence", 2020. https://doi.org/10.1007/978-981-15-7571-6_32
10. Vinoop, P. et al.: PSO-NN-based hybrid model for long-term wind speed prediction: a study on 67 Cities of India. In: Book chapter in Applications of Artificial Intelligence Techniques in Engineering, Advances in Intelligent Systems and Computing vol. 697, pp. 319–327 (2018). https://doi.org/10.1007/978-981-13-1822-1_29
11. Mukherji, V. et al.: Fractional order control and simulation of wind-biomass isolated hybrid power system using particle swarm optimization. In: Book chapter in Applications of Artificial Intelligence Techniques in Engineering, Advances in Intelligent Systems and Computing, vol. 698, pp. 277–287 (2018). https://doi.org/10.1007/978-981-13-1819-1_28
12. Faiz Minai, A. et al.: Metaheuristics paradigms for renewable energy systems: advances in optimization algorithms. In: Springer Nature Book: Metaheuristic and Evolutionary Computation: Algorithms and Applications, under book series "Studies in Computational Intelligence", 2020. https://doi.org/10.1007/978-981-15-7571-6_2
13. Mahto, T., et al.: Load frequency control of a solar-diesel based isolated hybrid power system by fractional order control using particle swarm optimization. J. Intell. Fuzzy Syst. **35**(5), 5055–5061 (2018). https://doi.org/10.3233/JIFS-169789

A Novel Lossless Image Cryptosystem for Binary Images Using Feed-Forward Back-Propagation Neural Networks

Harsha Vardhan Sahoo, Sumitra Kisan, and Gargi Bhattacharjee

Abstract Currently, one of the most challenging areas of research in communication systems is to build a secure communication channel. The existing public key cryptosystem appears to be more complex owing to the consumption of greater computational power. The neural net application is one of the promising developments in cryptography. This chapter examines the application of neural networks in binary image security. The proposed methodology works by encrypting individual sets of binary values for enhanced security with no loss in image quality. We have termed this novel scheme as *Individual Pixel Encryption*. The presented approach yields more security than the existing methods, which simply generate the cipher using neural networks by performing mix operations on the plaintext. Generally, working with individual pixels has its own share of complexity in terms of implementation and execution, which is why, it has yet to gain traction in the field of image encryption. But with our approach, we have tried to overcome this limitation using neural networks which are best suited for this purpose. The goal of this work is to realize an image cryptosystem using neural networks which is simple and efficient enough to be executed on a daily driver, robust enough that it does not compromise on security aspects and powerful enough that there is no loss in image quality. The proposed work finds its application in the fields of satellite imaging systems, medical imaging systems, military communications systems, social media and peer-to-peer image sharing, confidential imaging systems for civilian and enterprise and other such applications.

H. V. Sahoo (✉) · S. Kisan
Computer Science & Engineering, Veer Surendra Sai University of Technology, Burla, Odisha, India
e-mail: harshasahoo76730@gmail.coms

S. Kisan
e-mail: sumitrakisan.ism@gmail.com

G. Bhattacharjee
Information Technology, Veer Surendra Sai University of Technology, Burla, Odisha, India
e-mail: gbhattacharjee_it@vssut.ac.in

© The Author(s), under exclusive license to Springer Nature Singapore Pte Ltd. 2021   491
H. Malik et al. (eds.), *AI and Machine Learning Paradigms for Health Monitoring System*, Studies in Big Data 86,
https://doi.org/10.1007/978-981-33-4412-9_34

Keywords Binary image · Lossless image cryptography · Feed-forward neural network · Back-propagation · Image security · Image cryptosystem · Image encryption · Individual pixel encryption

1 Introduction

The Internet governs today's information exchange, resulting in huge volumes of data being shared in seconds. With the escalation in the volume of information being shared, it becomes a requisite to protect the integrity of the data being shared. As the data shared is highly confidential in nature, any information leak can lead to serious security problems. Cryptography [1] converts the sensitive information to some indiscernible text using various techniques. This conversion of information to an indiscernible form is called encryption, and the reverse is called decryption. Unlike text encryption, image encryption is difficult both because of its large size and complexity. Many image encryption algorithms have been proposed, in the past two decades using various techniques like DNA substitutions, DNA sequencing and genetic algorithm, chaotic maps, transforms like discrete cosine transform (DCT) and discrete wavelet transform (DWT), etc.

Some of the existing methods employ random numbers in the encryption and pre-encryption process. But the random numbers employed are not purely random since most of the random number generator algorithms repeat the sequence after some iterations. It is just that the field or range of each iteration is so large (exponential) that humans are not able to perceive it. So, the use of random numbers in cryptography is also to some extent vulnerable. Image encryption using discrete cosine transform [2] is simple and fast but the image quality degrades to some extent, i.e., it is not lossless. A few image encryption techniques, viz. [3], especially in computer forensic science, employ the concept of hiding the main image among layer(s) of dummy images. Here the layer(s) of images are encrypted in such a way that the actual image to be sent gets embedded in the dummy images, and it becomes indiscernible. Some other image encryption techniques, viz. [4–9] and [10] employ the use of chaotic maps. In mathematical terms, a chaotic map is an evolutionary function that exhibits some type of chaotic behavior. Usage of chaotic maps supports in achieving chaos as a mathematical function which is better than using random numbers. However, using chaotic maps results in noise and blurring effects on the decrypted image.

Some techniques, viz. [4, 8, 9, 11–14] and [15] employ DNA operations which include DNA addition, concatenation, union, reverse, complement, substitution and encoding. The union and concatenation operations play the roles of addition and multiplication, respectively, in some algebraic structures. These operations are used for pixel substitutions and encryptions. Some other techniques, viz. [16–18] and [19] also employ genetic algorithms which are adaptive heuristics search algorithms based on the evolutionary concepts of genetics and natural selection. Genetic algorithms are used to achieve pixel scrambling and reduce the correlation among the scrambled pixels.

One of the promising approaches, which has not been explored much in the past two decades, is the use of neural networks for encryption (cryptography) and decryption (crypt-analysis). This branch of cryptography dedicated to analyzing the application of neural networks, especially artificial neural networks, in encryption and decryption is called neural cryptography. Artificial neural networks offer a novel approach based on the fundamental principle that any possible function that exists and can exist can be successfully replicated by the use of a neural network, thus making it a powerful computational tool in finding the inverse function of any existing cryptographic algorithm. This feature when combined with the ability of neural networks of selectively exploring the solution space of a given problem makes neural networks a mainstay in the field of crypt-analysis. These implications of using neural networks in the field of cryptography and crypt-analysis have influenced the proposal of this novel image cryptosystem.

The organization of the remaining chapter is as follows: Sect. 2 focuses on the literature survey and its analysis, followed by Sect. 3 focusing on our proposed approach *Individual Pixel-based Lossless Image Cryptosystem*. In Sect. 4, we analyze our results along with comparing it with the existing approaches. Finally, the last section concludes our work.

2 Literature Survey and Analysis

There has been a limited number of researches during the past two decades on the application of neural networks in image cryptography. The first work that is known in this field can be traced back to 1995. This has been followed by numerous works proposed by many others using different types of neural networks like the Hopfield neural network, which is a form of recurrent neural networks (RNN), multi-layer feed-forward networks (MLFF), which are a class of feed-forward neural networks, chaotic neural networks (CNN), the perceptron model, all of which are variations or evolutionary offshoots of the artificial neural network.

References [20–25] and [26] use chaotic neural networks, whereas [27] and [28] use hyper-chaotic and chaotic fuzzy cellular neural networks, respectively. These neural network models exhibit chaotic behavior. Chaotic neural networks possess a significant advantage over random number generators. Unlike random number generators which give different outputs for the same set of inputs, a chaotic neural network always gives the same correct output for the same set of inputs. However, one cannot predict how the output will vary if there is a slight change in the input. This is what makes chaotic neural networks so powerful as compared to random number generators whose output can theoretically be predicted. [29, 30] and [26] use the Hopfield neural network. It is a type of recurrent neural network which works by first learning several binary patterns and then returns the one that matches the given input the most. The purpose of a Hopfield network is to store binary patterns and recall them based on given partial input. This makes them quite useful in crypt-analysis for pattern recognition. Some of the approaches use a multi-layer feed-forward neural network, a form of artificial neural network, where the connections that are present between the multiple layers of computational units or nodes do not form a cycle. The key benefit of this class of neural networks over the others is that the output values after being compared to the desired output is fed back into the network. Now, using these values, the weight of each connection is then adjusted by the algorithm to reduce the error function's value. After multiple iterations, the error becomes very small. Thus, unlike others, this class of neural networks is self-learning. However, the simplest of them all is the perceptron model which was used by Wang et al. [31]. A perceptron is a single neuron and multiple layers of perceptron form a neural network. A perceptron is a linear classifier and helps to classify the given input data.

Lian et al. [22] in their work have proposed a cryptographic algorithm derived from chaotic neural networks which is used to encode JPEG2000 images. Yu and Cao [26] in their study present a novel cryptographic approach with time-varying delay based on Hopfield chaotic neural networks. Lian [23] in his research has proposed a chaotic neural network-based block cipher. Peng et al. [27] have proposed an image encryption scheme that employs a hyper-chaotic cellular neural network. Wang et al. [31] have proposed a perceptron model based on a high-dimensional Lorenz chaotic system for their image cryptosystem. Bigdeli et al. [29] in their work introduce a hybrid image encryption algorithm which is based on chaotic control parameters and a hyper-chaotic Hopfield neural network. In yet another research by Bigdeli et al. [20], they have proposed a chaotic neural network by combining the characteristics of a neural network and a chaotic system. Cheng and Cheng [32] in their study have put forth an image cryptosystem that is asymmetric and based on the synchronization of a cellular neural network and a unified chaotic system. Xing-Yuan and Xue-Mei [25] have proposed a new block cryptographic scheme based on a chaotic neural network derived from a spatiotemporal chaotic system. Zhang et al. [33] in their study have proposed an image encryption scheme that is built around a hybrid of logistic map and cellular neural network. Joshi et al. [34] in their work have proposed an artificial neural network-based secure image transmission technique using randomness in the encryption scheme by adding impurities to the original cipher. Some application-based image encryption works include Hua et al.'s work [35] in the encryption of medical images using high-speed pixel scrambling and adaptive pixel diffusion and Ismail et al.'s work [36] in the encryption of satellite images using back-propagation neural networks.

However, after studying and analyzing the aforementioned works, we have found that there are some trade-offs that many of the approaches perform in order to achieve their intended objective. Nakajima and Yamaguchi's work [3] suffers from two problems. First, the image quality gets deteriorated. Second, even if the approach provides a way to improve the image quality, there is a trade-off of security. Similarly, Seethalakshmi et al.'s work [37], which is also based on visual cryptography like [3], focuses on enhancing the security in image steganography using neural networks but loses out on image quality. Tedmori and Al-Najdawi's approach [2] is lossless even though it uses discrete cosine transform, but this quality is achieved at the expense of substantial encryption.

Singh and Kaur's approach [9] which employs chaotic maps and DNA operations has a major flaw. The decrypted image suffers from the effects of noise and blur which must be removed using suitable filtering schemes. However, Chakraborty et al.'s work [4], which also employs chaotic maps and DNA substitution, is quite robust and highly resilient against cryptographic attacks. Also, their approach leads to lossless images. Although Pujari et al.'s work [17] yields a robust hybridized model using genetic algorithm and DNA sequence, this approach suffers from many setbacks suffered by traditional cryptographic systems. First, even though genetic algorithm and DNA cryptography enhance the security, it is still based on a conventional symmetric key cryptosystem, i.e., it uses a single key for both encryption and decryption, which is not secure. Second, since this encryption algorithm is key-based, it naturally suffers from the problems of secure key exchange that plague key-dependent cryptosystems. Zhu et al.'s work [38], which is based on chaos and SHA-256, a novel hash function of the SHA-2 family (SHA: Secure Hash Algorithm), and Patel et al.'s work [8], which uses 3D chaotic maps with DNA encoding techniques, also suffer from the above two problems that affect symmetric key cryptosystems. The only drawback to Lian et al.'s approach [22] is the time consumed in the encryption process. This is because this approach suffers from the same drawbacks as those suffered by stream ciphers, one of which is the time consumed to encrypt a very long stream of bits. Even though experimental results for Wang et al.'s approach [31] show that the algorithm has enhanced security and a strong resistance to the existing methods of attack, the rate at which crypt-analysis attacks and techniques are advancing, a key-dependent cryptosystem is far from safe. The modern age of cryptography requires keyless cryptosystems which do not suffer from the problems of key-dependent cryptosystems. Kumar and Dhiman's work [39], even with all its merits of shorter execution time and higher security, has its own limitation. It results in lossy decrypted images, although it achieves the least distortion as compared to other algorithms.

Using neural networks helps tackle two significant problems that plague the present cryptographic algorithms and other proposed approaches; first, neural networks provide fast, secure and often lossless encryption. Second, the neural key exchange protocol solves the problem of key exchange faced by traditional cryptographic algorithms using the Diffie–Hellman key exchange protocol. In modern cryptography, neural networks have made significant strides toward the security and efficiency of cryptographic algorithms, while at the same time providing crypt-analysts a powerful tool to "test" the security of those algorithms. However, with all the benefits also come a couple of deterrents to the application of neural networks, viz. bad input selection and inadequate learning rate. Utilizing the maximum potential of neural networks means overcoming the above two shortcomings as well.

3 Proposed Approach: *Individual Pixel-Based Lossless Image Cryptosystem*

In response to the problems encountered by most of the modern image encryption techniques, we have proposed a novel image cryptosystem named *Individual Pixel-based Lossless Image Cryptosystem*. This is based on our novel scheme of *Individual Pixel Encryption*, which provides high-speed encryption and decryption of binary images without compromising on the security and quality aspects of the image. Our proposed cryptosystem works by encrypting individual bits or pixels which is far more secure than the rest of the methods that simply generate the cipher using neural networks and perform mix operations. The concept of *Individual Pixel Encryption* has not yet gained traction in the field of image encryption as almost all other approaches steer clear of it due to the sheer complexity associated with implementing it. With the application of neural networks, we have overcome the shortcomings of encrypting individual pixels in real time, hence, greatly reducing the operational complexity. Also, the algorithm/cryptosystem is *keyless,* i.e., it does not require a key.

The algorithm can be very easily adapted for multi-core and multi-processor systems to benefit from the additional computing units. This exponentially increases the efficiency while reducing the execution time. This image cryptosystem is capable of processing binary images irrespective of their formats. Also, the algorithm can be tweaked to accept binary images of all sizes. This makes our cryptosystem highly scalable. Also, binary images carry much less data as compared to grayscale and color images. So, the use of complex traditional encryption algorithms becomes unnecessary as it increases the operational overhead of the system. So, the proposed cryptosystem entirely focuses only on binary images to significantly lower the operational overhead.

The algorithm can be thought of as combining the elements of both asymmetric key cryptosystems and digital signatures. Our work is based on the fundamental principle that it is easier to encrypt something as a summation, e.g., $1 + 2 + 3 + 4 = 10$. But it is extremely difficult to decrypt the sum to get the inputs, e.g., 10 can be $5 + 5$ or $1 + 2 + 3 + 4$ or $8 + 2$ or $7 + 3$ and so on.

3.1 Binary Image Encryption

For binary image encryption, the input to our algorithm will be a binary image, also known as a 1-bit image. Then using the *imread( )* MATLAB function, the pixel values from the image will be extracted in sets of four and written into a text file. This text file will then be read by a Python script which will store the pixel values in lists of size four each. This will act as the input to the neural network. Prior to all of this, the neural network will be trained using similar datasets of binary images which will be in the form of pixel values stored in lists. The input data will then be fed into the trained neural network for encryption which will be developed using Python. Based on the training, it will convert the sets of four pixel values into sets of three pixel values, which will then be stored in a text file consisting of lists of size three each. This text file, when read by MATLAB and converted to an image, will result in a highly distorted and low-resolution encrypted image which can then be sent to the receiver over a secure channel.

Input—Original Image (256 × 256)
Output—Encrypted Image (192 × 256) + Guiding Image (512 × 32)

3.1.1 Pixel Extraction Using MATLAB

Step 1: Read the binary image using the *imread( )* function to get the pixel values and store them in a 256 × 256 matrix.
Step 2: Convert the 256 × 256 matrix into a 65,536 × 1 column matrix.
Step 3: Write the matrix entities into a text file named **Pixels.txt** using the *fprintf( )* function.

3.1.2 Individual Pixel Encryption Using Python

Step 1: Read the text file named **Pixels.txt** using the *readlines( )* function to get the pixel values and store them in a string.
Step 2: Get the length of the string and create an empty list named *pixels* of the same length and initialize the list with the pixel values contained in the string by iteration.
Step 3: Read the first four values in the list and assign those values to four variables w, x, y and z.
Step 4: Use the trained neural network to encrypt four pixel values at a time to get three encrypted pixel values, until the iteration reaches the end of the list.
Step 5: Store the encrypted pixel values in a list named *enc* which 3/4th the size of the original *pixels* list.
Step 6: Extract the guiding bits from the pixels and store them in a list named *guide* which is 1/4th the size of the original *pixels* list.
Step 7: Write the encrypted pixel values into a text file named **Encrypted.txt**.
Step 8: Write the guiding bits into a text file named **Guide.txt**.

3.1.3 Construction of Encrypted and Guiding Image Using MATLAB

Step 1: Read the text file named **Encrypted.txt** using the *fscanf( )* function to get the encrypted pixel values and store them in a 49,152 × 1 column matrix.
Step 2: Reshape the matrix using the *reshape( )* function.
Step 3: Convert the reshaped matrix into a gray image using the *mat2gray( )* function.

Step 4: Binarize the gray image using the *imbinarize()* function and then save it as the encrypted image.
Step 5: Read the text file named **Guide.txt** using the *fscanf()* function to get the guiding bits and store them in a 16,384 × 1 column matrix.
Step 6: Reshape the matrix using the *reshape()* function.
Step 7: Convert the reshaped matrix into a gray image using the *mat2gray()* function.
Step 8: Binarize the gray image using the *imbinarize()* function and then save it as the guiding image.

3.2   Binary Image Decryption

For binary image decryption, the encrypted image is first converted into a text file containing the pixel values. This text file consisting of lists of size three will be read by another trained neural network which will be the inverse of the neural network used for encryption. The encrypted pixel values in the form of lists of size three each will then be decoded back to the original pixel values in the form of lists of size four each and then written into a MATLAB readable text file. These pixel values when read and converted by MATLAB into their corresponding color values will give the original image.

Input—Encrypted Image (192 × 256) + Guiding Image (512 × 32)
Output—Original Image (256 × 256).

3.2.1   Extraction of Encrypted Pixel Values and Guiding Bits Using MATLAB

Step 1: Read the encrypted image using the *imread()* function to get the encrypted pixel values and store them in a 49,152 × 1 column matrix.
Step 2: Write the encrypted pixel values into a text file named **Encrypted.txt** using the *fprintf()* function.
Step 3: Read the guiding image using the *imread()* function to get the guiding bits and store them in a 16,384 × 1 column matrix.
Step 4: Write the guiding bits into a text file named **Guide.txt** using the *fprintf()* function.

3.2.2   Individual Pixel Decryption Using Python

Step 1: Read the text file named **Encrypted.txt** using the *readlines()* function to get the encrypted pixel values and store them in a string.
Step 2: Get the length of the string to create an empty list named *enc* of the same length and initialize the list with the pixel values contained in the string by iteration.

Step 3:   Read the text file named **Guide.txt** using the *readlines( )* function to get the guiding bits and store them in a string.

Step 4:   Get the length of the string and create an empty list named *guide* of the same length and initialize the list with the guiding bits contained in the string by iteration.

Step 5:   Read the first three values in the list and assign those values to three variables x, y and z.

Step 6:   Use the trained neural network to decrypt three pixel values at a time to get four decrypted pixel values, until the iteration reaches the end of the list.

Step 7:   Store the decrypted pixel values in a list named *dec* which is 4/3rd the size of the *enc* list.

Step 8:   Use the guiding bits to replace every offset bit in the *dec* list to remove the randomness associated with neural networks.

Step 9:   Write the decrypted pixel values into a text file named Decrypted.txt (Figs. 1 and 2).

3.2.3   Original Image Reconstruction Using MATLAB

Step 1:   Read the text file named **Decrypted.txt** using the *fscanf( )* function to get the decrypted pixel values and store them in a $65,536 \times 1$ column matrix.

Step 2:   Reshape the matrix using the *reshape( )* function.

Step 3:   Convert the reshaped matrix into a gray image using the *mat2gray( )* function.

Step 4:   Binarize the gray image using the *imbinarize( )* function and then save it as the decrypted image.

3.3   *Training the Neural Network*

We have used a two-layer feed-forward back-propagation neural network for our approach which uses the *Sigmoid Function* as the transfer function. The neural network for encryption consists of *four*-input nodes and *three* output nodes, and the neural network for decryption consists of *three*-input nodes and *four*-output nodes. The reason for using separate neural networks is to make it harder for the attacker to decipher the images sent over the channel. Using separate neural networks for encryption and decryption, which are mathematically related, also helps us achieve the security benefits of asymmetric key cryptosystems and digital signatures. The feed-forward back-propagation neural network is also the most basic form of neural networks after the perceptron model, which makes it more flexible as compared to other types of neural networks and thus can be modified to a much higher degree to suit our needs.

The neural network for encryption has been implemented as *three two-layer four-input one-output* neural networks, and the neural network for decryption has been

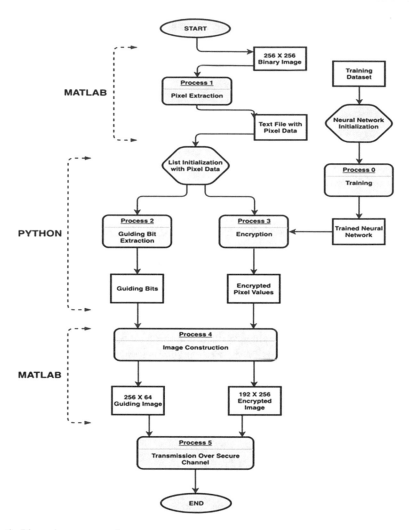

Fig. 1 Binary image encryption

implemented as *four two-layer three-input one-output* neural networks. The reason for implementing each neural network as multiple smaller neural networks is to reduce the correlation among the output bits, which leads to *confusion*, and to reduce the operational complexity of training the neural network. This is because splitting the neural network removes the correlation of errors between the output bits, which in turn results in much faster training times due to reduced error calculation and learning times. For the better understanding of the ANN design and implementation, reader may refer [40–44].

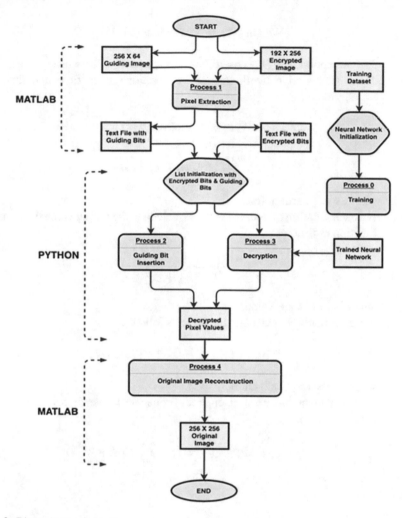

Fig. 2 Binary image decryption

3.3.1 Neural Network Training Using Python

Step 1: The training set inputs consist of sets of *four bits for encryption* and sets of *three bits for decryption* which are fed into the network.

Step 2: The training set outputs consist of the expected outputs for each set of input which are fed into the network.

Step 3: A seed value of 1 is provided to the *random()* function whose task is to assign weights randomly to the nodes.

Step 4: Assign random weights to the nodes using the function:

$$\text{Weight (W)} = 2 * \text{random} ((4, 1)) - 1 \tag{1}$$

$$\text{Weight (W)} = 2 * \text{random} ((3, 1)) - 1 \qquad (2)$$

For encryption, Eq. (1) is used. For decryption, Eq. (2) is used.

Step 5: Train the neural network for 10,000 iterations, each time updating the weights as follows:

$$W\text{new} = W\text{old} + \Delta W i j \qquad (3)$$

$$\Delta W i j = l * \text{Err} j * O i \qquad (4)$$

where, l = Learning Rate.

Step 6: For each iteration of updated weights, calculate the output using the transfer function as follows:

$$O j = \frac{1}{(1 + e^{-I_j})} \qquad (1)$$

where, $I j$ = Node Value

Step 7: For each iteration, calculate the error as follows:

$$\text{Err} = O j * (1 - O j) * (T - O j) \qquad (2)$$

where, T = Expected Output

Step 8: Once the error has been calculated, propagate the error back as follows (Figs. 3 and 4):

$$\text{Err} j = O j * (1 - O j) * \sum_{k} (\text{Err} k * W j k) \qquad (7)$$

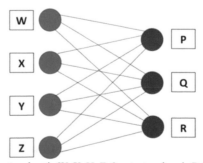

4 Input nodes viz W, X, Y, Z; 3 output nodes viz P, Q, R

Fig. 3 Neural network for encryption

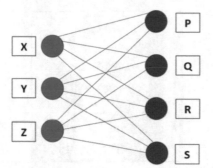

3 Input nodes viz X, Y, Z; 3 output nodes viz P, Q, R, S

Fig. 4 Neural network for decryption

4 Results and Discussion

The cryptosystem has been validated on an experimental database and tested on the *Miscellaneous Dataset (a.k.a. Volume 3)* of the *USC-SIPI Image Database* [45] consisting of a total of forty standard test binary images of size 256 × 256. For experimental purposes, six standard test binary images from the above database, namely Lenna, Female, Male, Cameraman, Mandrill and Peppers, each of size 256 × 256, have been considered.

The proposed image cryptosystem has been implemented in MATLAB R2019a, and the neural network implementation has been done using Anaconda3 (Python Distribution) in Spyder 4.0 Integrated Development Environment (IDE), running on Windows 10 Pro. The algorithm was executed on a personal desktop computer with an Intel(R) Core™ i7-5775C quad-core processor and 16 GB of primary memory.

4.1 Binary Image Encryption

See Figs. 5, 6, 7, 8, 9, 10, 11, 12, 13, 14, 15, 16, 17, 18, 19, 20, 21 and 22.

4.2 Binary Image Decryption

See Figs. 23, 24, 25, 26, 27 and 28.

The execution of the algorithm results in highly complex and robust encrypted images along with guiding images. There was no error or noise introduced into the cipher images while encryption, i.e., the mean square error (MSE) values were found to be zero. Thus, the peak signal-to-noise ratio (PSNR) values in each case were found to be infinity. These PSNR values imply a *Lossless Image Cryptosystem*. This makes

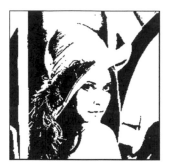

Fig. 5 Lenna (original image) (256 × 256)

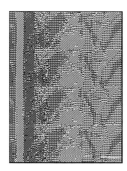

Fig. 6 Lenna (encrypted image) (192 × 256)

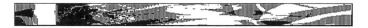

Fig. 7 Lenna (guiding image) (512 × 32)

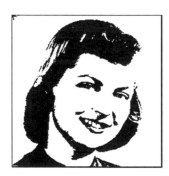

Fig. 8 Female (original image) (256 × 256)

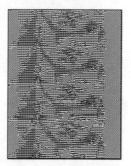

Fig. 9 Female (encrypted image) (192 × 256)

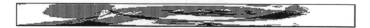

Fig. 10 Female (guiding image) (512 × 32)

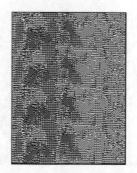

Fig. 11 Male (original image) (256 × 256)

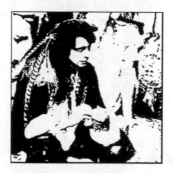

Fig. 12 Male (encrypted image) (192 × 256)

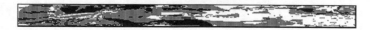

Fig. 13 Male (guiding image) (512 × 32)

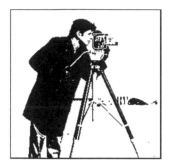

Fig. 14 Cameraman (original image) (256 × 256)

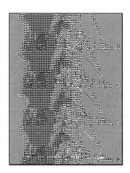

Fig. 15 Cameraman (encrypted image) (192 × 256)

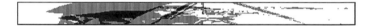

Fig. 16 Cameraman (guiding image) (512 × 32)

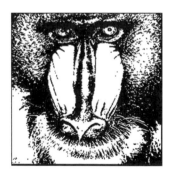

Fig. 17 Mandrill (original image) (256 × 256)

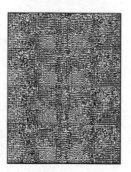

Fig. 18 Mandrill (encrypted image) (192 × 256)

Fig. 19 Mandrill (guiding image) (512 × 32)

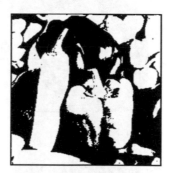

Fig. 20 Peppers (original image) (256 × 256)

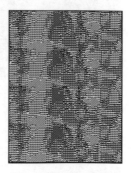

Fig. 21 Peppers (encrypted image) (192 × 256)

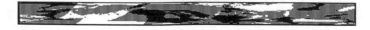

Fig. 22 Peppers (guiding image) (512 × 32)

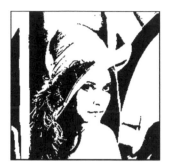

Fig. 23 Lenna (decrypted image) (256 × 256)

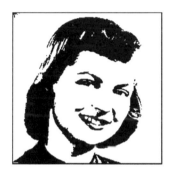

Fig. 24 Female (decrypted image) (256 × 256)

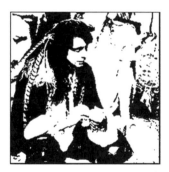

Fig. 25 Male (decrypted image) (256 × 256)

our algorithm one of the very few, if not, the only lossless image encryption algorithm with a PSNR value of infinity (Table 1).

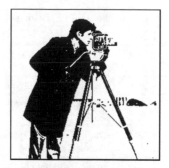

Fig. 26   Cameraman (decrypted image) (256 × 256)

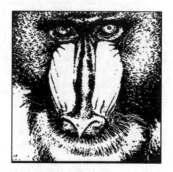

Fig. 27   Mandrill (decrypted image) (256 × 256)

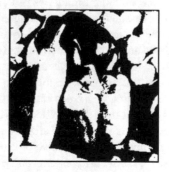

Fig. 28   Peppers (decrypted image) (256 × 256)

5   Conclusion

The algorithm proposed in this chapter is based on the novel concept of *Individual Pixel Encryption*. Individual Pixel Encryption, implemented through feed-forward back-propagation neural networks, greatly enhances the security of the cryptosystem as individual pixels are encrypted in real time without compromising on the security

Table 1 Comparative study of existing methods for binary images

Author	Year	Approach used	PSNR
Lian et al. [22]	2004	Chaotic neural network-based cipher	32.63–39.42 dB
Yu and Cao [26]	2006	Hopfield chaotic neural networks	30.91–37.13 dB
Lian [23]	2009	Chaotic neural network-based block cipher	45.12–49.23 dB
Wang et al. [31]	2010	Chaotic image encryption system based on perceptron model	41.87–34.26 dB
Xing-Yuan and Xue-Mei [25]	2013	Spatio-temporal chaotic neural network	38.33–42.19 dB
Kumar and Dhiman [39]	2015	Multilayer feed-forward network	36.11–43.72 dB
Ratnavelu et al. [28]	2017	Chaotic fuzzy cellular neural networks	71.28–91.68 dB
Sahoo et al. (our approach)	2020	2-layer feed-forward back-propagation neural network-based individual pixel encryption	∞

and quality aspects, thus making true lossless encryption and decryption a reality. This means it is *virtually impossible* to decrypt the encrypted image even though the attacker has a copy of the trained neural network. The main advantage of our algorithm/cryptosystem over others is that it is *keyless,* i.e., it does not require a key. Thus, the proposed method does not suffer from the problem of key exchange. Using neural networks, we have overcome the limitations of encrypting individual pixels in real time. The complexity exhibited in terms of implementation and execution has been greatly reduced with the application of neural networks.

The algorithm was validated on an experimental database and tested on a collection of standard test images, and the resulting encrypted images obtained were completely different from the original images. Also, the original images were completely indistinguishable from the corresponding decrypted images, thereby validating that the process is lossless, which is evident from the PSNR values of infinity. From the experimental results, we can conclude that we have realized a novel image cryptosystem which is *simple* and *efficient* enough to be executed on a daily driver, *robust* enough that it does not compromise on the security aspects and *powerful* enough that there is no loss in image quality. This effective image cryptosystem can very well be put forth in practice for satellite imaging systems, medical imaging systems, military communications systems, social media and peer-to-peer confidential image sharing, confidential imaging systems for civilian and enterprise and other such applications.

Conflict of Interest The authors declare that they have no conflict of interest.

References

1. Mollin, R.A.: An Introduction to Cryptography. CRC Press (2000). Accessed on 10-09-2020 at https://books.google.co.in/books/about/An_Introduction_to_Cryptography.html?id=MsxSygPO_fwC

2. Tedmori, S., Al-Najdawi, N.: Lossless image cryptography algorithm based on discrete cosine transform. Int. Arab. J. Inf. Technol. **9**(5), 471–478 (2012). Accessed on 10-09-2020 at https://iajit.org/PDF/vol.9,no.5/3007-11.pdf

3. Nakajima, M., Yamaguchi, Y.: Extended visual cryptography for natural images (2002). Accessed on 10-09-2020 at http://wscg.zcu.cz/wscg2002/Papers_2002/A73.pdf

4. Chakraborty, S., Seal, A., Roy, M., Mali, K.: A novel lossless image encryption method using DNA substitution and chaotic logistic map. Int. J. Secur. Its Appl. **10**(2), 205–216 (2016). https://doi.org/10.14257/ijsia.2016.10.2.19

5. Khanzadi, H., Eshghi, M., Borujeni, S.E.: Image encryption using random bit sequence based on chaotic maps. Arab. J. Sci. Eng. **39**(2), 1039–1047 (2014). https://doi.org/10.1007/s13369-013-0713-z

6. Li, C., Xie, T., Liu, Q., Cheng, G.: Cryptanalyzing image encryption using chaotic logistic map. Nonlinear Dyn. **78**(2), 1545–1551 (2014). https://doi.org/10.1007/s11071-014-1533-8

7. Pareek, N.K., Patidar, V., Sud, K.K.: Image encryption using chaotic logistic map. Image Vis. Comput. **24**(9), 926–934 (2006). https://doi.org/10.1016/j.imavis.2006.02.021

8. Patel, S., Bharath, K.P., Kumar, R.: Symmetric keys image encryption and decryption using 3D chaotic maps with DNA encoding technique. Multim. Tools Appl., pp. 1–19 (2020). https://doi.org/10.1007/s11042-020-09551-9

9. Singh, K., Kaur, K.: Image encryption using chaotic maps and DNA addition operation and noise effects on it. Int. J. Comput. Appl. **23**(6), 17–24 (2011). https://doi.org/10.5120/2892-3779

10. Xu, L., Li, Z., Li, J., Hua, W.: A novel bit-level image encryption algorithm based on chaotic maps. Opt. Lasers Eng. **78**, 17–25 (2016). https://doi.org/10.1016/j.optlaseng.2015.09.007

11. Akhavan, A., Samsudin, A., Akhshani, A.: Cryptanalysis of an image encryption algorithm based on DNA encoding. Opt. Laser Technol. **95**, 94–99 (2017). https://doi.org/10.1016/j.optlastec.2017.04.022

12. Wang, X.Y., Zhang, Y.Q., Bao, X.M.: A novel chaotic image encryption scheme using DNA sequence operations. Opt. Lasers Eng. **73**, 53–61 (2015). https://doi.org/10.1016/j.optlaseng.2015.03.022

13. Wang, X.Y., Zhang, Y.Q., Zhao, Y.Y.: A novel image encryption scheme based on 2-D logistic map and DNA sequence operations. Nonlinear Dyn. **82**(3), 1269–1280 (2015). https://doi.org/10.1007/s11071-015-2234-7

14. Zhang, Q., Guo, L., Xue, X., Wei, X.: An image encryption algorithm based on DNA sequence addition operation. In: 2009 Fourth International on Conference on Bio-Inspired Computing, pp. 1–5. IEEE (2009). https://doi.org/10.1109/bicta.2009.5338151

15. Zhang, Q., Xue, X., Wei, X.: A novel image encryption algorithm based on DNA subsequence operation. Sci. World J. **2012** (2012). https://doi.org/10.1100/2012/286741

16. Mousa, H.M.: DNA-genetic encryption technique. Int. J. Comput. Netw. Inf. Secur. **8**(7), 1 (2016). https://doi.org/10.5815/ijcnis.2016.07.01

17. Pujari, S.K., Bhattacharjee, G., Bhoi, S.: A hybridized model for image encryption through genetic algorithm and DNA sequence. Procedia Comput. Sci. **125**, 165–171 (2018). https://doi.org/10.1016/j.procs.2017.12.023

18. Saranya, M.R., Mohan, A.K., Anusudha, K.: A composite image cipher using DNA sequence and genetic algorithm. In: 2014 International Conference on Contemporary Computing and Informatics (IC3I), pp. 1022–1026. IEEE (2014). https://doi.org/10.1109/ic3i.2014.7019805

19. Saranya, M.R., Mohan, A.K., Anusudha, K.: Algorithm for enhanced image security using DNA and genetic algorithm. In: 2015 IEEE International Conference on Signal Processing, Informatics, Communication and Energy Systems (SPICES), pp. 1–5. IEEE (2015). https://doi.org/10.1109/spices.2015.7091462

20. Bigdeli, N., Farid, Y., Afshar, K.: A novel image encryption/decryption scheme based on chaotic neural networks. Eng. Appl. Artif. Intell. **25**(4), 753–765 (2012). https://doi.org/10.1016/j.eng appai.2012.01.007

21. Jain, A., Rajpal, N.: A two layer chaotic network based image encryption technique. In: 2012 National Conference on Computing and Communication Systems, pp. 1–5. IEEE (2012). https://doi.org/10.1109/ncccs.2012.6413005

22. Lian, S., Chen, G., Cheung, A., Wang, Z.: A chaotic-neural-network-based encryption algorithm for JPEG2000 encoded images. In: International Symposium on Neural Networks, pp. 627–632. Springer, Berlin, Heidelberg (2004). https://doi.org/10.1007/978-3-540-28648-6_100

23. Lian, S.: A block cipher based on chaotic neural networks. Neurocomputing **72**(4–6), 1296–1301 (2009). https://doi.org/10.1016/j.neucom.2008.11.005

24. Shukla, N., & Tiwari, A.: An empirical investigation of using ANN based N-state sequential machine and chaotic neural network in the field of cryptography. Glob. J. Comput. Sci. Technol. (2012). Accessed on 10-09-2020 at https://computerresearch.org/index.php/computer/article/view/516/516

25. Xing-Yuan, W., Xue-Mei, B.: A novel image block cryptosystem based on a spatio-temporal chaotic system and a chaotic neural network. Chin. Phys. B **22**(5), 050508 (2013). https://doi.org/10.1088/1674-1056/22/5/050508

26. Yu, W., Cao, J.: Cryptography based on delayed chaotic neural networks. Phys. Lett. A **356**(4–5), 333–338 (2006). https://doi.org/10.1016/j.physleta.2006.03.069

27. Peng, J., Zhang, D., Liao, X.: A digital image encryption algorithm based on hyper-chaotic cellular neural network. Fundam. Inf. **90**(3), 269–282 (2009). https://doi.org/10.3233/FI-2009-0018

28. Ratnavelu, K., Kalpana, M., Balasubramaniam, P., Wong, K., Raveendran, P.: Image encryption method based on chaotic fuzzy cellular neural networks. Sig. Process. **140**, 87–96 (2017). https://doi.org/10.1016/j.sigpro.2017.05.002

29. Bigdeli, N., Farid, Y., Afshar, K.: A robust hybrid method for image encryption based on Hopfield neural network. Comput. Electr. Eng. **38**(2), 356–369 (2012). https://doi.org/10.1016/j.compeleceng.2011.11.019

30. Lakshmi, C., Thenmozhi, K., Rayappan, J.B.B., Amirtharajan, R.: Hopfield attractor-trusted neural network: an attack-resistant image encryption. Neural Comput. Appl. **32**(15), 11477–11489 (2020). https://doi.org/10.1007/s00521-019-04637-4

31. Wang, X.Y., Yang, L., Liu, R., Kadir, A.: A chaotic image encryption algorithm based on perceptron model. Nonlinear Dyn. **62**(3), 615–621 (2010). https://doi.org/10.1007/s11071-010-9749-8

32. Cheng, C.J., Cheng, C.B.: An asymmetric image cryptosystem based on the adaptive synchronization of an uncertain unified chaotic system and a cellular neural network. Commun. Nonlinear Sci. Numer. Simul. **18**(10), 2825–2837 (2013). https://doi.org/10.1016/j.cnsns.2013.02.011

33. Zhang, W., Peng, J., Yang, H., Wei, P.: A digital image encryption scheme based on the hybrid of cellular neural network and logistic map. In: International Symposium on Neural Networks, pp. 860–867. Springer, Berlin, Heidelberg (2005). https://doi.org/10.1007/11427445_138

34. Joshi, S.D., Udupi, V.R., Joshi, D.R.: A novel neural network approach for digital image data encryption/decryption. In: 2012 International Conference on Power, Signals, Controls and Computation, pp. 1–4. IEEE (2012). https://doi.org/10.1109/epscicon.2012.6175229

35. Hua, Z., Yi, S., Zhou, Y.: Medical image encryption using high-speed scrambling and pixel adaptive diffusion. Sig. Process. **144**, 134–144 (2018). https://doi.org/10.1016/j.sigpro.2017.10.004

36. Ismail, I.A., Galal-Edeen, G.H., Khattab, S., Mohamed Abd Elhamid, M.: Satellite image encryption using neural networks backpropagation. In: 2012 22nd International Conference on Computer Theory and Applications (ICCTA), pp. 148–152. IEEE (2012). https://doi.org/10.1109/iccta.2012.6523561

37. Seethalakshmi, K.S., Usha, B.A., Sangeetha, K.N.: Security enhancement in image steganography using neural networks and visual cryptography. In: 2016 International Conference on Computation System and Information Technology for Sustainable Solutions (CSITSS), pp. 396–403. IEEE (2016). https://doi.org/10.1109/csitss.2016.7779393
38. Zhu, S., Zhu, C., Wang, W.: A new image encryption algorithm based on chaos and secure hash SHA-256. Entropy **20**(9), 716 (2018). https://doi.org/10.3390/e20090716
39. Kumar, R., Dhiman, M.: Secured image transmission using a novel neural network approach and secret image sharing technique. Int. J. Signal Process., Image Process. Pattern Recognit. **8**(1), 161–192 (2015). https://doi.org/10.14257/ijsip.2015.8.1.16
40. Fatema, N. et al.: Data-driven occupancy detection hybrid model using particle swarm optimization based artificial neural network. In: Springer Nature Book: Metaheuristic and Evolutionary Computation: Algorithms and Applications, under book series "Studies in Computational Intelligence", 2020. https://doi.org/10.1007/978-981-15-7571-6_13
41. Mishra, S. et al.: Artificial neural network and empirical mode decomposition based imbalance fault diagnosis of wind turbine using TurbSim, FAST and simulink. IET Renew. Power Gener. **11**(6), 889–902 (2017). https://doi.org/10.1049/iet-rpg.2015.0382
42. Yadav, A.K. et al.: Application of neuro-fuzzy scheme to investigate the winding insulation paper deterioration in oil-immersed power transformer. Electr. Power Energy Syst. **53**, 256–271 (2013). https://doi.org/10.1016/j.ijepes.2013.04.023
43. Sharma, V. et al.: Daily array yield prediction of grid-interactive photovoltaic plant using relief attribute evaluator based radial basis function neural network. Renew. Sustain. Energy Rev. **81**(Part 2), 2115–2127 (2018). Doi:https://doi.org/10.1016/j.rser.2017.06.023
44. Chandel, S.S. et al.: Selection of most relevant input parameters using WEKA for artificial neural network based solar radiation prediction models. Renew. Sustain. Energy Rev. **31**, 509–519 (2014). https://doi.org/10.1016/j.rser.2013.12.008
45. The USC-SIPI Image Database: Accessed on 10-09-2020 at http://sipi.usc.edu/database/database.php

Printed in the United States
by Baker & Taylor Publisher Services